FUNDAMENTALS FOOD MICROBIOLOGY

Edited by
Patricia Marques

ArclerPress

Fundamentals Food Microbiology

Edited by Patricia Marques

Edition 2018

ArclerPress

Published by
Arcler Press LLC
708 3rd Avenue, 6th Floor
New York
NY 10017
United States of America
www.arclerpress.com

ISBN: 978-1-68094-577-5 (Hardback)

Printed in United States of America

Library of Congress Control Number: 2017933142

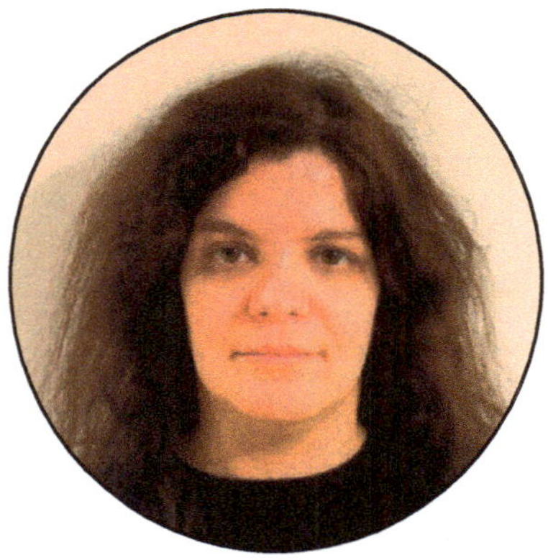

About the Editor

Patricia Marques

Patricia obtained her PhD form University College Dublin in 2010. Her interests are on Microbiology and Parasitology. She is currently working as a Postdoc at University of Maryland Baltimore, USA on Chlamydia infections

Table of Contents

List of Abbreviations xi
Preface xiii

1 FOOD MICROBIOLOGY GENERAL OVERVIEW

Introduction 1
Food Safety 2
- Fermentation 2
- Microbial Biopolymers 2
- Food Authenticity 3

Food sampling 3
- Sampling by Manufacturers 3
- Testing and Methods of Analysis 4
- Food Law Enforcement (UK) 4
- Food Testing 5

References 6

2 INTRODUCTION TO THE STUDY OF MICROORGANISM

Introduction 7
- Evolution 9
- Pre-Microbiology 9
- History of Discovery 10
- Classification and Structure 13

Prokaryote 13
- Structure 14
- Morphology 15
- Reproduction 16
- DNA Transfer 16
- Sociality 16
- Environment 17

Classification....18
Evolution....18
Relationship to Eukaryotes....19
Bacteria....21
Etymology....22
Origin and early Evolution....22
Morphology....22
Cellular Structure....24
Metabolism....29
Growth and Reproduction....31
Genomes....33
Genetics....33
DNA Transfer....33
Bacteriophages....34
Behaviour....34
Movement....35
Interactions with other Organisms....39
Predators....39
Mutualists....40
Significance in Technology and Industry....41
History of Bacteriology....42
Archaea....43
Classification....44
Origin and Evolution....46
Morphology....50
Structure, Composition Development, and Operation....50
Metabolism....53
Genetics....55
Reproduction....57
Ecology....57
Mutualism....60
Commensalism....60
Significance in Technology and Industry....60
Eukaryote....61
Cell Features....62
Differences among Eukaryotic Cells....66
Reproduction....69
Classification....70
Phylogeny....72
Origin of Eukaryotes....75
Protist....79
Subdivisions....80

Classification 81
Metabolism 82
Reproduction 83
Ecology 84
Fossil Record 84
Fungus 85
Etymology 86
Characteristics 86
Fungal hyphae cells 86
Diversity 89
Mycology 90
Morphology 91
Growth and Physiology 93
Reproduction 94
Evolution 98
Taxonomy 99
Ecology 104
Mycotoxins 109
Pathogenic Mechanisms 109
Human Use 110
Therapeutic Uses 111
Soil Microorganisms 116
Symbiotic Microorganisms 116
Applications 116
Food Production 117
Soil 117
Fermentation 117
Hygiene 117
Water Treatment 118
Energy 118
Chemicals, Enzymes 118
Science 118
Warfare 119
Human Health 119
Etymology and Pronunciation 119
Microorganisms Used in Food and Beverage Preparation 120
References 129

3 THE MICROBIOLOGY OF FOOD PRESERVATION

Introduction 137
Traditional Techniques 138

Drying 138
Cooling 138
Freezing 139
Boiling 139
Heating 139
Salting 139
Sugaring 140
Smoking 140
Pickling 141
Lye 141
Canning 141
Jellying 142
Jugging 142
Burial 143
Curing 143
Fermentation 143
Industrial/Modern Techniques 144
Pasteurization 144
Vacuum Packing 144
Artificial Food Additives 144
Radiation 144
Pulsed Electric Field Electroporation 145
Modified Atmosphere 145
Nonthermal Plasma 146
High-Pressure Food Preservation 146
Biopreservation 147
Hurdle Technology 147
References 148

4 MICROBIAL FOOD SPOILAGE

Introduction 151
Reasons 152
Bacteria 152
Yeasts 152
Signs 153
Consequences 153
Prevention 153
Food Rotation System 153
Preservative 154
Antimicrobial Preservatives 154

Antioxidants 155
Nonsynthetic Compounds for Food Preservation 156
Public Awareness of Food Preservation 157
Lactic Acid Fermentation 157
Applications 158
References 159

5 MICROBIAL FOOD CULTURES

Introduction 163
Milestones 164
Function of Microbial Food Cultures In Food 164
Bacteria 164
Yeasts 165
Moulds 166
Production of Microbial Food Cultures 166
Safety and Regulatory Aspects 167
Microorganisms with Documented History of Safe Use in Food 167
US 167
European Union 167
Denmark 168
References 168

6 FERMENTATION IN FOOD PROCESSING

Introduction 175
Uses 177
Fermented Foods by Region 178
List of Fermented Foods 179
Fermented Foods by Type 198
Vegetable-Based 198
Fruit-Based 199
Honey-Based 199
Dairy-Based 199
Fish-Based 200
Meat-Based 200
Tea-Based 200
Risks 200
References 201

7 FOODBORNE ILLNESS FOOD PATHOGENS

Introduction 204
Causes 204
Bacteria 205
Enterotoxins 206
Emerging Foodborne Pathogens 206
Preventing Bacterial Food Poisoning 207
Mycotoxins and Alimentary Mycotoxicoses 208
Viruses 209
Parasites 210
Natural Toxins 211
Other Pathogenic Agents 212
"Ptomaine Poisoning" 212
Mechanism 212
Infectious Dose 213
Epidemiology 213
United States 213
France 214
Australia 214
Comparison between Countries 215
Outbreaks 215
Society and Culture 216
United Kingdom 216
United States 216
Organizations 217
International Food Safety Authorities Network (INFOSAN) 217
Regulatory Steps 218
References 218

8 IMPEDANCE MICROBIOLOGY

Introduction 223
Principle of Operation 224
Instrumentation 227
Applications 227
References 227

Index 231

List of Abbreviations

ATP	Adenosine Triphosphate
AGWP	Aanthropogenic Global Warming Potential
ARMAN	Archaeal Richmond Mine Acidophilic Nanoorganisms
CO	Carbon Dioxide
CDC	Center for Disease Control
CFU	Colony-Forming Units
DON	Deoxynivalenol
DT	Detect Time
DAS	Fiacetoxyscirpenol
EGT	Endosymbiotic Gene Transfer
EHEC	Enterohemorrhagic
EFFCA	European Food and Feed Cultures Association
EFSA	European Food Safety Authority
FIFO	First in First Out Method
GRAS	Generally Recognized by Experts as Safe
IDF	International Dairy Federation
LAB	Lactic Acid Bacteria
LEM	Leukoencephalomalacia
OTA	Ochratoxin A
PCR	Polymerase Chain Reaction
PCR	Polymerase Chain Reaction
γ-PGA	Poly-γ-Glutamic Acid
PEF	Pulsed Electric Field

QPS	Qualified Presumption of Safety
RAD	Radicinin
rRNA	Ribosomal RNA
SET	Serial Endosymbiotic Theory
TeA	Tenuazonic Acid
WHO	World Health Organization

Preface

Food microbiology is the scientific study of microorganisms, both in food and used for the production of food. Food microbiology focuses on the general biology of the microorganisms that are found in foods including: their growth characteristics, identification, and pathogenesis. Specifically, areas of interest which concern food microbiology are food poisoning, food spoilage, food preservation, and food legislation. Pathogens in product, or harmful microorganisms, result in major public health problems worldwide and are the leading causes of illnesses and death. Bacteria are the most important microorganisms to the food processor. Most are harmless, many are highly beneficial, some indicate the probable presence of filth, disease organisms, spoilage and a few cause disease. There are thousands of species of bacteria, but all are single-celled and fall into three basic shapes: spherical, straight rods, and spiral rods. Yeasts are oval-shaped and slightly larger than bacteria. They reproduce most often by budding. In budding each cell can produce several buds, or swellings, which break away to form new, fully formed daughter cells. Molds as found on bread, fruit, damp paper, or other surfaces are actually composed of millions of microscopic cells joined together to form chains. The chains usually have numerous branches, called hyphae. Molds can thrive in conditions too adverse for bacteria or yeasts. They reproduce by spores that are frequently present as green or black masses on the protruding hyphae. Yeasts and molds grow on most foods, on equipment, and building surfaces where there are small amounts of nutrient and moisture. Since bacteria grow faster, they greatly outnumber yeasts and molds in most foods. However, bacteria find conditions of low pH, moisture, or temperature and high salt or sugar unfavorable. In such environments, yeasts or molds predominate. Thus, they can be a problem in dry foods, salted fish, bread, pickles, fruits, jams, jellies, and similar commodities. Microorganisms can cause a variety of effects in food products including spoilage, which primarily affects product quality, and food poisoning, which is generally caused by pathogens. As regulators, we are most concerned with the effects that microorganisms have on food that leads to food borne illness, because this affects public health. A food borne illness (or disease) is exactly what the term indicates - a disease or illness caused by the consumption of contaminated foods or beverages. It would seem rather obvious that a food borne microbial pathogen, or a preformed microbial toxic product, or another poison such as a poisonous chemical that has somehow contaminated the food and/or beverage, leads to one of the many different food borne illnesses. There is no one "syndrome" that is representative of food borne illness/disease. Different diseases have many different symptoms. However, the microbe or toxin enters the body through the gastrointestinal tract, and often causes the first clinical signs such as nausea, vomiting, abdominal cramps and diarrhea, which are common symptoms in many food borne disease.

Content Coverage

Chapters One and *Two* present an overview of food microbiology and microorganism, correspondingly. Microorganisms are very diverse and include all bacteria, archaea and most protozoa. This group also contains some species of fungi, algae, and certain microscopic animals, such as rotifers

Chapters Three and *Four* present a coverage of microbiology of food preservation and food spoilage, respectively. Food preservation may also include processes that inhibit visual deterioration, such as the enzymatic browning reaction in apples after they are cut during food preparation.

Chapter Five presents emphasis on microbial food cultures are live bacteria, yeasts or moulds used in food production. Microbial food cultures carry out the fermentation process in foodstuffs. Used by humans since the Neolithic period fermentation helps to preserve perishable foods and to improve their nutritional and organoleptic qualities.

Chapter Six focuses on fermentation in food processing, which is the process of converting carbohydrates to alcohol or organic acids using microorganisms—yeasts or bacteria—under anaerobic conditions.

Chapters Seven and *Eight* present an outline of food pathogens and impedance microbiology, separately. Vegetables and fruits are not immune to contamination with foodborne pathogens, despite the fact that they are picked, not slaughtered. Impedance microbiology, however, is a rapid microbiological technique used to measure the microbial concentration (mainly bacteria but also yeasts) of a sample by monitoring the electrical parameters of the growth medium.

CHAPTER 1

Food Microbiology General Overview

Chapter Contents

- **Introduction**
- **Food Safety**
- **Food Sampling**

Food Microbiology does not have a precise beginning. Events which stretched over several centuries ultimately led to the recognition of the significance and role of microorganisms in foods. Food borne disease and food spoilage have been part of the human experience since the dawn of our race. Although the actual cause of these problems would remain a mystery for thousands of years, many early civilizations discovered and applied effective methods to preserve and protect their food:

INTRODUCTION

Food microbiology is the study of the microorganisms that inhabit, create, or contaminate food, including the study of microorganisms causing food spoilage. "Good" bacteria, however, such as probiotics, are becoming increasingly important in food science. In addition, microorganisms are essential for the production of foods such as cheese, yogurt, bread, beer, wine and, other fermented foods.

FOOD SAFETY

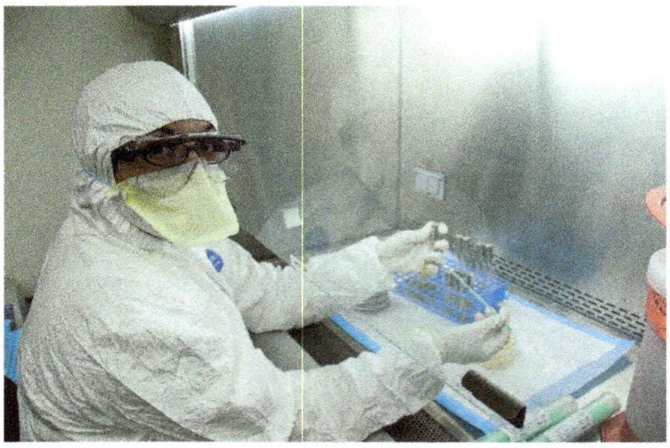

A microbiologist working in a biosafety laboratory tests for high risk pathogens in food.

Food safety is a major focus of food microbiology. Pathogenic bacteria, viruses and toxins produced by microorganisms are all possible contaminants of food. However, microorganisms and their products can also be used to combat these pathogenic microbes. Probiotic bacteria, including those that produce bacteriocins, can kill and inhibit pathogens. Alternatively, purified bacteriocins such as nisin can be added directly to food products. Finally, bacteriophages, viruses that only infect bacteria, can be used to kill bacterial pathogens. Thorough preparation of food, including proper cooking, eliminates most bacteria and viruses. However, *toxins produced* by contaminants may not be liable to change to non-toxic forms by heating or cooking the contaminated food due to other safety conditions.

Fermentation

Fermentation is one of the methods to preserve food and alter its quality. Yeast, especially *Saccharomyces cerevisiae*, is used to leaven bread, brew beer and make wine. Certain bacteria, including lactic acid bacteria, are used to make yogurt, cheese, hot sauce, pickles, fermented sausages and dishes such as kimchi. A common effect of these fermentations is that the food product is less hospitable to other microorganisms, including pathogens and spoilage-causing microorganisms, thus extending the food's shelf-life. Some cheese varieties also require molds to ripen and develop their characteristic flavors.

Microbial Biopolymers

Several microbially produced biopolymers are used in the food industry.

Alginate

Alginates can be used as thickening agents. Although listed here under the category 'Microbial polysaccharides', commercial alginates are currently only produced by extraction from brown seaweeds such as *Laminaria hyperborea* or *L. japonica*.

Poly-γ-Glutamic Acid

Poly-γ-glutamic acid (γ-PGA) produced by various strains of *Bacillus* has potential applications as a thickener in the food industry.

Food Authenticity

It is important to be able to detect microorganisms in food, in particular pathogenic microorganisms or genetically modified microorganisms.

FOOD SAMPLING

Food sampling is a process used to check that a food is safe and that it does not contain harmful contaminants, or that it contains only permitted additives at acceptable levels, or that it contains the right levels of key ingredients and its label declarations are correct, or to know the levels of nutrients present.

A food sample is carried out by subjecting the product to physical analysis. Analysis may be undertaken by or on behalf of a manufacturer regarding their own product, or for official food law enforcement or control purposes, or for research or public information.

To undertake any analysis, unless the whole amount of food to be considered is very small so that the food can be used for testing in its entirety, it is usually necessary for a portion of it to be taken (e.g. a small quantity from a full production batch, or a portion of what is on sale in a shop) – this process is known as food sampling.

In most cases with food to be analysed there are two levels of sampling – the first being selection of a portion from the whole, which is then submitted to a laboratory for testing, and the second being the laboratory's taking of the individual amounts necessary for individual tests that may be applied. It is the former that is 'food sampling': the latter is analytical laboratory 'sub-sampling', often relying upon initial homogenisation of the entire submitted sample.

Where it is intended that the results of any analysis to relate to the food as a whole it is crucially important that the sample is representative of that whole – and the results of any analysis can only be meaningful if the sampling is undertaken effectively. This is true whether the 'whole' is a manufacturer's entire production batch, or where it is a single item but too large to all be used for the test.

Factors relevant in considering the representativeness of a sample include the homogeneity of the food, the relative sizes of the sample to be taken and the whole, the potential degree of variation of the parameter(s) in question through the whole, and the significance and intended use of the analytical result.

Sampling by Manufacturers

Food manufacturers and producers would need to satisfy themselves that any sample taken for analysis is sufficiently representative of the food for the analytical result to be meaningful. This is true whether the data are to be used as the basis of labelling declarations, assurance of compliance with legislative or other standards, monitoring of production as part of HACCP (Hazard Analysis and Critical Control Points), or for routine quality control.

In the United Kingdom although various guidance is available, either from manufacturers' associations or from sources of standards such as British Standards Institution (such as British Standard BS6001), some of which may be relevant to certain food types. It is largely down to manufacturers to make their own evaluations of need and suitability. This must be translated into an assessment both of sample portion size and number, and the frequency of taking samples.

Testing and Methods of Analysis

To ensure food safety and quality, some food samples which are perishable require certain tests and analyses. The following tests and analyses can be conducted:

- Food allergen testing
- Food chemical analysis
- Food contact tests
- Food contaminant testing
- Nutritional analysis and testing
- GMO testing
- Melamine contamination testing
- Microbiological tests
- Spiral plating for bacterial count
- Pesticide residue testing
- Veterinary drug residue testing
- PCR food testing

Food Law Enforcement (UK)

In the United Kingdom, enforcement is under the Food Safety Act 1990. Food sampling is undertaken primarily by local authorities and port health authorities for submission to public analysts for analysis. Much of the legislation relates to food as supplied to a consumer, meaning that every portion of a size of perishable food and foods at risk as may be supplied to a consumer has to comply, so that in such cases the sample submitted for analysis could simply be an entire consumer-sized portion. There are exceptions, however, such as the sampling of nut products for the presence of aflatoxins, which stipulate a primary sample size related to the size of the consignment – with associated requirements for initial homogenisation to produce a smaller sample to be sent for analysis.

The Food Safety Act 1990 affords a right for defence analysis, and for referee analysis in case of disputed analytical results, by stipulating that except where to do so would prevent effective analysis the sample must be divided into three parts. The UK

Food Standards Agency provides supplementary guidance to the enforcement authorities to assist with the sampling process and associated decisions by sampling officers.

There is no set frequency or rate for the sampling of food for law enforcement in the UK. Between the 1930s and 1990s there had been a guideline minimum rate for sampling for chemical analysis (not including samples for microbiological examination) of 2.5 samples per annum per 1000 head of population, however that was an arbitrary figure and more recent thinking suggested that the selection of a frequency for sampling should be based on risk. In this context risk includes all 'consumer protection' issues such as pecuniary disadvantage from substandard or counterfeit products, as well as risk to health. The Association of Public Analysts was commissioned by the Food Standards Agency to look into this, culminating in a scheme for *Risk Based Sampling*, though it has not yet been adopted by the enforcement authorities.

Food Testing

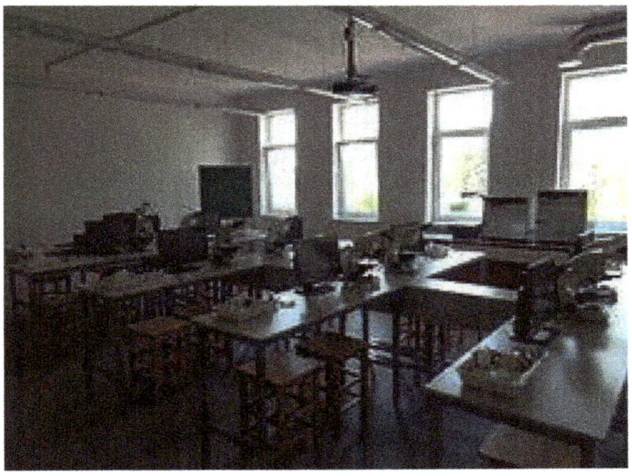

Food microbiology laboratory at the Faculty of Food Technology, Latvia University of Agriculture.

To ensure safety of food products, microbiological tests such as testing for pathogens and spoilage organisms are required. This way the risk of contamination under normal use conditions can be examined and food poisoning outbreaks can be prevented. Testing of food products and ingredients is important along the whole supply chain as possible flaws of products can occur at every stage of production. Apart from detecting spoilage, microbiological tests can also determine germ content, identify yeasts and molds, and salmonella. For salmonella, scientists are also developing rapid and portable technologies capable of identifying unique variants of Salmonella .

Polymerase Chain Reaction (PCR) is a quick and inexpensive method to generate numbers of copies of a DNA fragment at a specific band ("PCR (Polymerase Chain Reaction)," 2008). For that reason, scientists are using PCR to detect different kinds of viruses or bacteria, such as HIV and anthrax based on their unique DNA patterns. Various kits are commercially available to help in food pathogen nucleic acids extraction, PCR detection, and differentiation.The detection of bacterial strands in food products is very important to everyone in the world, for it helps prevent the occurrence of food borne illness. Therefore, PCR is recognized as a DNA detector in order to amplify and trace the presence of pathogenic strands in different processed food.

REFERENCES

1. Fratamico PM (2005). Bayles DO, ed. Foodborne Pathogens: Microbiology and Molecular Biology. Caister Academic Press. ISBN 978-1-904455-00-4.
2. Tannock GW, ed. (2005). Probiotics and Prebiotics: Scientific Aspects. Caister Academic Press. ISBN 978-1-904455-01-1.
3. Ljungh A, Wadstrom T, eds. (2009). Lactobacillus Molecular Biology: From Genomics to Probiotics. Caister Academic Press. ISBN 978-1-904455-41-7.
4. Mayo, B (2010). van Sinderen, D, ed. Bifidobacteria: Genomics and Molecular Aspects. Caister Academic Press. ISBN 978-1-904455-68-4.
5. Sillankorva, Sanna M.; Oliveira, Hugo; Azeredo, Joana (2012). "Bacteriophages and Their Role in Food Safety". International Journal of Microbiology. 2012: 1–13. doi:10.1155/2012/863945. Retrieved 28 September 2016.
6. Rehm BHA, ed. (2009). Microbial Production of Biopolymers and Polymer Precursors: Applications and Perspectives. Caister Academic Press. ISBN 978-1-904455-36-3.
7. Remminghorst & Rehm (2009). "Microbial Production of Alginate: Biosynthesis and Applications". Microbial Production of Biopolymers and Polymer Precursors. Caister Academic Press. ISBN 978-1-904455-36-3.
8. Shih & Wu (2009). "Biosynthesis and Application of Poly(gamma-glutamic acid)". Microbial Production of Biopolymers and Polymer Precursors. Caister Academic Press. ISBN 978-1-904455-36-3.
9. Food Testing Laboratories
10. Rapid Testing and Identification of Salmonella in Foods
11. FOOD PATHOGEN DNA EXTRACTION filter paper card
12. "UK Food Safety Act 1990".
13. "Food Standards Agency - Homepage".
14. "Risk Based Sampling - Vol 1:Risk Assessment for Sampling"
15. "Risk Based Sampling - Vol 2:Background and support"

CHAPTER 2

The Study of Microorganism

Chapter Contents

- **Introduction**
- **Prokaryote**
- **Bacteria**
- **Archaea**
- **Eukaryote**
- **Protist**
- **Fungus**
- **Microorganisms Used in Food and Beverage Preparations**

Microorganisms are manifold. Microorganisms include bacteria, fungi, archaea or protists, but not viruses and prions, which are generally classified as non-living.

INTRODUCTION

A microorganism or microbe is a microscopic living organism, which may be single-celled or multicellular. The study of microorganisms is called microbiology, a subject that began with the discovery of microorganisms in 1674 by Antonie van Leeuwenhoek, using a microscope of his own design.

Microorganisms are very diverse and include all bacteria, archaea and most protozoa. This group also contains some species of fungi, algae, and certain microscopic animals, such as rotifers. Many macroscopic animals and plants have microscopic juvenile stages. Some microbiologists also classify viruses (and viroids) as microorganisms, but others consider these as nonliving. In July 2016, scientists reported identifying a set of 355 genes from the last universal common ancestor of all life, including microorganisms, living on Earth.

Microorganisms live in every part of the biosphere, including soil, hot springs, "seven miles deep" in the ocean, "40 miles high" in the atmosphere and inside rocks far down within the Earth's crust. Microorganisms, under certain test conditions, have been observed to thrive in the vacuum of outer space. According to some estimates, microorganisms outweigh "all other living things combined thousands of times over". The mass of prokaryote microorganisms — which includes bacteria and archaea, but not the nucleated eukaryote microorganisms — may be as much as 0.8 trillion tons of carbon (of the total biosphere mass, estimated at between 1 and 4 trillion tons). On 17 March 2013, researchers reported data that suggested microbial life forms thrive in the Mariana Trench. the deepest spot in the Earth's oceans. Other researchers reported related studies that microorganisms thrive inside rocks up to 580 m (1,900 ft; 0.36 mi) below the sea floor under 2,590 m (8,500 ft; 1.61 mi) of ocean off the coast of the northwestern United States, as well as 2,400 m (7,900 ft; 1.5 mi) beneath the seabed off Japan. On 20 August 2014, scientists confirmed the existence of microorganisms living 800 m (2,600 ft; 0.50 mi) below the ice of Antarctica. According to one researcher, "You can find microbes everywhere — they're extremely adaptable to conditions, and survive wherever they are."

Microorganisms are crucial to nutrient recycling in ecosystems as they act as decomposers. As some microorganisms can fix nitrogen, they are a vital part of the nitrogen cycle, and recent studies indicate that airborne microorganisms may play a role in precipitation and weather. Microorganisms are also exploited in biotechnology, both in traditional food and beverage preparation, and in modern technologies based on genetic engineering. A small proportion of microorganisms are pathogenic, causing disease and even death in plants and animals.

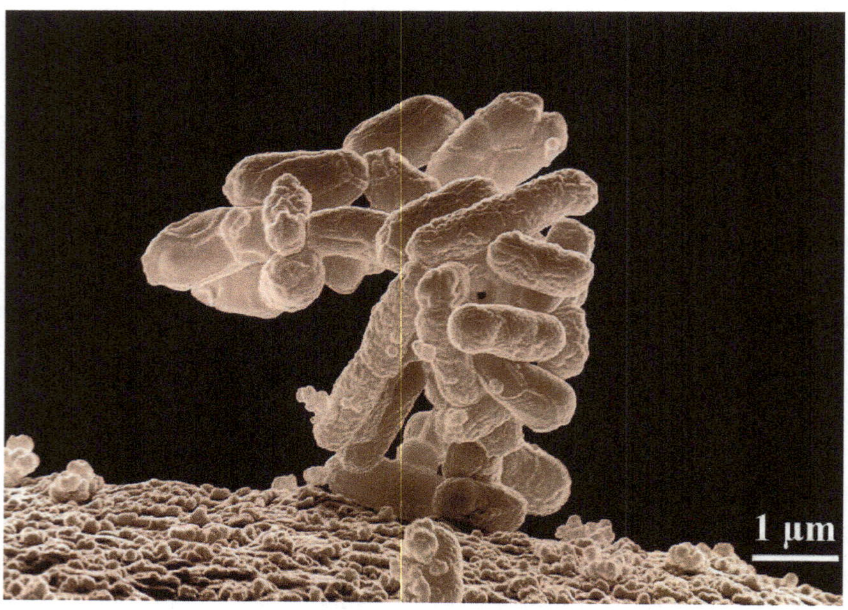

A cluster of Escherichia coli bacteria magnified 10,000 times

Evolution

Single-celled microorganisms were the first forms of life to develop on Earth, approximately 3–4 billion years ago. Further evolution was slow, and for about 3 billion years in the Precambrian eon, all organisms were microscopic. So, for most of the history of life on Earth, the only forms of life were microorganisms.Bacteria, algae and fungi have been identified in amber that is 220 million years old, which shows that the morphology of microorganisms has changed little since the Triassic period. The newly discovered biological role played by nickel, however — especially that engendered by volcanic eruptions from the Siberian Traps (site of the modern city of Norilsk) — is thought to have accelerated the evolution of methanogens towards the end of the Permian–Triassic extinction event.

Microorganisms tend to have a relatively fast rate of evolution. Most microorganisms can reproduce rapidly, and bacteria are also able to freely exchange genes through conjugation, transformation and transduction, even between widely divergent species. This horizontal gene transfer, coupled with a high mutation rate and many other means of genetic variation, allows microorganisms to swiftly evolve (via natural selection) to survive in new environments and respond to environmental stresses. This rapid evolution is important in medicine, as it has led to the recent development of "super-bugs", pathogenic bacteria that are resistant to modern antibiotics.

Pre-Microbiology

The possibility that microorganisms exist was discussed for many centuries before their discovery in the 17th century. The existence of unseen microbiological life was postulated by Jainism, which is based on Mahavira's teachings as early as 6th century BCE. Paul Dundas notes that Mahavira asserted the existence of unseen microbiological creatures living in earth, water, air and fire. The Jain scriptures also describe nigodas, which are sub-microscopic creatures living in large clusters and having a very short life, which are said to pervade every part of the universe, even the tissues of plants and animals. The earliest known idea to indicate the possibility of diseases spreading by yet unseen organisms was that of the Roman scholar Marcus Terentius Varro in a 1st-century BC book titled *On Agriculture* in which he warns against locating a homestead near swamps:... and because there are bred certain minute creatures that cannot be seen by the eyes, which float in the air and enter the body through the mouth and nose and they cause serious diseases.

In *The Canon of Medicine* (1020), Abū Alī ibn Sīnā (Avicenna) hypothesized that tuberculosis and other diseases might be contagious.

In 1546, Girolamo Fracastoro proposed that epidemic diseases were caused by transferable seedlike entities that could transmit infection by direct or indirect contact, or even without contact over long distances.

All these early claims about the existence of microorganisms were speculative and while grounded on indirect observations, they were not based on direct observation of microorganisms or systematized empirical investigation, e.g. experimentation. Microorganisms were neither proven, observed, nor accurately described until the 17th century. The reason for this was that all these early studies lacked the microscope.

History of Discovery

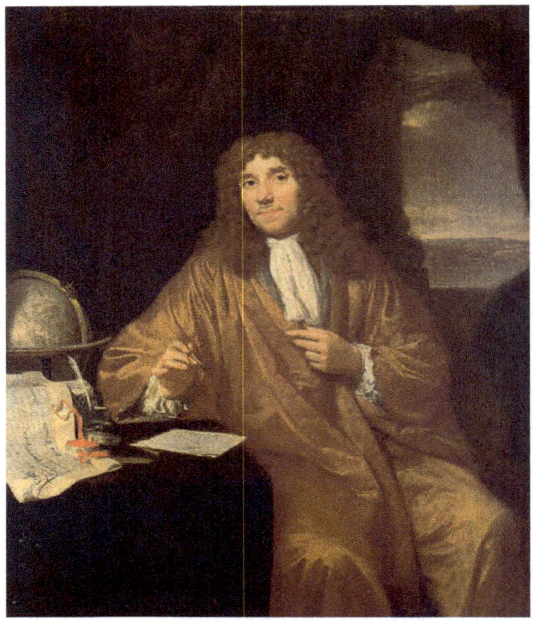

Antonie van Leeuwenhoek, the first person to observe microorganisms using a microscope

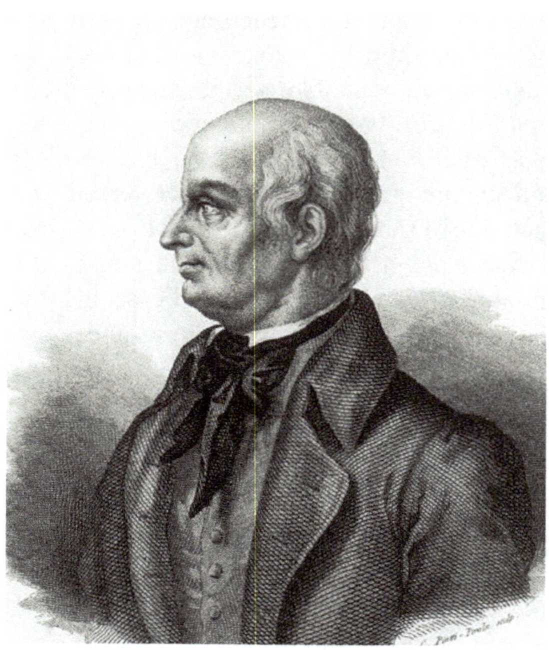

Lazzaro Spallanzani showed that boiling a broth stopped it from decaying.

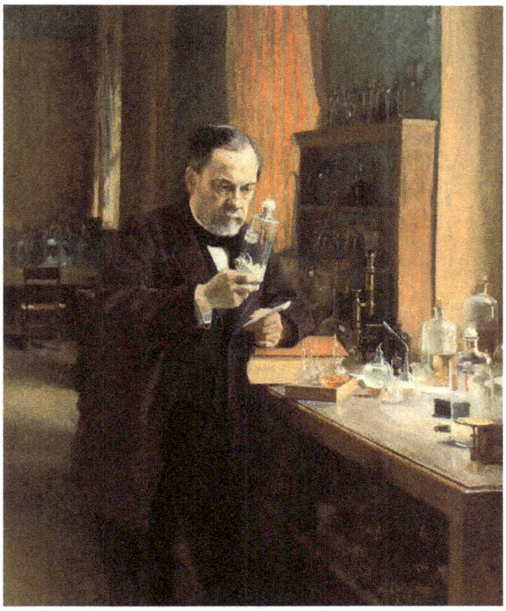

Louis Pasteur showed that Spallanzani's findings held even if air could enter through a filter that kept particles out.

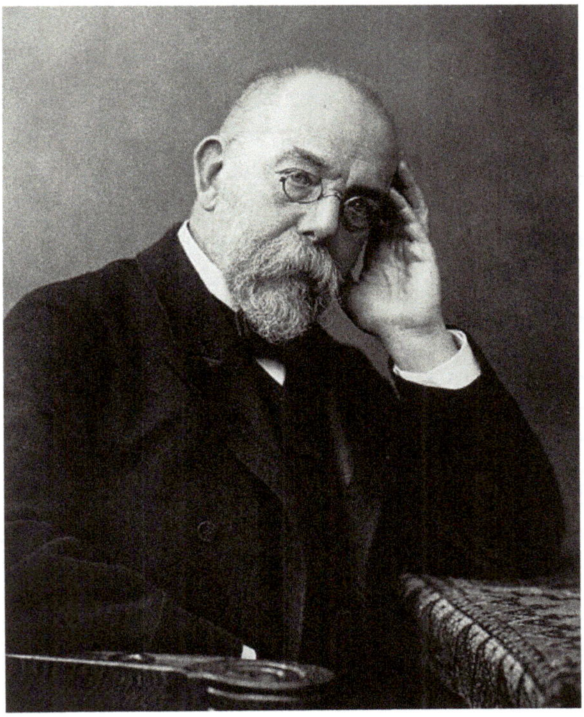

Robert Koch showed that microorganisms caused disease.

Antonie Van Leeuwenhoek (1632–1723) was one of the first people to observe microorganisms, using microscopes of his own design. Robert Hooke, a contemporary of Leeuwenhoek, also used microscopes to observe microbial life; his 1665 book *Micrographia* describes these observations and coined the term *cell*.

Before Leeuwenhoek's discovery of microorganisms in 1675, it had been a mystery why grapes could be turned into wine, milk into cheese, or why food would spoil. Leeuwenhoek did not make the connection between these processes and microorganisms, but using a microscope, he did establish that there were signs of life that were not visible to the naked eye. Leeuwenhoek's discovery, along with subsequent observations by Spallanzani and Pasteur, ended the long-held belief that life spontaneously appeared from non-living substances during the process of spoilage.

Lazzaro Spallanzani (1729–1799) found that boiling broth would sterilise it, killing any microorganisms in it. He also found that new microorganisms could only settle in a broth if the broth was exposed to air.

Louis Pasteur (1822–1895) expanded upon Spallanzani's findings by exposing boiled broths to the air, in vessels that contained a filter to prevent all particles from passing through to the growth medium, and also in vessels with no filter at all, with air being admitted via a curved tube that would not allow dust particles to come in contact with the broth. By boiling the broth beforehand, Pasteur ensured that no microorganisms survived within the broths at the beginning of his experiment. Nothing grew in the broths in the course of Pasteur's experiment. This meant that the living organisms that grew in such broths came from outside, as spores on dust, rather than spontaneously generated within the broth. Thus, Pasteur dealt the death blow to the theory of spontaneous generation and supported germ theory.

In 1876, Robert Koch (1843–1910) established that microorganisms can cause disease. He found that the blood of cattle which were infected with anthrax always had large numbers of *Bacillus anthracis*. Koch found that he could transmit anthrax from one animal to another by taking a small sample of blood from the infected animal and injecting it into a healthy one, and this caused the healthy animal to become sick. He also found that he could grow the bacteria in a nutrient broth, then inject it into a healthy animal, and cause illness. Based on these experiments, he devised criteria for establishing a causal link between a microorganism and a disease and these are now known as Koch's postulates. Although these postulates cannot be applied in all cases, they do retain historical importance to the development of scientific thought and are still being used today.

On 8 November 2013, scientists reported the discovery of what may be the earliest signs of life on Earth—the oldest complete fossils of a microbial mat (associated with sandstone in Western Australia) estimated to be 3.48 billion years old.

Classification and Structure

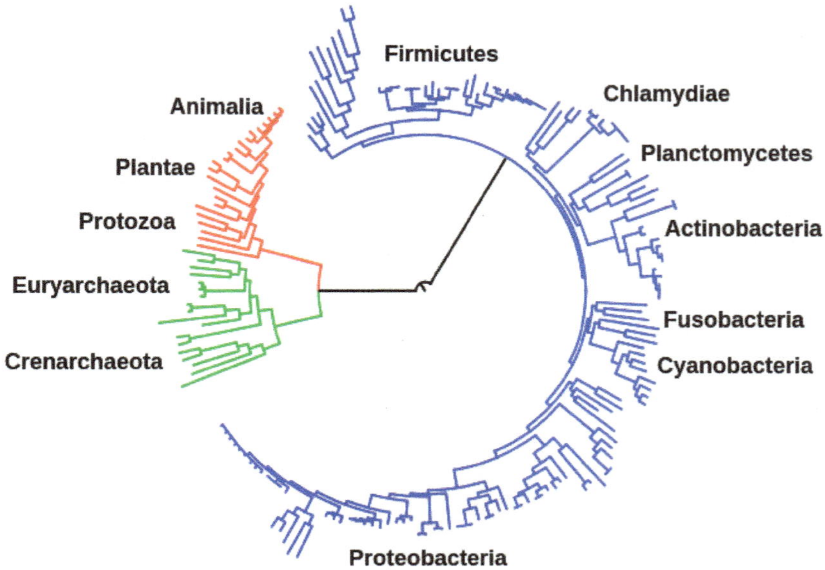

Evolutionary tree showing the common ancestry of all three domains of life. Bacteria are colored blue, eukaryotes red, and archaea green. Relative positions of some phyla are shown around the tree.

Microorganisms can be found almost anywhere in the taxonomic organization of life on the planet. Bacteria and archaea are almost always microscopic, while a number of eukaryotes are also microscopic, including most protists, some fungi, as well as some animals and plants. Viruses are generally regarded as not living and therefore not considered as microorganisms, although the field of microbiology also encompasses the study of viruses.

PROKARYOTE

A prokaryote is a unicellular organism that lacks a membrane-bound nucleus (karyon), mitochondria, or any other membrane-bound organelle. The word prokaryote comes from the Greek πρό (pro) "before" and καρυόν (karyon) "nut or kernel". Prokaryotes can be divided into two domains, Archaea and bacteria. In contrast, species with nuclei and organelles are placed in the domain Eukaryota.

In the prokaryotes, all the intracellular water-soluble components (proteins, DNA and metabolites) are located together in the cytoplasm enclosed by the cell membrane, rather than in separate cellular compartments. Bacteria, however, do possess protein-based bacterial microcompartments, which are thought to act as primitive organelles enclosed in protein shells. Some prokaryotes, such as cyanobacteria may form large colonies. Others, such as myxobacteria, have multicellular stages in their life cycles.

Molecular studies have provided insight into the evolution and interrelationships of the three domains of biological species. Eukaryotes are organisms, including humans, whose cells have a well defined membrane-bound nucleus (containing chromosomal DNA) and organelles. The division between prokaryotes and eukaryotes reflects the existence of two very different levels of cellular organization. Distinctive types of prokaryotes include extremophiles and methanogens; these are common in some extreme environments.

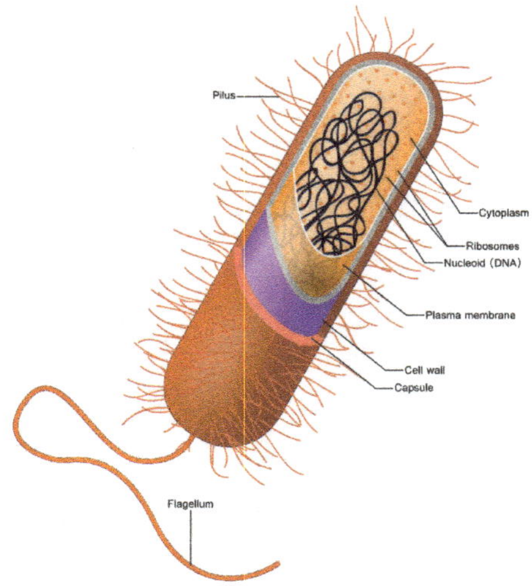

A diagram of a typical prokaryotic bacteria cell.

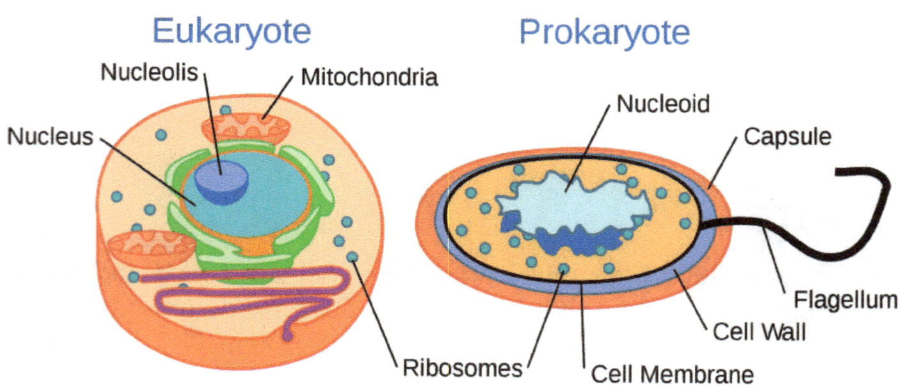

Comparison of eukaryotes vs. prokaryotes

Structure

Prokaryotes have a prokaryotic cytoskeleton, albeit more primitive than that of the eukaryotes. Besides homologues of actin and tubulin (MreB and FtsZ), the helically arranged building-block of the flagellum, flagellin, is one of the most significant cytoskeletal proteins of bacteria, as it provides structural backgrounds of chemotaxis, the basic cell physiological response of bacteria. At least some prokaryotes also contain intracellular structures that can be seen as primitive organelles. Membranous organelles (or intracellular membranes) are known in some groups of prokaryotes, such as vacuoles or membrane systems devoted to special metabolic properties, such as photosynthesis or chemolithotrophy. In addition, some species also contain carbohydrate-enclosed microcompartments, which have distinct physiological roles (e.g. carboxysomes or gas vacuoles).

Most prokaryotes are between 1 µm and 10 µm, but they can vary in size from 0.2 µm (*Mycoplasma genitalium*) to 750 µm (*Thiomargarita namibiensis*).

Prokaryotic cell structure
Flagellum (only in some types of prokaryotes) Long, whip-like protrusion that aids cellular locomotion.
Cell membrane Surrounds the cell's cytoplasm and regulates the flow of substances in and out of the cell.
Cell wall (except genera Mycoplasma and Thermoplasma) Outer covering of most cells that protects the bacterial cell and gives it shape.
Cytoplasm A gel-like substance composed mainly of water that also contains enzymes, salts, cell components, and various organic molecules.
Ribosome Cell structures responsible for protein production.
Nucleoid Area of the cytoplasm that contains the single bacterial DNA molecule.
Glycocalyx (only in some types of prokaryotes) A glycoprotein-polysaccharide covering that surrounds the cell membranes.
Inclusions

Morphology

Prokaryotic cells have various shapes; the four basic shapes of bacteria are:

- Cocci – spherical
- Bacilli – rod-shaped
- Spirochaete – spiral-shaped
- Vibrio – comma-shaped

The archaeon Haloquadratum has flat square-shaped cells.

Reproduction

Bacteria and archaea reproduce through asexual reproduction, usually by binary fission. Genetic exchange and recombination still occur, but this is a form of horizontal gene transfer and is not a replicative process, simply involving the transference of DNA between two cells, as in bacterial conjugation.

DNA Transfer

DNA transfer between prokaryotic cells occurs in bacteria and archaea, although it has been mainly studied in bacteria. In bacteria, gene transfer occurs by three processes. These are (1) bacterial virus (bacteriophage)-mediated transduction, (2) plasmid-mediated conjugation, and (3) natural transformation. Transduction of bacterial genes by bacteriophage appears to reflect an occasional error during intracellular assembly of virus particles, rather than an adaptation of the host bacteria. The transfer of bacterial DNA is under the control of the bacteriophage's genes rather than bacterial genes. Conjugation in the well-studied *E. coli* system is controlled by plasmid genes, and is an adaptation for distributing copies of a plasmid from one bacterial host to another. Infrequently during this process, a plasmid may integrate into the host bacterial chromosome, and subsequently transfer part of the host bacterial DNA to another bacterium. Plasmid mediated transfer of host bacterial DNA (conjugation) also appears to be an accidental process rather than a bacterial adaptation.

Natural bacterial transformation involves the transfer of DNA from one bacterium to another through the intervening medium. Unlike transduction and conjugation, transformation is clearly a bacterial adaptation for DNA transfer, because it depends on numerous bacterial gene products that specifically interact to perform this complex process. For a bacterium to bind, take up and recombine donor DNA into its own chromosome, it must first enter a special physiological state called competence. About 40 genes are required in *Bacillus subtilis* for the development of competence. The length of DNA transferred during *B. subtilis* transformation can be as much as a third to the whole chromosome. Transformation is a common mode of DNA transfer, and 67 prokaryotic species are thus far known to be naturally competent for transformation.

Among archaea, *Halobacterium volcanii* forms cytoplasmic bridges between cells that appear to be used for transfer of DNA from one cell to another. Another archaeon, *Sulfolobus solfataricus*, transfers DNA between cells by direct contact. Frols et al. found that exposure of *S. solfataricus* to DNA damaging agents induces cellular aggregation, and suggested that cellular aggregation may enhance DNA transfer among cells to provide increased repair of damaged DNA via homologous recombination.

Sociality

While prokaryotes are considered strictly unicellular, most can form stable aggregate communities. When such communities are encased in a stabilizing polymer matrix ("slime"), they may be called "biofilms". Cells in biofilms often show distinct patterns of gene expression (phenotypic differentiation) in time and space. Also, as with multicellular eukaryotes, these changes in expression often appear to result from cell-to-cell signaling, a phenomenon known as quorum sensing.

Biofilms may be highly heterogeneous and structurally complex and may attach to solid surfaces, or exist at liquid-air interfaces, or potentially even liquid-liquid interfaces. Bacterial biofilms are often made up of microcolonies (approximately dome-shaped masses of bacteria and matrix) separated by "voids" through which the medium (e.g., water) may flow easily. The microcolonies may join together above the substratum to form a continuous layer, closing the network of channels separating microcolonies. This structural complexity—combined with observations that oxygen limitation (a ubiquitous challenge for anything growing in size beyond the scale of diffusion) is at least partially eased by movement of medium throughout the biofilm—has led some to speculate that this may constitute a circulatory system and many researchers have started calling prokaryotic communities multicellular (for example). Differential cell expression, collective behavior, signaling, programmed cell death, and (in some cases) discrete biological dispersal events all seem to point in this direction. However, these colonies are seldom if ever founded by a single founder (in the way that animals and plants are founded by single cells), which presents a number of theoretical issues. Most explanations of co-operation and the evolution of multicellularity have focused on high relatedness between members of a group (or colony, or whole organism). If a copy of a gene is present in all members of a group, behaviors that promote cooperation between members may permit those members to have (on average) greater fitness than a similar group of selfish individuals (see inclusive fitness and Hamilton's rule).

Should these instances of prokaryotic sociality prove to be the rule rather than the exception, it would have serious implications for the way we view prokaryotes in general, and the way we deal with them in medicine. Bacterial biofilms may be 100 times more resistant to antibiotics than free-living unicells and may be nearly impossible to remove from surfaces once they have colonized them. Other aspects of bacterial cooperation—such as bacterial conjugation and quorum-sensing-mediated pathogenicity, present additional challenges to researchers and medical professionals seeking to treat the associated diseases.

Environment

Prokaryotes have diversified greatly throughout their long existence. The metabolism of prokaryotes is far more varied than that of eukaryotes, leading to many highly distinct prokaryotic types. For example, in addition to using photosynthesis or organic compounds for energy, as eukaryotes do, prokaryotes may obtain energy from inorganic compounds such as hydrogen sulfide. This enables prokaryotes to thrive in harsh environments as cold as the snow surface of Antarctica, studied in cryobiology or as hot as undersea hydrothermal vents and land-based hot springs.

Prokaryotes live in nearly all environments on Earth. Some archaea and bacteria thrive in harsh conditions, such as high temperatures (thermophiles) or high salinity (halophiles). Organisms such as these are referred to as extremophiles. Many archaea grow as plankton in the oceans. Symbiotic prokaryotes live in or on the bodies of other organisms, including humans.

Classification

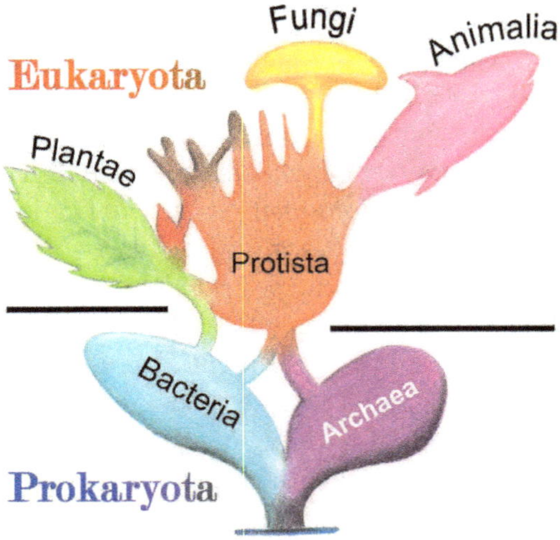

Phylogenetic and symbiogenetic tree of living organisms, showing the origins of eukaryotes and prokaryotes

In 1977, Carl Woese proposed dividing prokaryotes into the Bacteria and Archaea (originally Eubacteria and Archaebacteria) because of the major differences in the structure and genetics between the two groups of organisms. Archaea were originally thought to be extremophiles, living only in inhospitable conditions such as extremes of temperature, pH, and radiation but have since been found in all types of habitats. The resulting arrangement of Eukaryota (also called "Eukarya"), Bacteria, and Archaea is called the three-domain system, replacing the traditional two-empire system.

One criticism of the dichotomous prokaryote-eukaryote distinction points out that the word "prokaryote" is based on what these organisms are not (they are not eukaryotic), rather than what they are (either archaea or bacteria).

Evolution

The current model of the evolution of the first living organisms is that these were some form of prokaryotes, which may have evolved out of protocells. In general, the eukaryotes are thought to have evolved later in the history of life.

However, some authors have questioned this conclusion, arguing that the current set of prokaryotic species may have evolved from more complex eukaryotic ancestors through a process of simplification.

Others have argued that the three domains of life arose simultaneously, from a set of varied cells that formed a single gene pool.

This controversy was summarized in 2005:

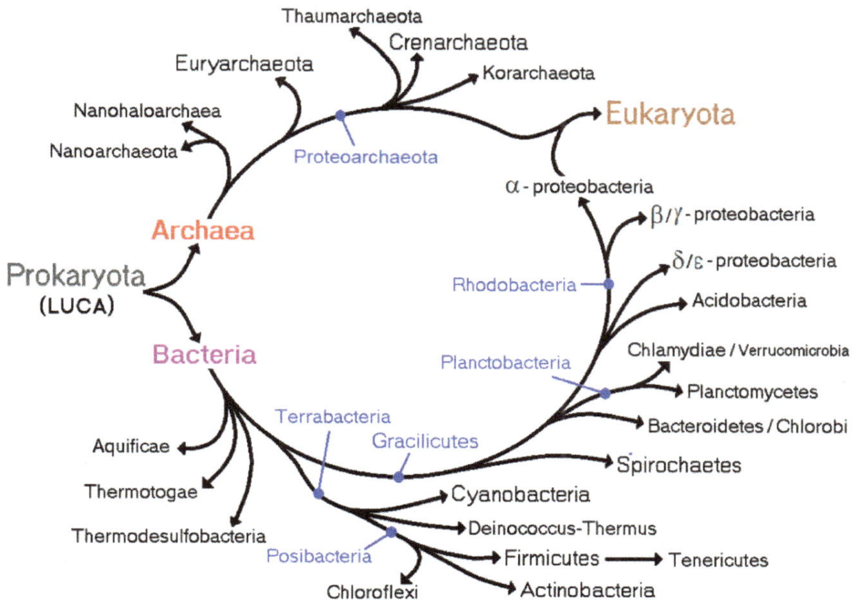

Phylogenetic ring showing the diversity of prokaryotes, and symbiogenetic origins of eukaryotes

There is no consensus among biologists concerning the position of the eukaryotes in the overall scheme of cell evolution. Current opinions on the origin and position of eukaryotes span a broad spectrum including the views that eukaryotes arose first in evolution and that prokaryotes descend from them, that eukaryotes arose contemporaneously with eubacteria and archeabacteria and hence represent a primary line of descent of equal age and rank as the prokaryotes, that eukaryotes arose through a symbiotic event entailing an endosymbiotic origin of the nucleus, that eukaryotes arose without endosymbiosis, and that eukaryotes arose through a symbiotic event entailing a simultaneous endosymbiotic origin of the flagellum and the nucleus, in addition to many other models, which have been reviewed and summarized elsewhere.

The oldest known fossilized prokaryotes were laid down approximately 3.5 billion years ago, only about 1 billion years after the formation of the Earth's crust. Eukaryotes only appear in the fossil record later, and may have formed from endosymbiosis of multiple prokaryote ancestors. The oldest known fossil eukaryotes are about 1.7 billion years old. However, some genetic evidence suggests eukaryotes appeared as early as 3 billion years ago.

While Earth is the only place in the universe where life is known to exist, some have suggested that there is evidence on Mars of fossil or living prokaryotes.However, this possibility remains the subject of considerable debate and skepticism.

Relationship to Eukaryotes

The division between prokaryotes and eukaryotes is usually considered the most important distinction or difference among organisms. The distinction is that eukaryotic cells have a "true" nucleus containing their DNA, whereas prokaryotic cells do not have a nucleus. Both eukaryotes and prokaryotes contain large RNA/protein structures called ribosomes, which produce protein.

Another difference is that ribosomes in prokaryotes are smaller than in eukaryotes. However, two organelles found in many eukaryotic cells, mitochondria and chloroplasts, contain ribosomes similar in size and makeup to those found in prokaryotes. This is one of many pieces of evidence that mitochondria and chloroplasts are themselves descended from free-living bacteria. This theory holds that early eukaryotic cells took in primitive prokaryotic cells by phagocytosis and adapted themselves to incorporate their structures, leading to the mitochondria we see today.

The genome in a prokaryote is held within a DNA/protein complex in the cytosol called the nucleoid, which lacks a nuclear envelope. The complex contains a single, cyclic, double-stranded molecule of stable chromosomal DNA, in contrast to the multiple linear, compact, highly organized chromosomes found in eukaryotic cells. In addition, many important genes of prokaryotes are stored in separate circular DNA structures called plasmids.

Prokaryotes lack mitochondria and chloroplasts. Instead, processes such as oxidative phosphorylation and photosynthesis take place across the prokaryotic cell membrane. However, prokaryotes do possess some internal structures, such as prokaryotic cytoskeletons. It has been suggested that the bacterial order Planctomycetes have a membrane around their nucleoid and contain other membrane-bound cellular structures. However, further investigation revealed that Planctomycetes cells are not compartmentalized or nucleated and like the other bacterial membrane systems are all interconnected.

Prokaryotic cells are usually much smaller than eukaryotic cells. Therefore, prokaryotes have a larger surface-area-to-volume ratio, giving them a higher metabolic rate, a higher growth rate, and as a consequence, a shorter generation time than eukaryotes.

Prokaryotes are organisms that lack a cell nucleus and the other membrane bound organelles. They are almost always unicellular, although some species such as myxobacteria can aggregate into complex structures as part of their life cycle.

Consisting of two domains, bacteria and archaea, the prokaryotes are the most diverse and abundant group of organisms on Earth and inhabit practically all environments where the temperature is below +140 °C. They are found in water, soil, air, animals' gastrointestinal tracts, hot springs and even deep beneath the Earth's crust in rocks. Practically all surfaces that have not been specially sterilized are covered by prokaryotes. The number of prokaryotes on Earth is estimated to be around five million trillion trillion, or 5×10^{30}, accounting for at least half the biomass on Earth.

The biodiversity of the prokaryotes is unknown, but may be very large. A May 2016 estimate, based on laws of scaling from known numbers of species against the size of organism, gives an estimate of perhaps 1 trillion species on the planet, of which most would be microorganisms. Currently, only one-thousandth of one percent of that total have been described.

BACTERIA

Bacteria constitute a large domain of prokaryoticmicroorganisms. Typically a few micrometres in length, bacteria have a number of shapes, ranging from spheres to rods and spirals. Bacteria were among the first life forms to appear on Earth, and are present in most of its habitats. Bacteria inhabit soil, water, acidic hot springs, radioactive waste, and the deep portions of Earth's crust. Bacteria also live in symbiotic and parasitic relationships with plants and animals.

There are typically 40 million bacterial cells in a gram of soil and a million bacterial cells in a millilitre of fresh water. There are approximately 5×10^{30} bacteria on Earth, forming a biomass which exceeds that of all plants and animals. Bacteria are vital in recycling nutrients, with many of the stages in nutrient cycles dependent on these organisms, such as the fixation of nitrogen from the atmosphere and putrefaction. In the biological communities surrounding hydrothermal vents and cold seeps, bacteria provide the nutrients needed to sustain life by converting dissolved compounds, such as hydrogen sulphide and methane, to energy. On 17 March 2013, researchers reported data that suggested bacterial life forms thrive in the Mariana Trench, which with a depth of up to 11 kilometres is the deepest part of the Earth's oceans. Other researchers reported related studies that microbes thrive inside rocks up to 580 metres below the sea floor under 2.6 kilometres of ocean off the coast of the northwestern United States. According to one of the researchers, "You can find microbes everywhere—they're extremely adaptable to conditions, and survive wherever they are."

Most bacteria have not been characterised, and only about half of the bacterial phyla have species that can be grown in the laboratory. The study of bacteria is known as bacteriology, a branch of microbiology.

There are approximately ten times as many bacterial cells in the human flora as there are human cells in the body, with the largest number of the human flora being in the gut flora, and a large number on the skin. The vast majority of the bacteria in the body are rendered harmless by the protective effects of the immune system, and some are beneficial. However, several species of bacteria are pathogenic and cause infectious diseases, including cholera, syphilis, anthrax, leprosy, and bubonic plague. The most common fatal bacterial diseases are respiratory infections, with tuberculosis alone killing about 2 million people per year, mostly in sub-Saharan Africa. In developed countries, antibiotics are used to treat bacterial infections and are also used in farming, making antibiotic resistance a growing problem. In industry, bacteria are important in sewage treatment and the breakdown of oil spills, the production of cheese and yogurt through fermentation, and the recovery of gold, palladium, copper and other metals in the mining sector, as well as in biotechnology, and the manufacture of antibiotics and other chemicals.

Once regarded as plants constituting the class *Schizomycetes*, bacteria are now classified as prokaryotes. Unlike cells of animals and other eukaryotes, bacterial cells do not contain a nucleus and rarely harbour membrane-bound organelles. Although the term *bacteria* traditionally included all prokaryotes, the scientific classification changed after the discovery in the 1990s that prokaryotes consist of two very different groups of organisms that evolved from an ancient common ancestor. These evolutionary domains are called *Bacteria* and *Archaea*.

Etymology

The word *bacteria* is the plural of the New Latin *bacterium*, which is the latinisation of the Greek βακτήριον (*bakterion*), the diminutive of βακτηρία (*bakteria*), meaning "staff, cane", because the first ones to be discovered were rod-shaped.

Origin and early Evolution

The ancestors of modern bacteria were unicellular microorganisms that were the first forms of life to appear on Earth, about 4 billion years ago. For about 3 billion years, most organisms were microscopic, and bacteria and archaea were the dominant forms of life. In 2008, fossils of macroorganisms were discovered and named as the Francevillian biota. Although bacterial fossils exist, such as stromatolites, their lack of distinctive morphology prevents them from being used to examine the history of bacterial evolution, or to date the time of origin of a particular bacterial species. However, gene sequences can be used to reconstruct the bacterial phylogeny, and these studies indicate that bacteria diverged first from the archaeal/eukaryotic lineage.Bacteria were also involved in the second great evolutionary divergence, that of the archaea and eukaryotes. Here, eukaryotes resulted from the entering of ancient bacteria into endosymbiotic associations with the ancestors of eukaryotic cells, which were themselves possibly related to the Archaea. This involved the engulfment by proto-eukaryotic cells of alphaproteobacterial symbionts to form either mitochondria or hydrogenosomes, which are still found in all known Eukarya (sometimes in highly reduced form, e.g. in ancient "amitochondrial" protozoa). Later on, some eukaryotes that already contained mitochondria also engulfed cyanobacterial-like organisms. This led to the formation of chloroplasts in algae and plants. There are also some algae that originated from even later endosymbiotic events. Here, eukaryotes engulfed a eukaryotic algae that developed into a "second-generation" plastid. This is known as secondary endosymbiosis.

Morphology

Bacteria display a wide diversity of shapes and sizes, called *morphologies*. Bacterial cells are about one-tenth the size of eukaryotic cells and are typically 0.5–5.0 micrometres in length. However, a few species are visible to the unaided eye—for example, *Thiomargarita namibiensis* is up to half a millimetre long and *Epulopiscium fishelsoni* reaches 0.7 mm. Among the smallest bacteria are members of the genus *Mycoplasma*, which measure only 0.3 micrometres, as small as the largest viruses. Some bacteria may be even smaller, but these ultramicrobacteria are not well-studied.

Most bacterial species are either spherical, called *cocci* (*sing*. coccus, from Greek *kókkos*, grain, seed), or rod-shaped, called *bacilli* (*sing*. bacillus, from Latin *baculus*, stick). Elongation is associated with swimming. Some bacteria, called *vibrio*, are shaped like slightly curved rods or comma-shaped; others can be spiral-shaped, called *spirilla*, or tightly coiled, called *spirochaetes*. A small number of species even have tetrahedral or cuboidal shapes. More recently, some bacteria were discovered deep under Earth's crust that grow as branching filamentous types with a star-shaped cross-section. The large surface area to volume ratio of this morphology may give these bacteria an advantage in nutrient-poor environments. This wide variety of shapes is determined by the bacterial cell wall and cytoskeleton, and is important because it can influence the ability of bacteria to acquire nutrients, attach to surfaces, swim through liquids and escape predators.

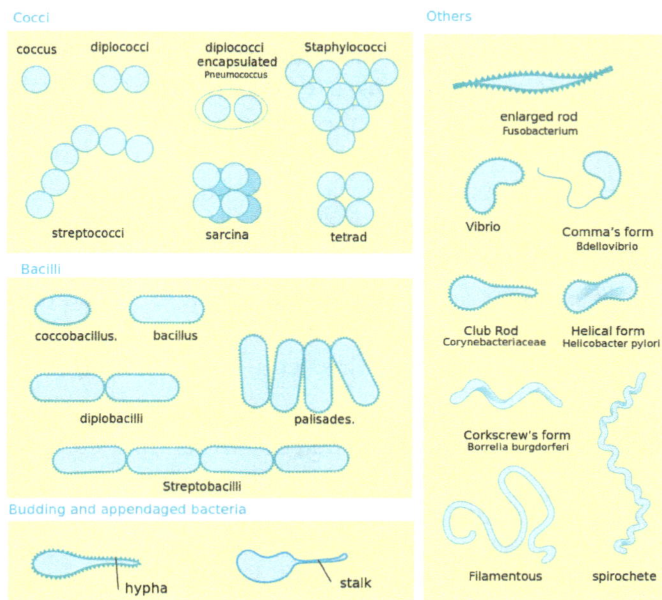

Bacteria display many cell morphologies and arrangements

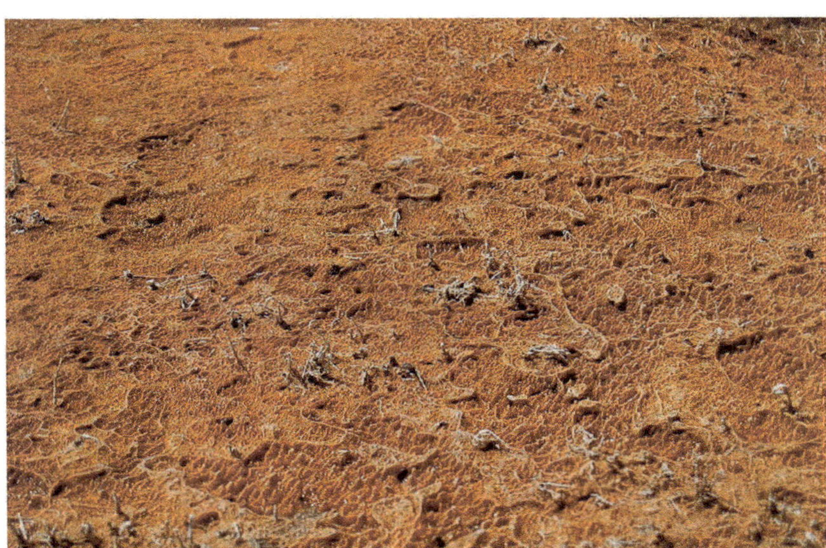

A biofilm of thermophilic bacteria in the outflow of Mickey Hot Springs, Oregon, approximately 20 mm thick.

Many bacterial species exist simply as single cells, others associate in characteristic patterns: *Neisseria* form diploids (pairs), *Streptococcus* form chains, and *Staphylococcus* group together in "bunch of grapes" clusters. Bacteria can also be elongated to form filaments, for example the Actinobacteria. Filamentous bacteria are often surrounded by a sheath that contains many individual cells. Certain types, such as species of the genus *Nocardia*, even form complex, branched filaments, similar in appearance to fungal mycelia.

Bacteria often attach to surfaces and form dense aggregations called *biofilms* or bacterial mats. These films can range from a few micrometres in thickness to up to half a metre in depth, and may contain multiple species of bacteria, protists and archaea. Bacteria living in biofilms display a complex arrangement of cells and extracellular components, forming secondary structures, such as microcolonies, through which there are networks of channels to enable better diffusion of nutrients.In natural environments, such as soil or the surfaces of plants, the majority of bacteria are bound to surfaces in biofilms.Biofilms are also important in medicine, as these structures are often present during chronic bacterial infections or in infections of implanted medical devices, and bacteria protected within biofilms are much harder to kill than individual isolated bacteria.

Even more complex morphological changes are sometimes possible. For example, when starved of amino acids, Myxobacteria detect surrounding cells in a process known as quorum sensing, migrate towards each other, and aggregate to form fruiting bodies up to 500 micrometres long and containing approximately 100,000 bacterial cells. In these fruiting bodies, the bacteria perform separate tasks; this type of cooperation is a simple type of multicellular organisation. For example, about one in 10 cells migrate to the top of these fruiting bodies and differentiate into a specialised dormant state called myxospores, which are more resistant to drying and other adverse environmental conditions than are ordinary cells.

Cellular Structure

Intracellular Structures

The bacterial cell is surrounded by a cell membrane (also known as a lipid, cytoplasmic or plasma membrane). This membrane encloses the contents of the cell and acts as a barrier to hold nutrients, proteins and other essential components of the *cytoplasm* within the cell. As they are prokaryotes, bacteria do not usually have membrane-bound organelles in their cytoplasm, and thus contain few large intracellular structures. They lack a true nucleus, mitochondria, chloroplasts and the other organelles present in eukaryotic cells. Bacteria were once seen as simple bags of cytoplasm, but structures such as the *prokaryotic cytoskeleton* and the localisation of proteins to specific locations within the cytoplasm that give bacteria some complexity have been discovered. These subcellular levels of organisation have been called "bacterial hyperstructures".

Bacterial microcompartments, such as carboxysomes, provide a further level of organisation; they are compartments within bacteria that are surrounded by polyhedral protein shells, rather than by lipid membranes. These "polyhedral organelles" localise and compartmentalise bacterial metabolism, a function performed by the membrane-bound organelles in eukaryotes.

Many important biochemical reactions, such as energy generation, use concentration gradients across membranes. The general lack of internal membranes in bacteria means reactions such as electron transport occur across the cell membrane between the cytoplasm and the *periplasmic space*. However, in many photosynthetic bacteria the plasma membrane is highly folded and fills most of the cell with layers of light-gathering membrane. These light-gathering complexes may even form lipid-enclosed structures called chlorosomes in green sulfur bacteria.Other proteins import nutrients across the cell membrane, or expel undesired molecules from the cytoplasm.

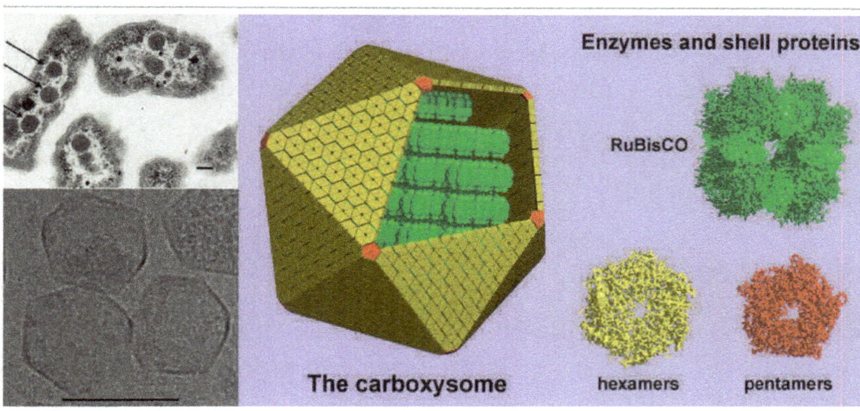

Carboxysomes are protein-enclosed bacterial organelles. Top left is an electron microscope image of carboxysomes in *Halothiobacillus neapolitanus*, below is an image of purified carboxysomes. On the right is a model of their structure. Scale bars are 100 nm.

Bacteria do not have a membrane-bound nucleus, and their genetic material is typically a single circular DNA chromosome located in the cytoplasm in an irregularly shaped body called the *nucleoid*. The nucleoid contains the chromosome with its associated proteins and RNA. The phylum Planctomycetes and candidate phylum Poribacteria may be exceptions to the general absence of internal membranes in bacteria, because they appear to have a double membrane around their nucleoids and contain other membrane-bound cellular structures. Like all living organisms, bacteria contain *ribosomes*, often grouped in chains called polyribosomes, for the production of proteins, but the structure of the bacterial ribosome is different from that of eukaryotes and Archaea. Bacterial ribosomes have a sedimentation rate of 70S (measured in Svedberg units): their subunits have rates of 30S and 50S. Some antibiotics bind specifically to 70S ribosomes and inhibit bacterial protein synthesis. Those antibiotics kill bacteria without affecting the larger 80S ribosomes of eukaryotic cells and without harming the host.

Some bacteria produce intracellular nutrient storage granules for later use, such as glycogen, polyphosphate, sulfur or polyhydroxyalkanoates. Certain bacterial species, such as the photosynthetic Cyanobacteria, produce internal gas vesicles, which they use to regulate their buoyancy—allowing them to move up or down into water layers with different light intensities and nutrient levels.*Intracellular membranes* called *chromatophores* are also found in membranes of phototrophic bacteria. Used primarily for photosynthesis, they contain bacteriochlorophyll pigments and carotenoids. An early idea was that bacteria might contain membrane folds termed mesosomes, but these were later shown to be artefacts produced by the chemicals used to prepare the cells for electron microscopy. *Inclusions* are considered to be nonliving components of the cell that do not possess metabolic activity and are not bounded by membranes. The most common inclusions are glycogen, lipid droplets, crystals, and pigments. *Volutin granules* are cytoplasmic inclusions of complexed inorganic polyphosphate. These granules are called *metachromatic granules* due to their displaying the metachromatic effect; they appear red or blue when stained with the blue dyes methylene blue or toluidine blue. *Gas vacuoles*, which are freely permeable to gas, are membrane-bound vesicles present in some species of *Cyanobacteria*. They allow the bacteria to control their buoyancy. *Microcompartments* are widespread, membrane-bound organelles that are made of a protein shell that surrounds and encloses various enzymes. *Carboxysomes* are bacterial microcompartments that contain enzymes involved in carbon fixation. *Magnetosomes* are bacterial microcompartments, present in magnetotactic bacteria, that contain magnetic crystals.

Extracellular Structures

In most bacteria, a *cell wall* is present on the outside of the cell membrane. The cell membrane and cell wall comprise the *cell envelope*. A common bacterial cell wall material is *peptidoglycan* (called "murein" in older sources), which is made from polysaccharide chains cross-linked by peptides containing D-amino acids.Bacterial cell walls are different from the cell walls of plants and fungi, which are made of cellulose and chitin, respectively. The cell wall of bacteria is also distinct from that of Archaea, which do not contain peptidoglycan. The cell wall is essential to the survival of many bacteria, and the antibiotic penicillin is able to kill bacteria by inhibiting a step in the synthesis of peptidoglycan.

There are broadly speaking two different types of cell wall in bacteria, a thick one in the gram-positives and a thinner one in the gram-negatives. The names originate from the reaction of cells to the Gram stain, a long-standing test for the classification of bacterial species.

Gram-positive bacteria possess a thick cell wall containing many layers of peptidoglycan and *teichoic acids*. In contrast, *gram-negative bacteria* have a relatively thin cell wall consisting of a few layers of peptidoglycan surrounded by a second lipid membrane containing *lipopolysaccharides* and lipoproteins. Lipopolysaccharides, also called *endotoxins*, are composed of polysaccharides and *lipid A* that is responsible for much of the toxicity of gram-negative bacteria. Most bacteria have the gram-negative cell wall, and only the Firmicutes and Actinobacteria have the alternative gram-positive arrangement. These two groups were previously known as the low G+C and high G+C gram-positive bacteria, respectively. These differences in structure can produce differences in antibiotic susceptibility; for instance, vancomycin can kill only gram-positive bacteria and is ineffective against gram-negative pathogens, such as *Haemophilus influenzae* or *Pseudomonas aeruginosa*. If the bacterial cell wall is entirely removed, it is called a *protoplast*, whereas if it is partially removed, it is called a *spheroplast*. *β*-Lactam antibiotics, such as penicillin, inhibit the formation of peptidoglycan cross-links in the bacterial cell wall. The enzyme lysozyme, found in human tears, also digests the cell wall of bacteria and is the body's main defence against eye infections.

Acid-fast bacteria, such as *Mycobacteria*, are resistant to decolorisation by acids during staining procedures. The high mycolic acid content of *Mycobacteria*, is responsible for the staining pattern of poor absorption followed by high retention. The most common staining technique used to identify acid-fast bacteria is the Ziehl-Neelsen stain or acid-fast stain, in which the acid-fast bacilli are stained bright-red and stand out clearly against a blue background. *L-form bacteria* are strains of bacteria that lack cell walls. The main pathogenic bacteria in this class is *Mycoplasma* (not to be confused with *Mycobacteria*).

In many bacteria, an *S-layer* of rigidly arrayed protein molecules covers the outside of the cell. This layer provides chemical and physical protection for the cell surface and can act as a macromolecular diffusion barrier. S-layers have diverse but mostly poorly understood functions, but are known to act as virulence factors in *Campylobacter* and contain surface enzymes in *Bacillus stearothermophilus*.

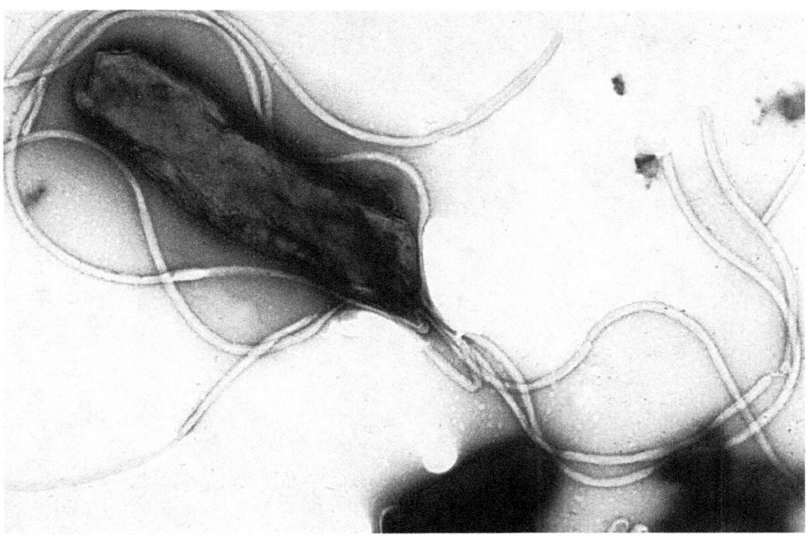

Helicobacter pylori electron micrograph, showing multiple flagella on the cell surface

Flagella are rigid protein structures, about 20 nanometres in diameter and up to 20 micrometres in length, that are used for motility. Flagella are driven by the energy released by the transfer of ions down an electrochemical gradient across the cell membrane.

Fimbriae (sometimes called "attachment pili") are fine filaments of protein, usually 2–10 nanometres in diameter and up to several micrometres in length. They are distributed over the surface of the cell, and resemble fine hairs when seen under the electron microscope. Fimbriae are believed to be involved in attachment to solid surfaces or to other cells, and are essential for the virulence of some bacterial pathogens. *Pili* (*sing.* pilus) are cellular appendages, slightly larger than fimbriae, that can transfer genetic material between bacterial cells in a process called conjugation where they are called *conjugation pili* or "sex pili" (see bacterial genetics, below). They can also generate movement where they are called *type IV pili* (see movement, below).

Glycocalyx are produced by many bacteria to surround their cells, and vary in structural complexity: ranging from a disorganised *slime layer* of extra-cellular polymer to a highly structured *capsule*. These structures can protect cells from engulfment by eukaryotic cells such as macrophages (part of the human immune system). They can also act as antigens and be involved in cell recognition, as well as aiding attachment to surfaces and the formation of biofilms.

The assembly of these extracellular structures is dependent on bacterial secretion systems. These transfer proteins from the cytoplasm into the periplasm or into the environment around the cell. Many types of secretion systems are known and these structures are often essential for the virulence of pathogens, so are intensively studied.

Endospores

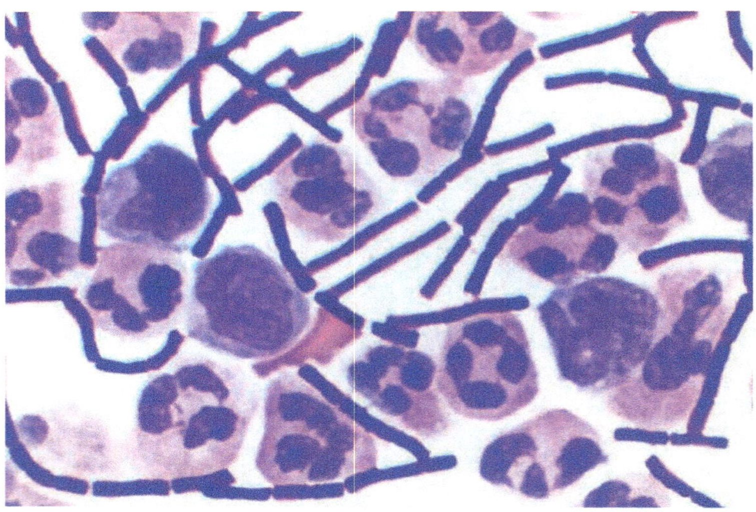

Bacillus anthracis (stained purple) growing in cerebrospinal fluid

Certain genera of gram-positive bacteria, such as *Bacillus*, *Clostridium*, *Sporohalobacter*, *Anaerobacter*, and *Heliobacterium*, can form highly resistant, dormant structures called *endospores*. In almost all cases, one endospore is formed and this is not a reproductive process, although *Anaerobacter* can make up to seven endospores in a single cell. Endospores have a central core of cytoplasm containing DNA and ribosomes surrounded by a cortex layer and protected by an impermeable and rigid coat. Dipicolinic acid is a chemical compound that composes 5% to 15% of the dry weight of bacterial spores. It is implicated as responsible for the heat resistance of the endospore.

Endospores show no detectable metabolism and can survive extreme physical and chemical stresses, such as high levels of UV light, gamma radiation, detergents, disinfectants, heat, freezing, pressure, and desiccation. In this dormant state, these organisms may remain viable for millions of years, and endospores even allow bacteria to survive exposure to the vacuum and radiation in space. According to scientist Dr. Steinn Sigurdsson, "There are viable bacterial spores that have been found that are 40 million years old on Earth—and we know they're very hardened to radiation." Endospore-forming bacteria can also cause disease: for example, anthrax can be contracted by the inhalation of *Bacillus anthracis* endospores, and contamination of deep puncture wounds with *Clostridium tetani* endospores causes tetanus.

Metabolism

Bacteria exhibit an extremely wide variety of metabolic types. The distribution of metabolic traits within a group of bacteria has traditionally been used to define their taxonomy, but these traits often do not correspond with modern genetic classifications. Bacterial metabolism is classified into nutritional groups on the basis of three major criteria: the kind of energy used for growth, the source of carbon, and the electron donors used for growth. An additional criterion of respiratory microorganisms are the electron acceptors used for aerobic or anaerobic respiration.

Nutritional types in bacterial metabolism

Nutritional type	Source of energy	Source of carbon	Examples
Phototrophs	Sunlight	Organic compounds (photoheterotrophs) or carbon fixation (photoautotrophs)	Cyanobacteria, Green sulfur bacteria, Chloroflexi, or Purple bacteria
Lithotrophs	Inorganic compounds	Organic compounds (lithoheterotrophs) or carbon fixation (lithoautotrophs)	Thermodesulfobacteria, *Hydrogenophilaceae*, or Nitrospirae
Organotrophs	Organic compounds	Organic compounds (chemoheterotrophs) or carbon fixation (chemoautotrophs)	*Bacillus*, *Clostridium* or *Enterobacteriaceae*

Carbon metabolism in bacteria is either *heterotrophic*, where organic carbon compounds are used as carbon sources, or *autotrophic*, meaning that cellular carbon is obtained by fixing carbon dioxide. Heterotrophic bacteria include parasitic types. Typical autotrophic bacteria are phototrophic cyanobacteria, green sulfur-bacteria and some purple bacteria, but also many chemolithotrophic species, such as nitrifying or sulfur-oxidising bacteria. Energy metabolism of bacteria is either based on *phototrophy*, the use of light through photosynthesis, or based on *chemotrophy*, the use of chemical substances for energy, which are mostly oxidised at the expense of oxygen or alternative electron acceptors (aerobic/anaerobic respiration).

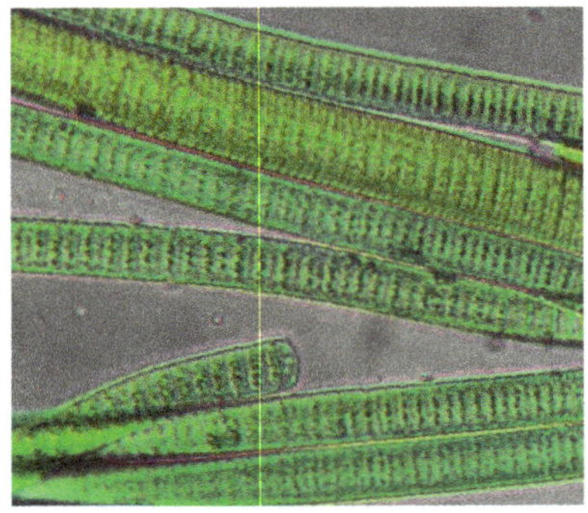

Filaments of photosyntheticcyanobacteria

Bacteria are further divided into *lithotrophs* that use inorganic electron donors and *organotrophs* that use organic compounds as electron donors. Chemotrophic organisms use the respective electron donors for energy conservation (by aerobic/anaerobic respiration or fermentation) and biosynthetic reactions (e.g., carbon dioxide fixation), whereas phototrophic organisms use them only for biosynthetic purposes. Respiratory organisms use chemical compounds as a source of energy by taking electrons from the reduced substrate and transferring them to a terminal electron acceptor in a redox reaction. This reaction releases energy that can be used to synthesise ATP and drive metabolism. In *aerobic organisms*, oxygen is used as the electron acceptor. In *anaerobic organisms* other inorganic compounds, such as nitrate, sulfate or carbon dioxide are used as electron acceptors. This leads to the ecologically important processes of denitrification, sulfate reduction, and acetogenesis, respectively.

Another way of life of chemotrophs in the absence of possible electron acceptors is fermentation, wherein the electrons taken from the reduced substrates are transferred to oxidised intermediates to generate reduced fermentation products (e.g., lactate, ethanol, hydrogen, butyric acid). Fermentation is possible, because the energy content of the substrates is higher than that of the products, which allows the organisms to synthesise ATP and drive their metabolism.

These processes are also important in biological responses to pollution; for example, sulfate-reducing bacteria are largely responsible for the production of the highly toxic forms of mercury (methyl- and dimethylmercury) in the environment. Non-respiratory anaerobes use fermentation to generate energy and reducing power, secreting metabolic by-products (such as ethanol in brewing) as waste. Facultative anaerobes can switch between fermentation and different terminal electron acceptors depending on the environmental conditions in which they find themselves.

Lithotrophic bacteria can use inorganic compounds as a source of energy. Common inorganic electron donors are hydrogen, carbon monoxide, ammonia (leading to nitrification), ferrous iron and other reduced metal ions, and several reduced sulfur compounds. In unusual circumstances, the gas methane can be used by methanotrophic bacteria as both a source of electrons and a substrate for carbon anabolism. In both aerobic phototrophy and chemolithotrophy, oxygen is used as a terminal electron acceptor, whereas under anaerobic conditions inorganic compounds are used instead. Most lithotrophic organisms are autotrophic, whereas organotrophic organisms are heterotrophic.

In addition to fixing carbon dioxide in photosynthesis, some bacteria also fix nitrogen gas (nitrogen fixation) using the enzyme nitrogenase. This environmentally important trait can be found in bacteria of nearly all the metabolic types listed above, but is not universal.

Regardless of the type of metabolic process they employ, the majority of bacteria are able to take in raw materials only in the form of relatively small molecules, which enter the cell by diffusion or through molecular channels in cell membranes. The Planctomycetes are the exception (as they are in possessing membranes around their nuclear material). It has recently been shown that *Gemmata obscuriglobus* is able to take in large molecules via a process that in some ways resembles endocytosis, the process used by eukaryotic cells to engulf external items.

Growth and Reproduction

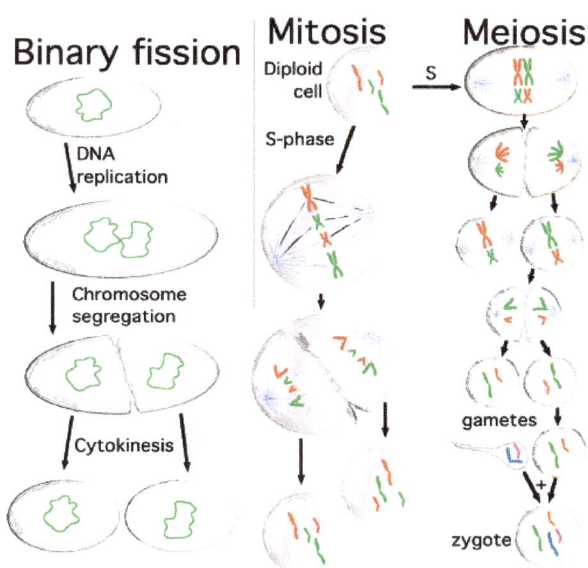

Many bacteria reproduce through binary fission, which is compared to mitosis and meiosis in this image.

Unlike in multicellular organisms, increases in cell size (cell growth) and reproduction by cell division are tightly linked in unicellular organisms. Bacteria grow to a fixed size and then reproduce through *binary fission*, a form of asexual reproduction. Under optimal conditions, bacteria can grow and divide extremely rapidly, and bacterial populations can double as quickly as every 9.8 minutes. In cell division, two identical clone daughter cells are produced. Some bacteria, while still reproducing asexually, form more complex reproductive structures that help disperse the newly formed daughter cells. Examples include fruiting body formation by *Myxobacteria* and aerial hyphae formation by *Streptomyces*, or budding. Budding involves a cell forming a protrusion that breaks away and produces a daughter cell.

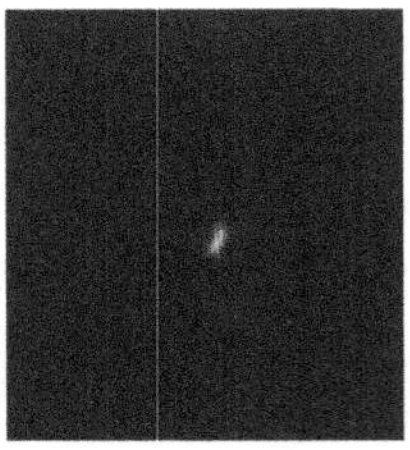

A colony of *Escherichia coli*

In the laboratory, bacteria are usually grown using solid or liquid media. Solid *growth media*, such as agar plates, are used to isolate pure cultures of a bacterial strain. However, liquid growth media are used when measurement of growth or large volumes of cells are required. Growth in stirred liquid media occurs as an even cell suspension, making the cultures easy to divide and transfer, although isolating single bacteria from liquid media is difficult. The use of selective media (media with specific nutrients added or deficient, or with antibiotics added) can help identify specific organisms.

Most laboratory techniques for growing bacteria use high levels of nutrients to produce large amounts of cells cheaply and quickly. However, in natural environments, nutrients are limited, meaning that bacteria cannot continue to reproduce indefinitely. This nutrient limitation has led the evolution of different growth strategies (see r/K selection theory). Some organisms can grow extremely rapidly when nutrients become available, such as the formation of algal (and cyanobacterial) blooms that often occur in lakes during the summer. Other organisms have adaptations to harsh environments, such as the production of multiple antibiotics by *Streptomyces* that inhibit the growth of competing microorganisms. In nature, many organisms live in communities (e.g., biofilms) that may allow for increased supply of nutrients and protection from environmental stresses. These relationships can be essential for growth of a particular organism or group of organisms (syntrophy).

Bacterial growth follows four phases. When a population of bacteria first enter a high-nutrient environment that allows growth, the cells need to adapt to their new environment. The first phase of growth is the *lag phase*, a period of slow growth when the cells are adapting to the high-nutrient environment and preparing for fast growth. The lag phase has high biosynthesis rates, as proteins necessary for rapid growth are produced. The second phase of growth is the *log phase*, also known as the *logarithmic or exponential phase*. The log phase is marked by rapid exponential growth. The rate at which cells grow during this phase is known as the *growth rate* (*k*), and the time it takes the cells to double is known as the *generation time* (*g*). During log phase, nutrients are metabolised at maximum speed until one of the nutrients is depleted and starts limiting growth. The third phase of growth is the *stationary phase* and is caused by depleted nutrients. The cells reduce their metabolic activity and consume non-essential cellular proteins. The stationary phase is a transition from rapid growth to a stress response state and there is increased expression of genes involved in DNA repair, antioxidant metabolism and nutrient transport. The final phase is the *death phase* where the bacteria run out of nutrients and die.

Genomes

The genomes of thousands of bacterial species have been sequenced, with at least 9,000 sequences completed and more than 42,000 left as "permanent" drafts (as of Sep 2016).

Most bacteria have a single circular chromosome that can range in size from only 160,000 base pairs in the endosymbiotic bacteria *Candidatus Carsonella ruddii*, to 12,200,000 base pairs in the soil-dwelling bacteria *Sorangium cellulosum*. The genes in bacterial genomes are usually a single continuous stretch of DNA and although several different types of introns do exist in bacteria, these are much rarer than in eukaryotes. Some bacteria, including the Spirochaetes of the genus *Borrelia* are a notable exception to this arrangement. *Borrelia burgdorferi*, the cause of Lyme disease, contains a single linear chromosome and several linear and circular plasmids.

Plasmids are small extra-chromosomal DNAs that may contain genes for antibiotic resistance or virulence factors. Plasmids replicate independently of chromosomes, so it is possible that plasmids could be lost in bacterial cell division. Against this possibility is the fact that a single bacterium can contain hundreds of copies of a single plasmid.

Genetics

Bacteria, as sexual organisms, inherit identical copies of their parent's genes (i.e., they are clonal). However, all bacteria can evolve by selection on changes to their genetic material DNA caused by genetic recombination or mutations. Mutations come from errors made during the replication of DNA or from exposure to mutagens. Mutation rates vary widely among different species of bacteria and even among different clones of a single species of bacteria. Genetic changes in bacterial genomes come from either random mutation during replication or "stress-directed mutation", where genes involved in a particular growth-limiting process have an increased mutation rate.

DNA Transfer

Some bacteria also transfer genetic material between cells. This can occur in three main ways. First, bacteria can take up exogenous DNA from their environment, in a process called *transformation*. Genes can also be transferred by the process of *transduction*, when the integration of a bacteriophage introduces foreign DNA into the chromosome. The third method of gene transfer is *conjugation*, whereby DNA is transferred through direct cell contact.

Transduction of bacterial genes by bacteriophage appears to be a consequence of infrequent errors during intracellular assembly of virus particles, rather than a bacterial adaptation. Conjugation, in the much-studied E. coli system is determined by plasmid genes, and is an adaptation for transferring copies of the plasmid from one bacterial host to another. It is seldom that a conjugative plasmid integrates into the host bacterial chromosome, and subsequently transfers part of the host bacterial DNA to another bacterium. Plasmid-mediated transfer of host bacterial DNA also appears to be an accidental process rather than a bacterial adaptation.

Transformation, unlike transduction or conjugation, depends on numerous bacterial gene products that specifically interact to perform this complex process, and thus transformation is clearly a bacterial adaptation for DNA transfer. In order for a bacterium to bind, take up and recombine donor DNA into its own chromosome, it must first enter a special physiological state termed competence (Natural competence). In *Bacillus subtilis*, about 40 genes are required for the development of competence. The length of DNA transferred during *B. subtilis* transformation can be between a third of a chromosome up to the whole chromosome.Transformation appears to be common among bacterial species, and thus far at least 60 species are known to have the natural ability to become competent for transformation. The development of competence in nature is usually associated with stressful environmental conditions, and seems to be an adaptation for facilitating repair of DNA damage in recipient cells.

In ordinary circumstances, transduction, conjugation, and transformation involve transfer of DNA between individual bacteria of the same species, but occasionally transfer may occur between individuals of different bacterial species and this may have significant consequences, such as the transfer of antibiotic resistance. In such cases, gene acquisition from other bacteria or the environment is called *horizontal gene transfer* and may be common under natural conditions. Gene transfer is particularly important in antibiotic resistance as it allows the rapid transfer of resistance genes between different pathogens.

Bacteriophages

Bacteriophages are viruses that infect bacteria. Many types of bacteriophage exist, some simply infect and lyse their host bacteria, while others insert into the bacterial chromosome. A bacteriophage can contain genes that contribute to its host's phenotype: for example, in the evolution of *Escherichia coli* O157:H7 and *Clostridium botulinum*, the toxin genes in an integrated phage converted a harmless ancestral bacterium into a lethal pathogen. Bacteria resist phage infection through restriction modification systems that degrade foreign DNA, and a system that uses CRISPR sequences to retain fragments of the genomes of phage that the bacteria have come into contact with in the past, which allows them to block virus replication through a form of RNA interference. This CRISPR system provides bacteria with acquired immunity to infection.

Behaviour

Secretion

Bacteria frequently secrete chemicals into their environment in order to modify it favourably. The secretions are often proteins and may act as enzymes that digest some form of food in the environment.

Bioluminescence

A few bacteria have chemical systems that generate light. This bioluminescence often occurs in bacteria that live in association with fish, and the light probably serves to attract fish or other large animals.

Multicellularity

Bacteria often function as multicellular aggregates known as biofilms, exchanging a variety of molecular signals for inter-cell communication, and engaging in coordinated multicellular behaviour.

The communal benefits of multicellular cooperation include a cellular division of labour, accessing resources that cannot effectively be used by single cells, collectively defending against antagonists, and optimising population survival by differentiating into distinct cell types. For example, bacteria in biofilms can have more than 500 times increased resistance to antibacterial agents than individual "planktonic" bacteria of the same species.

One type of inter-cellular communication by a molecular signal is called quorum sensing, which serves the purpose of determining whether there is a local population density that is sufficiently high that it is productive to invest in processes that are only successful if large numbers of similar organisms behave similarly, as in excreting digestive enzymes or emitting light.

Quorum sensing allows bacteria to coordinate gene expression, and enables them to produce, release and detect autoinducers or pheromones which accumulate with the growth in cell population.

Movement

Many bacteria can move using a variety of mechanisms: flagella are used for swimming through fluids; bacterial gliding and twitching motility move bacteria across surfaces; and changes of buoyancy allow vertical motion.

Swimming bacteria frequently move near 10 body lengths per second and a few as fast as 100. This makes them at least as fast as fish, on a relative scale.

In bacterial gliding and twitching motility, bacteria use their *type IV pili* as a grappling hook, repeatedly extending it, anchoring it and then retracting it with remarkable force (>80 pN).

Our observations redefine twitching motility as a rapid, highly organized mechanism of bacterial translocation by which Pseudomonas aeruginosa can disperse itself over large areas to colonize new territories. It is also now clear, both morphologically and genetically, that twitching motility and social gliding motility, such as occurs in Myxococcus xanthus, are essentially the same process.

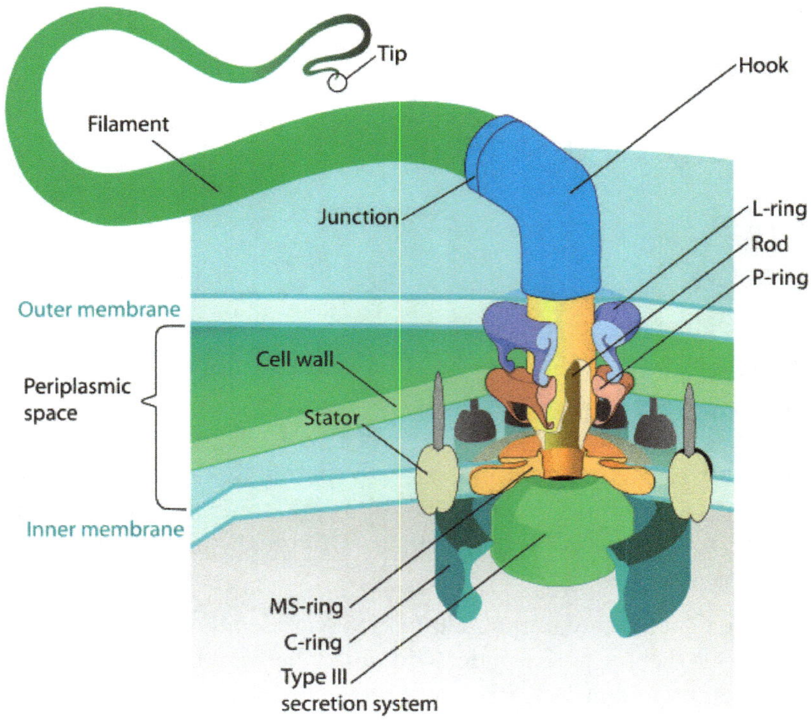

Flagellum of gram-negative bacteria. The base drives the rotation of the hook and filament.

—Semmler, Whitchurch & Mattick (1999)

Flagella are semi-rigid cylindrical structures that are rotated and function much like the propeller on a ship. Objects as small as bacteria operate a low Reynolds number and cylindrical forms are more efficient than the flat, paddle-like, forms appropriate at human-size scale.

Bacterial species differ in the number and arrangement of flagella on their surface; some have a single flagellum (*monotrichous*), a flagellum at each end (*amphitrichous*), clusters of flagella at the poles of the cell (*lophotrichous*), while others have flagella distributed over the entire surface of the cell (*peritrichous*). The bacterial flagella is the best-understood motility structure in any organism and is made of about 20 proteins, with approximately another 30 proteins required for its regulation and assembly. The flagellum is a rotating structure driven by a reversible motor at the base that uses the electrochemical gradient across the membrane for power. This motor drives the motion of the filament, which acts as a propeller.

Many bacteria (such as *E. coli*) have two distinct modes of movement: forward movement (swimming) and tumbling. The tumbling allows them to reorient and makes their movement a three-dimensional random walk. (See external links below for link to videos.) The flagella of a unique group of bacteria, the spirochaetes, are found between two membranes in the periplasmic space. They have a distinctive helical body that twists about as it moves.

Motile bacteria are attracted or repelled by certain stimuli in behaviours called **taxes**: these include chemotaxis, phototaxis, energy taxis, and magnetotaxis. In one peculiar group, the myxobacteria, individual bacteria move together to form waves of cells that then differentiate to form fruiting bodies containing spores. The myxobacteria move only when on solid surfaces, unlike *E. coli*, which is motile in liquid or solid media.

Several *Listeria* and *Shigella* species move inside host cells by usurping the cytoskeleton, which is normally used to move organelles inside the cell. By promoting actin polymerisation at one pole of their cells, they can form a kind of tail that pushes them through the host cell's cytoplasm.

Classification and Identification

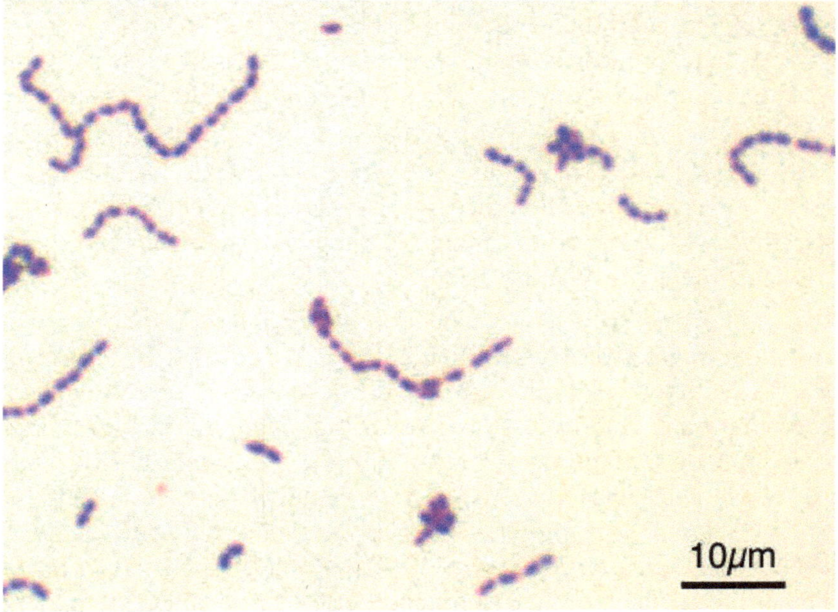

Streptococcus mutans visualised with a Gram stain

Classification seeks to describe the diversity of bacterial species by naming and grouping organisms based on similarities. Bacteria can be classified on the basis of cell structure, cellular metabolism or on differences in cell components, such as DNA, fatty acids, pigments, antigens and quinones. While these schemes allowed the identification and classification of bacterial strains, it was unclear whether these differences represented variation between distinct species or between strains of the same species. This uncertainty was due to the lack of distinctive structures in most bacteria, as well as lateral gene transfer between unrelated species. Due to lateral gene transfer, some closely related bacteria can have very different morphologies and metabolisms. To overcome this uncertainty, modern bacterial classification emphasises molecular systematics, using genetic techniques such as guanine cytosine ratio determination, genome-genome hybridisation, as well as sequencing genes that have not undergone extensive lateral gene transfer, such as the rRNA gene. Classification of bacteria is determined by publication in the International Journal of Systematic Bacteriology,and Bergey's Manual of Systematic Bacteriology. The International Committee on Systematic Bacteriology (ICSB) maintains international rules for the naming of bacteria and taxonomic categories and for the ranking of them in the International Code of Nomenclature of Bacteria.

The term "bacteria" was traditionally applied to all microscopic, single-cell prokaryotes. However, molecular systematics showed prokaryotic life to consist of two separate domains, originally called *Eubacteria* and *Archaebacteria*, but now called *Bacteria* and *Archaea* that evolved independently from an ancient common ancestor. The archaea and eukaryotes are more closely related to each other than either is to the bacteria. These two domains, along with Eukarya, are the basis of the three-domain system, which is currently the most widely used classification system in microbiolology. However, due to the relatively recent introduction of molecular systematics and a rapid increase in the number of genome sequences that are available, bacterial classification remains a changing and expanding field. For example, a few biologists argue that the Archaea and Eukaryotes evolved from gram-positive bacteria.

The identification of bacteria in the laboratory is particularly relevant in medicine, where the correct treatment is determined by the bacterial species causing an infection. Consequently, the need to identify human pathogens was a major impetus for the development of techniques to identify bacteria.

The *Gram stain*, developed in 1884 by Hans Christian Gram, characterises bacteria based on the structural characteristics of their cell walls. The thick layers of peptidoglycan in the "gram-positive" cell wall stain purple, while the thin "gram-negative" cell wall appears pink. By combining morphology and Gram-staining, most bacteria can be classified as belonging to one of four groups (gram-positive cocci, gram-positive bacilli, gram-negative cocci and gram-negative bacilli). Some organisms are best identified by stains other than the Gram stain, particularly mycobacteria or *Nocardia*, which show acid-fastness on Ziehl–Neelsen or similar stains. Other organisms may need to be identified by their growth in special media, or by other techniques, such as serology.

Culture techniques are designed to promote the growth and identify particular bacteria, while restricting the growth of the other bacteria in the sample. Often these techniques are designed for specific specimens; for example, a sputum sample will be treated to identify organisms that cause pneumonia, while stool specimens are cultured on selective media to identify organisms that cause diarrhoea, while preventing growth of non-pathogenic bacteria. Specimens that are normally sterile, such as blood, urine or spinal fluid, are cultured under conditions designed to grow all possible organisms. Once a pathogenic organism has been isolated, it can be further characterised by its morphology, growth patterns (such as aerobic or anaerobic growth), patterns of hemolysis, and staining.

As with bacterial classification, identification of bacteria is increasingly using molecular methods. Diagnostics using DNA-based tools, such as polymerase chain reaction, are increasingly popular due to their specificity and speed, compared to culture-based methods. These methods also allow the detection and identification of "viable but nonculturable" cells that are metabolically active but non-dividing. However, even using these improved methods, the total number of bacterial species is not known and cannot even be estimated with any certainty. Following present classification, there are a little less than 9,300 known species of prokaryotes, which includes bacteria and archaea; but attempts to estimate the true number of bacterial diversity have ranged from 10^7 to 10^9 total species—and even these diverse estimates may be off by many orders of magnitude.

Interactions with other Organisms

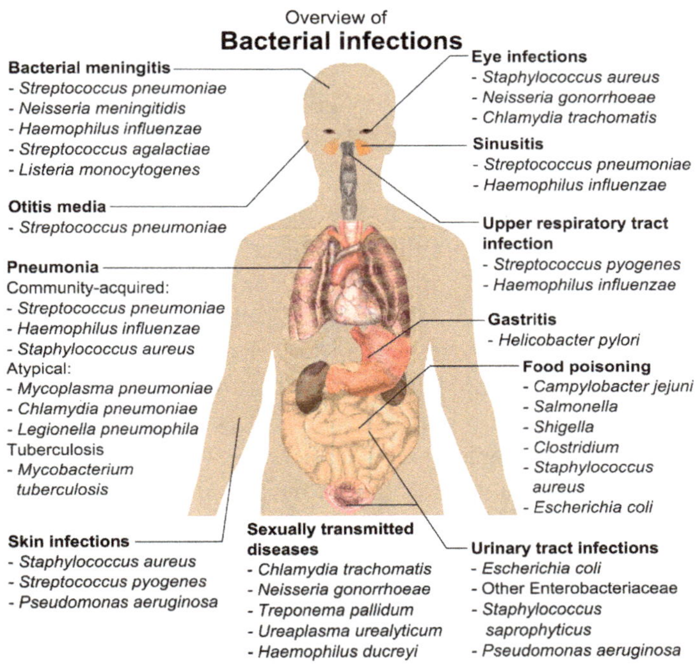

Overview of bacterial infections and main species involved.

Despite their apparent simplicity, bacteria can form complex associations with other organisms. These symbiotic associations can be divided into parasitism, mutualism and commensalism. Due to their small size, commensal bacteria are ubiquitous and grow on animals and plants exactly as they will grow on any other surface. However, their growth can be increased by warmth and sweat, and large populations of these organisms in humans are the cause of body odour.

Predators

Some species of bacteria kill and then consume other microorganisms, these species are called *predatory bacteria*. These include organisms such as *Myxococcus xanthus*, which forms swarms of cells that kill and digest any bacteria they encounter. Other bacterial predators either attach to their prey in order to digest them and absorb nutrients, such as *Vampirovibrio chlorellavorus*, or invade another cell and multiply inside the cytosol, such as *Daptobacter*. These predatory bacteria are thought to have evolved from saprophages that consumed dead microorganisms, through adaptations that allowed them to entrap and kill other organisms.

Mutualists

Certain bacteria form close spatial associations that are essential for their survival. One such mutualistic association, called interspecies hydrogen transfer, occurs between clusters of anaerobic bacteria that consume organic acids, such as butyric acid or propionic acid, and produce hydrogen, and methanogenic Archaea that consume hydrogen. The bacteria in this association are unable to consume the organic acids as this reaction produces hydrogen that accumulates in their surroundings. Only the intimate association with the hydrogen-consuming Archaea keeps the hydrogen concentration low enough to allow the bacteria to grow.

In soil, microorganisms that reside in the rhizosphere (a zone that includes the root surface and the soil that adheres to the root after gentle shaking) carry out nitrogen fixation, converting nitrogen gas to nitrogenous compounds. This serves to provide an easily absorbable form of nitrogen for many plants, which cannot fix nitrogen themselves. Many other bacteria are found as symbionts in humans and other organisms. For example, the presence of over 1,000 bacterial species in the normal human gut flora of the intestines can contribute to gut immunity, synthesise vitamins, such as folic acid, vitamin K and biotin, convert sugars to lactic acid (see *Lactobacillus*), as well as fermenting complex undigestible carbohydrates. The presence of this gut flora also inhibits the growth of potentially pathogenic bacteria (usually through competitive exclusion) and these beneficial bacteria are consequently sold as probiotic dietary supplements.

Pathogens

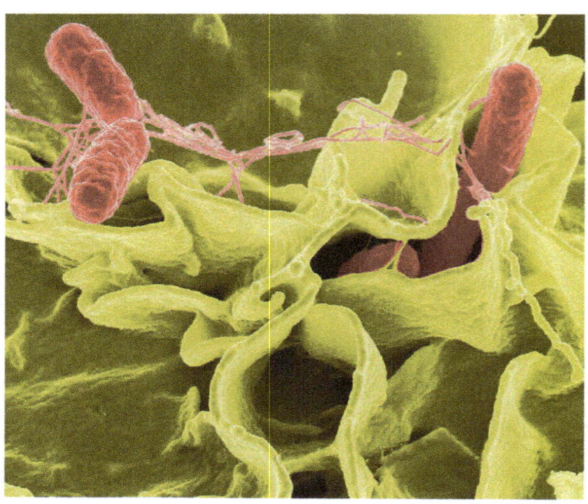

Colour-enhanced scanning electron micrograph showing *Salmonella typhimurium* (red) invading cultured human cells

If bacteria form a parasitic association with other organisms, they are classed as pathogens. Pathogenic bacteria are a major cause of human death and disease and cause infections such as tetanus, typhoid fever, diphtheria, syphilis, cholera, foodborne illness, leprosy and tuberculosis. A pathogenic cause for a known medical disease may only be discovered many years after, as was the case with *Helicobacter pylori* and peptic ulcer disease. Bacterial diseases are also important in agriculture, with bacteria causing leaf spot, fire blight and wilts in plants, as well as Johne's disease, mastitis, salmonella and anthrax in farm animals.

Each species of pathogen has a characteristic spectrum of interactions with its human hosts. Some organisms, such as *Staphylococcus* or *Streptococcus*, can cause skin infections, pneumonia, meningitis and even overwhelming sepsis, a systemic inflammatory response producing shock, massive vasodilation and death. Yet these organisms are also part of the normal human flora and usually exist on the skin or in the nose without causing any disease at all. Other organisms invariably cause disease in humans, such as the Rickettsia, which are obligate intracellular parasites able to grow and reproduce only within the cells of other organisms. One species of Rickettsia causes typhus, while another causes Rocky Mountain spotted fever. *Chlamydia*, another phylum of obligate intracellular parasites, contains species that can cause pneumonia, or urinary tract infection and may be involved in coronary heart disease. Finally, some species, such as *Pseudomonas aeruginosa*, *Burkholderia cenocepacia*, and *Mycobacterium avium*, are opportunistic pathogens and cause disease mainly in people suffering from immunosuppression or cystic fibrosis.

Bacterial infections may be treated with antibiotics, which are classified as bacteriocidal if they kill bacteria, or bacteriostatic if they just prevent bacterial growth. There are many types of antibiotics and each class inhibits a process that is different in the pathogen from that found in the host. An example of how antibiotics produce selective toxicity are chloramphenicol and puromycin, which inhibit the bacterial ribosome, but not the structurally different eukaryotic ribosome.Antibiotics are used both in treating human disease and in intensive farming to promote animal growth, where they may be contributing to the rapid development of antibiotic resistance in bacterial populations. Infections can be prevented by antiseptic measures such as sterilising the skin prior to piercing it with the needle of a syringe, and by proper care of indwelling catheters. Surgical and dental instruments are also sterilised to prevent contamination by bacteria. Disinfectants such as bleach are used to kill bacteria or other pathogens on surfaces to prevent contamination and further reduce the risk of infection.

Significance in Technology and Industry

Bacteria, often lactic acid bacteria, such as *Lactobacillus* and *Lactococcus*, in combination with yeasts and moulds, have been used for thousands of years in the preparation of fermented foods, such as cheese, pickles, soy sauce, sauerkraut, vinegar, wine and yogurt.

The ability of bacteria to degrade a variety of organic compounds is remarkable and has been used in waste processing and bioremediation. Bacteria capable of digesting the hydrocarbons in petroleum are often used to clean up oil spills. Fertiliser was added to some of the beaches in Prince William Sound in an attempt to promote the growth of these naturally occurring bacteria after the 1989 *Exxon Valdez* oil spill. These efforts were effective on beaches that were not too thickly covered in oil. Bacteria are also used for the bioremediation of industrial toxic wastes. In the chemical industry, bacteria are most important in the production of enantiomerically pure chemicals for use as pharmaceuticals or agrichemicals.

Bacteria can also be used in the place of pesticides in the biological pest control. This commonly involves *Bacillus thuringiensis* (also called BT), a gram-positive, soil dwelling bacterium. Subspecies of this bacteria are used as a Lepidopteran-specific insecticides under trade names such as Dipel and Thuricide. Because of their specificity, these pesticides are regarded as environmentally friendly, with little or no effect on humans, wildlife, pollinators and most other beneficial insects.

Because of their ability to quickly grow and the relative ease with which they can be manipulated, bacteria are the workhorses for the fields of molecular biology, genetics and biochemistry. By making mutations in bacterial DNA and examining the resulting phenotypes, scientists can determine the function of genes, enzymes and metabolic pathways in bacteria, then apply this knowledge to more complex organisms. This aim of understanding the biochemistry of a cell reaches its most complex expression in the synthesis of huge amounts of enzyme kinetic and gene expression data into mathematical models of entire organisms. This is achievable in some well-studied bacteria, with models of *Escherichia coli* metabolism now being produced and tested. This understanding of bacterial metabolism and genetics allows the use of biotechnology to bioengineer bacteria for the production of therapeutic proteins, such as insulin, growth factors, or antibodies.

Because of their importance for research in general, samples of bacterial strains are isolated and preserved in Biological Resource Centers. This ensures the availability of the strain to scientists worldwide.

History of Bacteriology

For the history of microbiology, see Microbiology. For the history of bacterial classification, see Bacterial taxonomy. For the natural history of Bacteria, see Last universal common ancestor.

Bacteria were first observed by the Dutch microscopist Antonie van Leeuwenhoek in 1676, using a single-lens microscope of his own design. He then published his observations in a series of letters to the Royal Society of London.Bacteria were Leeuwenhoek's most remarkable microscopic discovery. They were just at the limit of what his simple lenses could make out and, in one of the most striking hiatuses in the history of science, no one else would see them again for over a century. Only then were his by-then-largely-forgotten observations of bacteria—as opposed to his famous "animalcules" (spermatozoa)—taken seriously.

Christian Gottfried Ehrenberg introduced the word "bacterium" in 1828. In fact, his *Bacterium* was a genus that contained non-spore-forming rod-shaped bacteria, as opposed to *Bacillus*, a genus of spore-forming rod-shaped bacteria defined by Ehrenberg in 1835.

Louis Pasteur demonstrated in 1859 that the growth of microorganisms causes the fermentation process, and that this growth is not due to spontaneous generation. (Yeasts and moulds, commonly associated with fermentation, are not bacteria, but rather fungi.)

Along with his contemporary Robert Koch, Pasteur was an early advocate of the germ theory of disease.

Robert Koch, a pioneer in medical microbiology, worked on cholera, anthrax and tuberculosis. In his research into tuberculosis Koch finally proved the germ theory, for which he received a Nobel Prize in 1905. In *Koch's postulates*, he set out criteria to test if an organism is the cause of a disease, and these postulates are still used today.

Though it was known in the nineteenth century that bacteria are the cause of many diseases, no effective antibacterial treatments were available. In 1910, Paul Ehrlich developed the first antibiotic, by changing dyes that selectively stained *Treponema pallidum*—the spirochaete that causes syphilis—into compounds that selectively killed the pathogen. Ehrlich had been awarded a 1908 Nobel Prize for his work on immunology, and pioneered the use of stains to detect and identify bacteria, with his work being the basis of the Gram stain and the Ziehl–Neelsen stain.

A major step forward in the study of bacteria came in 1977 when Carl Woese recognised that archaea have a separate line of evolutionary descent from bacteria.This new phylogenetic taxonomy depended on the sequencing of 16S ribosomal RNA, and divided prokaryotes into two evolutionary domains, as part of the three-domain system.

Almost all bacteria are invisible to the naked eye, with a few extremely rare exceptions, such as *Thiomargarita namibiensis*. They lack a nucleus and other membrane-bound organelles, and can function and reproduce as individual cells, but often aggregate in multicellular colonies. Their genome is usually a single loop of DNA, although they can also harbor small pieces of DNA called plasmids. These plasmids can be transferred between cells through bacterial conjugation. Bacteria are surrounded by a cell wall, which provides strength and rigidity to their cells. They reproduce by binary fission or sometimes by budding, but do not undergo meiotic sexual reproduction. However, many bacterial species can transfer DNA between individual cells by a process referred to as natural transformation. Some species form extraordinarily resilient spores, but for bacteria this is a mechanism for survival, not reproduction. Under optimal conditions bacteria can grow extremely rapidly and can double as quickly as every 20 minutes.

ARCHAEA

The **Archaea** constitute a domain and kingdom of single-celledmicroorganisms. These microbes (archaea; singular archaeon) are prokaryotes, meaning that they have no cell nucleus or any other membrane-bound organelles in their cells.

Archaea were initially classified as bacteria, receiving the name archaebacteria (in the Archaebacteria kingdom), but this classification is outdated. Archaeal cells have unique properties separating them from the other two domains of life, Bacteria and Eukaryota. The Archaea are further divided into multiple recognized phyla. Classification is difficult because the majority have not been isolated in the laboratory and have only been detected by analysis of their nucleic acids in samples from their environment.

Archaea and bacteria are generally similar in size and shape, although a few archaea have very strange shapes, such as the flat and square-shaped cells of *Haloquadratum walsbyi*. Despite this morphological similarity to bacteria, archaea possess genes and several metabolic pathways that are more closely related to those of eukaryotes, notably the enzymes involved in transcription and translation. Other aspects of archaeal biochemistry are unique, such as their reliance on ether lipids in their cell membranes, including archaeols. Archaea use more energy sources than eukaryotes: these range from organic compounds, such as sugars, to ammonia, metal ions or even hydrogen gas. Salt-tolerant archaea (the Haloarchaea) use sunlight as an energy source, and other species of archaea fix carbon; however, unlike plants and cyanobacteria, no known species of archaea does both. Archaea reproduce asexually by binary fission, fragmentation, or budding; unlike bacteria and eukaryotes, no known species forms spores.

Archaea were initially viewed as extremophiles living in harsh environments, such as hot springs and salt lakes, but they have since been found in a broad range of habitats, including soils, oceans, marshlands and the human colon, oral cavity, and skin. Archaea are particularly numerous in the oceans, and the archaea in plankton may be one of the most abundant groups of organisms on the planet. Archaea are a major part of Earth's life and may play roles in both the carbon cycle and the nitrogen cycle. No clear examples of archaeal pathogens or parasites are known, but they are often mutualists or commensals. One example is the methanogens that inhabit human and ruminant guts, where their vast numbers aid digestion. Methanogens are also used in biogas production and sewage treatment, and enzymes from extremophile archaea that can endure high temperatures and organic solvents are exploited in biotechnology.

Classification

New Domain

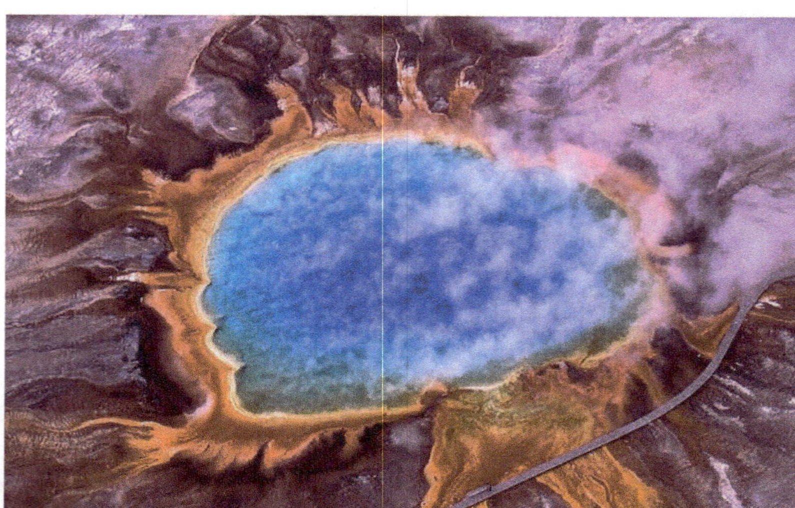

Archaea were first found in extreme environments, such as volcanic hot springs. Pictured here is Grand Prismatic Spring of Yellowstone National Park.

For much of the 20th century, prokaryotes were regarded as a single group of organisms and classified based on their biochemistry, morphology and metabolism. For example, microbiologists tried to classify microorganisms based on the structures of their cell walls, their shapes, and the substances they consume. In 1965, Emile Zuckerkandl and Linus Pauling proposed instead using the sequences of the genes in different prokaryotes to work out how they are related to each other. This approach, known as phylogenetics, is the main method used today.

Archaea were first classified as a separate group of prokaryotes in 1977 by Carl Woese and George E. Fox in phylogenetic trees based on the sequences of ribosomal RNA (rRNA) genes. These two groups were originally named the Archaebacteria and Eubacteria and treated as kingdoms or subkingdoms, which Woese and Fox termed *Urkingdoms*. Woese argued that this group of prokaryotes is a fundamentally different sort of life. To emphasize this difference, Woese later proposed a new natural system of organisms with three separate Domains: the Eukarya, the Bacteria and the Archaea, in what is now known as "The Woesian Revolution".

The word *archaea* comes from the Ancient Greek ρχαα, meaning "ancient things", as the first representatives of the domain Archaea were methanogens and it was assumed that their metabolism reflected Earth's primitive atmosphere and the organism's antiquity. For a long time, archaea were seen as extremophiles that only exist in extreme habitats such as hot springs and salt lakes. However, as new habitats were studied, more organisms were discovered. Extreme halophilic and hyperthermophilic microbes were also included in the Archaea. By the end of the 20th century, archaea had been identified in non-extreme environments as well. Today, they are known to be a large and diverse group of organisms that are widely distributed in nature and are common in all habitats. This new appreciation of the importance and ubiquity of archaea came from using polymerase chain reaction (PCR) to detect prokaryotes from environmental samples (such as water or soil) by multiplying their ribosomal genes. This allows the detection and identification of organisms that have not been cultured in the laboratory.

Current Classification

The classification of archaea, and of prokaryotes in general, is a rapidly moving and contentious field. Current classification systems aim to organize archaea into groups of organisms that share structural features and common ancestors. These classifications rely heavily on the use of the sequence of ribosomal RNA genes to reveal relationships between organisms (molecular phylogenetics). Most of the culturable and well-investigated species of archaea are members of two main phyla, the Euryarchaeota and Crenarchaeota. Other groups have been tentatively created. For example, the peculiar species *Nanoarchaeum equitans*, which was discovered in 2003, has been given its own phylum, the Nanoarchaeota. A new phylum Korarchaeota has also been proposed. It contains a small group of unusual thermophilic species that shares features of both of the main phyla, but is most closely related to the Crenarchaeota. Other recently detected species of archaea are only distantly related to any of these groups, such as the Archaeal Richmond Mine acidophilic nanoorganisms (ARMAN), which were discovered in 2006 and are some of the smallest organisms known.

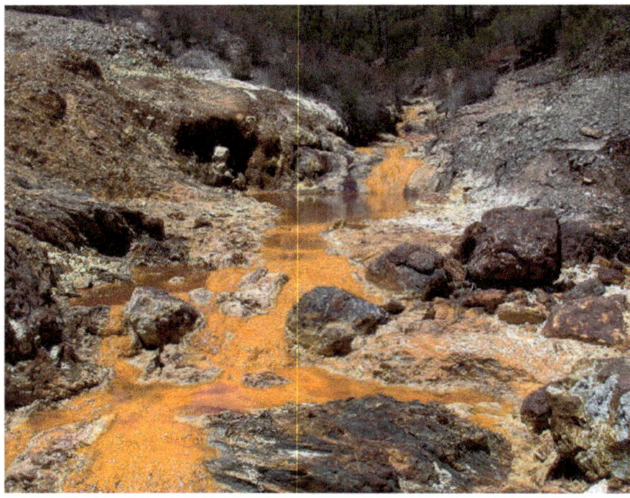

The ARMAN are a new group of archaea recently discovered in acid mine drainage.

A superphylum - TACK - has been proposed that includes the Thaumarchaeota, Aigarchaeota, Crenarchaeota, and Korarchaeota. This superphylum may be related to the origin of eukaryotes.

Concept of Species

The classification of archaea into species is also controversial. Biology defines a species as a group of related organisms. The familiar exclusive breeding criterion (organisms that can breed with each other but not with others) is of no help here because archaea reproduce asexually.

Archaea show high levels of horizontal gene transfer between lineages. Some researchers suggest that individuals can be grouped into species-like populations given highly similar genomes and infrequent gene transfer to/from cells with less-related genomes, as in the genus *Ferroplasma*. On the other hand, studies in *Halorubrum* found significant genetic transfer to/from less-related populations, limiting the criterion's applicability. A second concern is to what extent such species designations have practical meaning.

Current knowledge on genetic diversity is fragmentary and the total number of archaeal species cannot be estimated with any accuracy. Estimates of the number of phyla range from 18 to 23, of which only 8 have representatives that have been cultured and studied directly. Many of these hypothesized groups are known from a single rRNA sequence, indicating that the diversity among these organisms remains obscure. The Bacteria also contain many uncultured microbes with similar implications for characterization.

Origin and Evolution

The age of the Earth is about 4.54 billion years. Scientific evidence suggests that life began on Earth at least 3.5 billion years ago. The earliest evidence for life on Earth is graphite found to be biogenic in 3.7 billion-year-old metasedimentary rocks discovered in Western Greenland and microbial matfossils found in 3.48 billion-year-old sandstone discovered in Western Australia. More recently, in 2015, "remains of biotic life" were found in 4.1 billion-year-old rocks in Western Australia. An unrelated researcher, S. Blair Hedges, wrote in an email about the study saying, "If life arose relatively quickly on Earth ... then it could be common in the universe."

Although probable prokaryotic cell fossils date to almost 3.5 billion years ago, most prokaryotes do not have distinctive morphologies and fossil shapes cannot be used to identify them as archaea. Instead, chemical fossils of unique lipids are more informative because such compounds do not occur in other organisms.Some publications suggest that archaeal or eukaryotic lipid remains are present in shales dating from 2.7 billion years ago; such data have since been questioned. Such lipids have also been detected in even older rocks from west Greenland. The oldest such traces come from the Isua district, which include Earth's oldest known sediments, formed 3.8 billion years ago. The archaeal lineage may be the most ancient that exists on Earth.

Woese argued that the bacteria, archaea, and eukaryotes represent separate lines of descent that diverged early on from an ancestral colony of organisms.One possibility is that this occurred before the evolution of cells, when the lack of a typical cell membrane allowed unrestricted lateral gene transfer, and that the common ancestors of the three domains arose by fixation of specific subsets of genes. It is possible that the last common ancestor of the bacteria and archaea was a thermophile, which raises the possibility that lower temperatures are "extreme environments" in archaeal terms, and organisms that live in cooler environments appeared only later. Since the Archaea and Bacteria are no more related to each other than they are to eukaryotes, the term *prokaryote*'s only surviving meaning is "not a eukaryote", limiting its value.

Comparison to other Domains

The following table compares some major characteristics of the three domains, to illustrate their similarities and differences. Many of these characteristics are also discussed below.

Property	Archaea	Bacteria	Eukarya
Cell Membrane	Ether-linked lipids, pseudopeptidoglycan	Ester-linked lipids, peptidoglycan	Ester-linked lipids, various structures
Gene Structure	Circular chromosomes, similar translation and transcription to Eukarya	Circular chromosomes, unique translation and transcription	Multiple, linear chromosomes, similar translation and transcription to Archaea
Internal Cell Structure	No membrane-bound organelles or nucleus	No membrane-bound organelles or nucleus	Membrane-bound organelles and nucleus

Metabolism	Various, with methanogenesis unique to Archaea	Various, including photosynthesis, aerobic and anaerobic respiration, fermentation, and autotrophy	Photosynthesis and cellular respiration
Reproduction	Asexual reproduction, horizontal gene transfer	Asexual reproduction, horizontal gene transfer	Sexual and asexual reproduction

Archaea were split off as a third domain because of the large differences in their ribosomal RNA structure. The particular RNA molecule sequenced, known as 16s rRNA, is present in all organisms and always has the same vital function, the production of proteins. Because this function is so central to life, organisms with mutations of its 16s rRNA are unlikely to survive, leading to great stability in the structure of this nucleotide over many generations. 16s rRNA is also large enough to retain organism-specific information, but small enough to be sequenced in a manageable amount of time. In 1977, Carl Woese, a microbiologist studying the genetic sequencing of organisms, developed a new sequencing method that involved splitting the RNA into fragments that could be sorted and compared to other fragments from other organisms. The more similar the patterns between species were, the more closely related the organisms.

Woese used his new rRNA comparison method to categorize and contrast different organisms. He sequenced a variety of different species and happened upon a group of methanogens that had vastly different patterns than any known prokaryotes or eukaryotes. These methanogens were much more similar to each other than they were to other organisms sequenced, leading Woese to propose the new domain of Archaea. One of the interesting results of his experiments was that the Archaea were more similar to eukaryotes than prokaryotes, even though they were more similar to prokaryotes in structure. This led to the conclusion that Archaea and Eukarya shared a more recent common ancestor than Eukarya and Bacteria in general. The development of the nucleus occurred after the split between Bacteria and this common ancestor. Although Archaea are prokaryotic, they are more closely related to Eukarya and thus cannot be placed within either the Bacteria or Eukarya domains.

One property unique to Archaea is the abundant use of ether-linked lipids in their cell membranes. Ether linkages are more chemically stable than the ester linkages found in Bacteria and Eukarya, which may be a contributing factor to the ability of many Archaea to survive in extreme environments that place heavy stress on cell membranes, such as extreme heat and salinity. Another unique feature of Archaea is that no other known organisms are capable of methanogenesis (the metabolic production of methane). Methanogenic Archaea play a pivotal role in ecosystems with organisms that derive energy from oxidation of methane, many of which are Bacteria, as they are often a major source of methane in such environments and can play a role as primary producers. Methanogens also play a critical role in the carbon cycle, breaking down organic carbon into methane, which is also a major greenhouse gas.

Relationship to Bacteria

The relationship between the three domains is of central importance for understanding the origin of life. Most of the metabolic pathways, which comprise the majority of an organism's genes, are common between Archaea and Bacteria, while most genes involved in genome expression are common between Archaea and Eukarya. Within prokaryotes, archaeal cell structure is most similar to that of gram-positive bacteria, largely because both have a single lipid bilayer and usually contain a thick sacculus (exoskeleton) of varying chemical composition. In some phylogenetic trees based upon different gene/protein sequences of prokaryotic homologs, the archaeal homologs are more closely related to those of gram-positive bacteria. Archaea and gram-positive bacteria also share conserved indels in a number of important proteins, such as Hsp70 and glutamine synthetase I; however, the phylogeny of these genes was interpreted to reveal interdomain gene transfer, and might not reflect the organismal relationship(s).

It has been proposed that the archaea evolved from gram-positive bacteria in response to antibiotic selection pressure. This is suggested by the observation that archaea are resistant to a wide variety of antibiotics that are primarily produced by gram-positive bacteria, and that these antibiotics primarily act on the genes that distinguish archaea from bacteria. The proposal is that the selective pressure towards resistance generated by the gram-positive antibiotics was eventually sufficient to cause extensive changes in many of the antibiotics' target genes, and that these strains represented the common ancestors of present-day Archaea. The evolution of Archaea in response to antibiotic selection, or any other competitive selective pressure, could also explain their adaptation to extreme environments (such as high temperature or acidity) as the result of a search for unoccupied niches to escape from antibiotic-producing organisms; Cavalier-Smith has made a similar suggestion. This proposal is also supported by other work investigating protein structural relationships and studies that suggest that gram-positive bacteria may constitute the earliest branching lineages within the prokaryotes.

Relation to Eukaryotes

The evolutionary relationship between archaea and eukaryotes remains unclear. Aside from the similarities in cell structure and function that are discussed below, many genetic trees group the two.

Complicating factors include claims that the relationship between eukaryotes and the archaeal phylum Crenarchaeota is closer than the relationship between the Euryarchaeota and the phylum Crenarchaeota and the presence of archaea-like genes in certain bacteria, such as *Thermotoga maritima*, from horizontal gene transfer. The standard hypothesis states that the ancestor of the eukaryotes diverged early from the Archaea, and that eukaryotes arose through fusion of an archaean and eubacterium, which became the nucleus and cytoplasm; this explains various genetic similarities but runs into difficulties explaining cell structure. An alternative hypothesis, the eocyte hypothesis, posits that Eukaryota emerged relatively late from the Archaea.

A recently discovered lineage of archaea, *Lokiarchaeum*, named for a hydrothermal vent called Loki's Castle in the Arctic Ocean, has been found to be most closely related to eukaryotes. It has been called a transitional organism between prokaryotes and eukaryotes.

Morphology

Individual archaea range from 0.1 micrometers (μm) to over 15 μm in diameter, and occur in various shapes, commonly as spheres, rods, spirals or plates. Other morphologies in the Crenarchaeota include irregularly shaped lobed cells in *Sulfolobus*, needle-like filaments that are less than half a micrometer in diameter in *Thermofilum*, and almost perfectly rectangular rods in *Thermoproteus* and *Pyrobaculum*. Archaea in the genus *Haloquadratum* such as *Haloquadratum walsbyi* are flat, square archaea that live in hypersaline pools. These unusual shapes are probably maintained both by their cell walls and a prokaryotic cytoskeleton. Proteins related to the cytoskeleton components of other organisms exist in archaea, and filaments form within their cells, but in contrast to other organisms, these cellular structures are poorly understood. In *Thermoplasma* and *Ferroplasma* the lack of a cell wall means that the cells have irregular shapes, and can resemble amoebae.

Some species form aggregates or filaments of cells up to 200 μm long. These organisms can be prominent in biofilms. Notably, aggregates of *Thermococcus coalescens* cells fuse together in culture, forming single giant cells. Archaea in the genus *Pyrodictium* produce an elaborate multicell colony involving arrays of long, thin hollow tubes called *cannulae* that stick out from the cells' surfaces and connect them into a dense bush-like agglomeration. The function of these cannulae is not settled, but they may allow communication or nutrient exchange with neighbors. Multi-species colonies exist, such as the "string-of-pearls" community that was discovered in 2001 in a German swamp. Round whitish colonies of a novel Euryarchaeota species are spaced along thin filaments that can range up to 15 centimetres (5.9 in) long; these filaments are made of a particular bacteria species.

Structure, Composition Development, and Operation

Archaea and bacteria have generally similar cell structure, but cell composition and organization set the archaea apart. Like bacteria, archaea lack interior membranes and organelles. Like bacteria, archaea cell membranes are usually bounded by a cell wall and they swim using one or more flagella. Structurally, archaea are most similar to gram-positive bacteria. Most have a single plasma membrane and cell wall, and lack a periplasmic space; the exception to this general rule is *Ignicoccus*, which possess a particularly large periplasm that contains membrane-bound vesicles and is enclosed by an outer membrane.

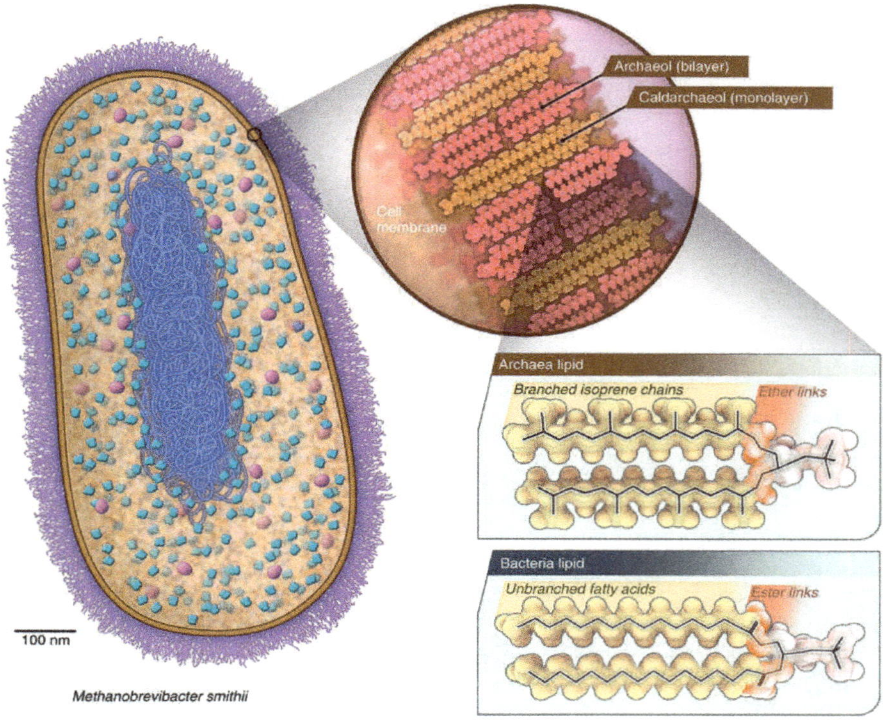

Diagrammatic view of *Methanobrevibacter smithii*, showing the cell membrane (ochre, with inset) and cell wall (purple).

Cell Wall and Flagella

Most archaea (but not *Thermoplasma* and *Ferroplasma*) possess a cell wall. In most archaea the wall is assembled from surface-layer proteins, which form an S-layer. An S-layer is a rigid array of protein molecules that cover the outside of the cell (like chain mail). This layer provides both chemical and physical protection, and can prevent macromolecules from contacting the cell membrane. Unlike bacteria, archaea lack peptidoglycan in their cell walls. Methanobacteriales do have cell walls containing pseudopeptidoglycan, which resembles eubacterial peptidoglycan in morphology, function, and physical structure, but pseudopeptidoglycan is distinct in chemical structure; it lacks D-amino acids and N-acetylmuramic acid.

Archaea flagella operate like bacterial flagella—their long stalks are driven by rotatory motors at the base. These motors are powered by the proton gradient across the membrane. However, archaeal flagella are notably different in composition and development. The two types of flagella evolved from different ancestors. The bacterial flagellum shares a common ancestor with the type III secretion system, while archaeal flagella appear to have evolved from bacterial type IV pili. In contrast to the bacterial flagellum, which is hollow and is assembled by subunits moving up the central pore to the tip of the flagella, archaeal flagella are synthesized by adding subunits at the base.

Membranes

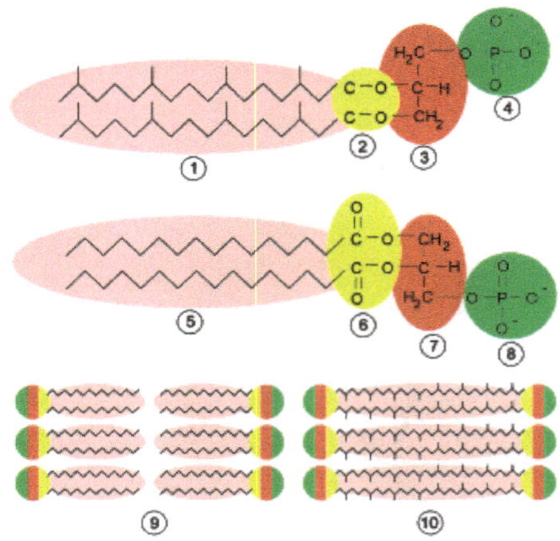

Membrane structures. **Top**, an archaeal phospholipid: **1**, isoprene chains; **2**, ether linkages; **3**, L-glycerol moiety; **4**, phosphate group. **Middle**, a bacterial or eukaryotic phospholipid: **5**, fatty acid chains; **6**, ester linkages; **7**, D-glycerol moiety; **8**, phosphate group. **Bottom**: **9**, lipid bilayer of bacteria and eukaryotes; **10**, lipid monolayer of some archaea.

Archaeal membranes are made of molecules that are distinctly different from those in all other life forms, showing that archaea are related only distantly to bacteria and eukaryotes. In all organisms, cell membranes are made of molecules known as phospholipids. These molecules possess both a polar part that dissolves in water (the phosphate "head"), and a "greasy" non-polar part that does not (the lipid tail). These dissimilar parts are connected by a glycerol moiety. In water, phospholipids cluster, with the heads facing the water and the tails facing away from it. The major structure in cell membranes is a double layer of these phospholipids, which is called a lipid bilayer.

The phospholipids of archaea are unusual in four ways:

- They have membranes composed of glycerol-ether lipids, whereas bacteria and eukaryotes have membranes composed mainly of glycerol-ester lipids. The difference is the type of bond that joins the lipids to the glycerol moiety; the two types are shown in yellow in the figure at the right. In ester lipids this is an ester bond, whereas in ether lipids this is an ether bond. Ether bonds are chemically more resistant than ester bonds. This stability might help archaea to survive extreme temperatures and very acidic or alkaline environments. Bacteria and eukaryotes do contain some ether lipids, but in contrast to archaea these lipids are not a major part of their membranes.
- The stereochemistry of the archaeal glycerol moiety is the reverse of that found in other organisms. The glycerol moiety can occur in two forms that are mirror images of one another, called the right-handed and left-handed forms or *enantiomers*. Just as a right hand does not fit easily into a left-handed glove, a right-handed phospholipid generally cannot be used or made by enzymes adapted for the left-handed form. This suggests that archaea use entirely different

enzymes for synthesizing phospholipids than do bacteria and eukaryotes. Such enzymes developed very early in life's history, indicating an early split from the other two domains.

- Archaeal lipid tails differ from those of other organisms in that they are based upon long isoprenoid chains with multiple side-branches, sometimes with cyclopropane or cyclohexane rings. By contrast, the fatty acids in the membranes of other organisms have straight chains without side branches or rings. Although isoprenoids play an important role in the biochemistry of many organisms, only the archaea use them to make phospholipids. These branched chains may help prevent archaeal membranes from leaking at high temperatures.
- In some archaea, the lipid bilayer is replaced by a monolayer. In effect, the archaea fuse the tails of two phospholipid molecules into a single molecule with two polar heads (a bolaamphiphile); this fusion may make their membranes more rigid and better able to resist harsh environments. For example, the lipids in *Ferroplasma* are of this type, which is thought to aid this organism's survival in its highly acidic habitat.

Metabolism

Archaea exhibit a great variety of chemical reactions in their metabolism and use many sources of energy. These reactions are classified into nutritional groups, depending on energy and carbon sources. Some archaea obtain energy from inorganic compounds such as sulfur or ammonia (they are lithotrophs). These include nitrifiers, methanogens and anaerobic methane oxidisers. In these reactions one compound passes electrons to another (in a redox reaction), releasing energy to fuel the cell's activities. One compound acts as an electron donor and one as an electron acceptor. The energy released generates adenosine triphosphate (ATP) through chemiosmosis, in the same basic process that happens in the mitochondrion of eukaryotic cells.

Other groups of archaea use sunlight as a source of energy (they are phototrophs). However, oxygen–generating photosynthesis does not occur in any of these organisms. Many basic metabolic pathways are shared between all forms of life; for example, archaea use a modified form of glycolysis (the Entner–Doudoroff pathway) and either a complete or partial citric acid cycle. These similarities to other organisms probably reflect both early origins in the history of life and their high level of efficiency.

Nutritional types in archaeal metabolism

Nutritional type	Source of energy	Source of carbon	Examples
Phototrophs	Sunlight	Organic compounds	*Halobacterium*
Lithotrophs	Inorganic compounds	Organic compounds or carbon fixation	*Ferroglobus*, *Methanobacteria* or *Pyrolobus*

Organotrophs	Organic compounds	Organic compounds or carbon fixation	*Pyrococcus*, *Sulfolobus* or *Methanosarcinales*

Some Euryarchaeota are methanogens living in anaerobic environments, such as swamps. This form of metabolism evolved early, and it is even possible that the first free-living organism was a methanogen. A common reaction involves the use of carbon dioxide as an electron acceptor to oxidize hydrogen. Methanogenesis involves a range of coenzymes that are unique to these archaea, such as coenzyme M and methanofuran. Other organic compounds such as alcohols, acetic acid or formic acid are used as alternative electron acceptors by methanogens. These reactions are common in gut-dwelling archaea. Acetic acid is also broken down into methane and carbon dioxide directly, by *acetotrophic* archaea. These acetotrophs are archaea in the order Methanosarcinales, and are a major part of the communities of microorganisms that produce biogas.

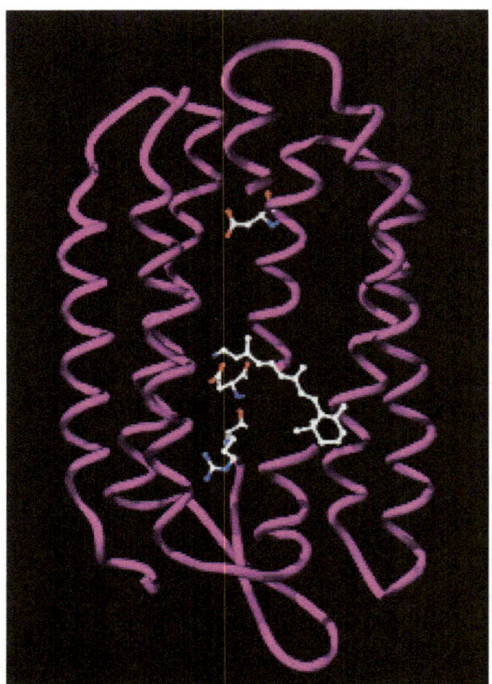

Bacteriorhodopsin from *Halobacterium salinarum*. The retinol cofactor and residues involved in proton transfer are shown as ball-and-stick models.

Other archaea use CO_2 in the atmosphere as a source of carbon, in a process called carbon fixation (they are autotrophs). This process involves either a highly modified form of the Calvin cycle or a recently discovered metabolic pathway called the 3-hydroxypropionate/4-hydroxybutyrate cycle. The Crenarchaeota also use the reverse Krebs cycle while the Euryarchaeota also use the reductive acetyl-CoA pathway. Carbon–fixation is powered by inorganic energy sources. No known archaea carry out photosynthesis. Archaeal energy sources are extremely diverse, and range from the oxidation of ammonia by the

Nitrosopumilales to the oxidation of hydrogen sulfide or elemental sulfur by species of *Sulfolobus*, using either oxygen or metal ions as electron acceptors.

Phototrophic archaea use light to produce chemical energy in the form of ATP. In the Halobacteria, light-activated ion pumps like bacteriorhodopsin and halorhodopsin generate ion gradients by pumping ions out of the cell across the plasma membrane. The energy stored in these electrochemical gradients is then converted into ATP by ATP synthase. This process is a form of photophosphorylation. The ability of these light-driven pumps to move ions across membranes depends on light-driven changes in the structure of a retinol cofactor buried in the center of the protein.

Genetics

Archaea usually have a single circular chromosome, with as many as 5,751,492 base pairs in *Methanosarcina acetivorans*, the largest known archaeal genome. The tiny 490,885 base-pair genome of *Nanoarchaeum equitans* is one-tenth of this size and the smallest archaeal genome known; it is estimated to contain only 537 protein-encoding genes. Smaller independent pieces of DNA, called *plasmids*, are also found in archaea. Plasmids may be transferred between cells by physical contact, in a process that may be similar to bacterial conjugation.

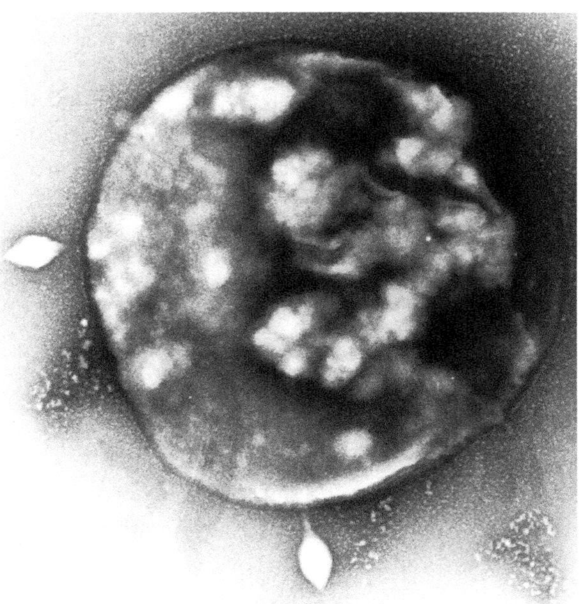

Sulfolobus infected with the DNA virus STSV1. Bar is 1 micrometer.

Archaea can be infected by double-stranded DNA viruses that are unrelated to any other form of virus and have a variety of unusual shapes, including bottles, hooked rods, or teardrops. These viruses have been studied in most detail in thermophilics, particularly the orders Sulfolobales and Thermoproteales. Two groups of single-stranded DNA viruses that infect archaea have been recently isolated. One group is exemplified by the *Halorubrum pleomorphic virus 1* ("Pleolipoviridae") infecting halophilic archaea and the other one by the Aeropyrum coil-shaped virus ("Spiraviridae") infecting a hyperthermophilic (optimal growth at 90–95 °C) host. Notably, the latter virus has the largest currently reported ssDNA genome. Defenses against these viruses may involve RNA interference from repetitive DNA sequences that are related to the genes of the viruses.

Archaea are genetically distinct from bacteria and eukaryotes, with up to 15% of the proteins encoded by any one archaeal genome being unique to the domain, although most of these unique genes have no known function. Of the remainder of the unique proteins that have an identified function, most belong to the Euryarchaea and are involved in methanogenesis. The proteins that archaea, bacteria and eukaryotes share form a common core of cell function, relating mostly to transcription, translation, and nucleotide metabolism. Other characteristic archaeal features are the organization of genes of related function—such as enzymes that catalyze steps in the same metabolic pathway into novel operons, and large differences in tRNA genes and their aminoacyl tRNA synthetases.

Transcription in archaea more closely resembles eukaryotic than bacterial transcription, with the archaeal RNA polymerase being very close to its equivalent in eukaryotes; while archaeal translation shows signs of both bacterial and eukaryal equivalents. Although archaea only have one type of RNA polymerase, its structure and function in transcription seems to be close to that of the eukaryotic RNA polymerase II, with similar protein assemblies (the general transcription factors) directing the binding of the RNA polymerase to a gene's promoter. However, other archaeal transcription factors are closer to those found in bacteria. Post-transcriptional modification is simpler than in eukaryotes, since most archaeal genes lack introns, although there are many introns in their transfer RNA and ribosomal RNA genes, and introns may occur in a few protein-encoding genes.

Gene Transfer and Genetic Exchange

Halobacterium volcanii, an extreme halophilic archaeon, forms cytoplasmic bridges between cells that appear to be used for transfer of DNA from one cell to another in either direction.

When the hyperthermophilic archaea *Sulfolobus solfataricus* and *Sulfolobus acidocaldarius* are exposed to the DNA damaging agents UV irradiation, bleomycin or mitomycin C, species-specific cellular aggregation is induced. Aggregation in *S. solfataricus* could not be induced by other physical stressors, such as pH or temperature shift, suggesting that aggregation is induced specifically by DNA damage. Ajon et al. showed that UV-induced cellular aggregation mediates chromosomal marker exchange with high frequency in *S. acidocaldarius*. Recombination rates exceeded those of uninduced cultures by up to three orders of magnitude. Frols et al. and Ajon et al. hypothesized that cellular aggregation enhances species specific DNA transfer between *Sulfolobus* cells in order to provide increased repair of damaged DNA by means of homologous recombination. This response may be a primitive form of sexual interaction similar to the more well-studied bacterial transformation systems that are also associated with species specific DNA transfer between cells leading to homologous recombinational repair of DNA damage.

Reproduction

Archaea reproduce asexually by binary or multiple fission, fragmentation, or budding; meiosis does not occur, so if a species of archaea exists in more than one form, all have the same genetic material. Cell division is controlled in a cell cycle; after the cell's chromosome is replicated and the two daughter chromosomes separate, the cell divides. In the genus *Sulfolobus*, the cycle has characteristics that are similar to both bacterial and eukaryotic systems. The chromosomes replicate from multiple starting-points (origins of replication) using DNA polymerases that resemble the equivalent eukaryotic enzymes.

In euryarchaea the cell division protein FtsZ, which forms a contracting ring around the cell, and the components of the septum that is constructed across the center of the cell, are similar to their bacterial equivalents. In cren- and thaumarchaea, however, the cell division machinery Cdv fulfills a similar role. This machinery is related to the eukaryotic ESCRT-III machinery which, while best known for its role in cell sorting, also has been seen to fulfill a role in separation between divided cell, suggesting an ancestral role in cell division.

Both bacteria and eukaryotes, but not archaea, make spores. Some species of Haloarchaea undergo phenotypic switching and grow as several different cell types, including thick-walled structures that are resistant to osmotic shock and allow the archaea to survive in water at low salt concentrations, but these are not reproductive structures and may instead help them reach new habitats.

Ecology

Habitats

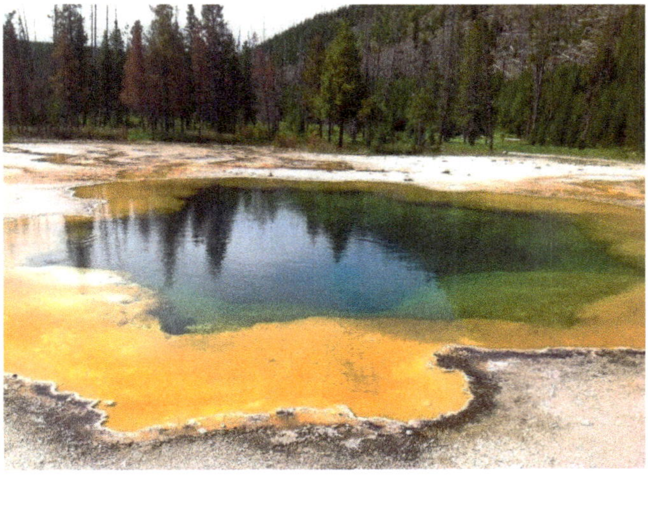

Archaea that grow in the hot water of the Morning Glory Hot Spring in Yellowstone National Park produce a bright colour

Archaea exist in a broad range of habitats, and as a major part of global ecosystems, may represent about 20% of microbial cells in the oceans. The first-discovered archaeans were extremophiles. Indeed, some archaea survive high temperatures, often above 100 °C (212 °F), as found in geysers, black smokers, and oil wells. Other common habitats include very cold habitats and highly saline, acidic, or alkaline water. However, archaea include mesophiles that grow in mild conditions, in swamps and marshland, sewage, the oceans, the intestinal tract of animals, and soils.

Extremophile archaea are members of four main physiological groups. These are the halophiles, thermophiles, alkaliphiles, and acidophiles. These groups are not comprehensive or phylum-specific, nor are they mutually exclusive, since some archaea belong to several groups. Nonetheless, they are a useful starting point for classification.

Halophiles, including the genus *Halobacterium*, live in extremely saline environments such as salt lakes and outnumber their bacterial counterparts at salinities greater than 20–25%. Thermophiles grow best at temperatures above 45 °C (113 °F), in places such as hot springs; *hyperthermophilic* archaea grow optimally at temperatures greater than 80 °C (176 °F). The archaeal *Methanopyrus kandleri* Strain 116 can even reproduce at 122 °C (252 °F), the highest recorded temperature of any organism.

Other archaea exist in very acidic or alkaline conditions. For example, one of the most extreme archaean acidophiles is *Picrophilus torridus*, which grows at pH 0, which is equivalent to thriving in 1.2 molar sulfuric acid.

This resistance to extreme environments has made archaea the focus of speculation about the possible properties of extraterrestrial life. Some extremophile habitats are not dissimilar to those on Mars, leading to the suggestion that viable microbes could be transferred between planets in meteorites.

Recently, several studies have shown that archaea exist not only in mesophilic and thermophilic environments but are also present, sometimes in high numbers, at low temperatures as well. For example, archaea are common in cold oceanic environments such as polar seas. Even more significant are the large numbers of archaea found throughout the world's oceans in non-extreme habitats among the plankton community (as part of the picoplankton). Although these archaea can be present in extremely high numbers (up to 40% of the microbial biomass), almost none of these species have been isolated and studied in pure culture.Consequently, our understanding of the role of archaea in ocean ecology is rudimentary, so their full influence on global biogeochemical cycles remains largely unexplored. Some marine Crenarchaeota are capable of nitrification, suggesting these organisms may affect the oceanic nitrogen cycle, although these oceanic Crenarchaeota may also use other sources of energy. Vast numbers of archaea are also found in the sediments that cover the sea floor, with these organisms making up the majority of living cells at depths over 1 meter below the ocean bottom. It has been demonstrated that in all oceanic surface sediments (from 1000- to 10,000-m water depth), the impact of viral infection is higher on archaea than on bacteria and virus-induced lysis of archaea accounts for up to one-third of the total microbial biomass killed, resulting in the release of ~0.3 to 0.5 gigatons of carbon per year globally.

Role in Chemical cycling

Archaea recycle elements such as carbon, nitrogen and sulfur through their various habitats. Although these activities are vital for normal ecosystem function, archaea can also contribute to human-made changes, and even cause pollution.

Archaea carry out many steps in the nitrogen cycle. This includes both reactions that remove nitrogen from ecosystems (such as nitrate-based respiration and denitrification) as well as processes that introduce nitrogen (such as nitrate assimilation and nitrogen fixation). Researchers recently discovered archaeal involvement in ammonia oxidation reactions. These reactions are particularly important in the oceans. The archaea also appear crucial for ammonia oxidation in soils. They produce nitrite, which other microbes then oxidize to nitrate. Plants and other organisms consume the latter.

In the sulfur cycle, archaea that grow by oxidizing sulfur compounds release this element from rocks, making it available to other organisms. However, the archaea that do this, such as *Sulfolobus*, produce sulfuric acid as a waste product, and the growth of these organisms in abandoned mines can contribute to acid mine drainage and other environmental damage.

In the carbon cycle, methanogen archaea remove hydrogen and play an important role in the decay of organic matter by the populations of microorganisms that act as decomposers in anaerobic ecosystems, such as sediments, marshes and sewage-treatment works.

Global methane levels in 2011 had increased by a factor of 2.5 since pre-industrial times: from 722 ppb to 1800 ppb, the highest value in at least 800,000 years.Methane has an anthropogenic global warming potential (AGWP) of 29, which means that it's 29 times stronger in heat-trapping than carbon dioxide is, over a 100-year time scale.

Interactions with other Organisms

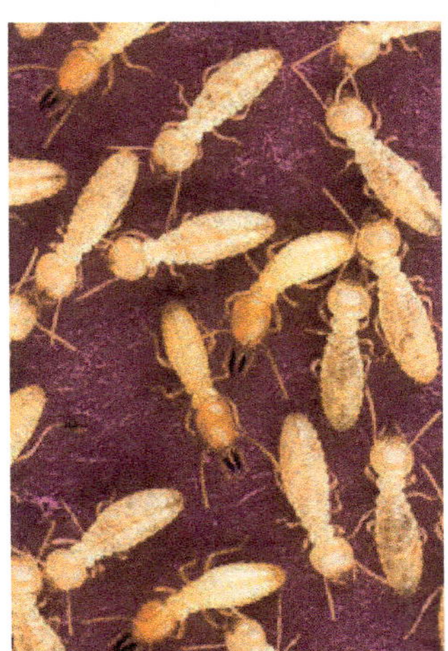

Methanogenic archaea form a symbiosis with termites.

The well-characterized interactions between archaea and other organisms are either mutual or commensal. There are no clear examples of known archaeal pathogens or parasites. However, some species of methanogens have been suggested to be involved in infections in the mouth, and *Nanoarchaeum equitans* may be a parasite of another species of archaea, since it only survives and reproduces within the cells of the Crenarchaeon *Ignicoccus hospitalis*, and appears to offer no benefit to its host. In contrast, Archaeal Richmond Mine Acidophilic Nanoorganisms (ARMAN) occasionally connect with other archaeal cells in acid mine drainage biofilms. The nature of this relationship is unknown. However, it is distinct from that of *Nanarchaeaum–Ignicoccus* in that the ultrasmall ARMAN cells are usually seen independent of the Thermoplasmatales cells.

Mutualism

One well-understood example of mutualism is the interaction between protozoa and methanogenic archaea in the digestive tracts of animals that digest cellulose, such as ruminants and termites. In these anaerobic environments, protozoa break down plant cellulose to obtain energy. This process releases hydrogen as a waste product, but high levels of hydrogen reduce energy production. When methanogens convert hydrogen to methane, protozoa benefit from more energy.

In anaerobic protozoa, such as *Plagiopyla frontata*, archaea reside inside the protozoa and consume hydrogen produced in their hydrogenosomes. Archaea also associate with larger organisms. For example, the marine archaean *Cenarchaeum symbiosum* lives within (is an endosymbiont of) the sponge *Axinella mexicana*.

Commensalism

Archaea can also be commensals, benefiting from an association without helping or harming the other organism. For example, the methanogen *Methanobrevibacter smithii* is by far the most common archaean in the human flora, making up about one in ten of all the prokaryotes in the human gut. In termites and in humans, these methanogens may in fact be mutualists, interacting with other microbes in the gut to aid digestion. Archaean communities also associate with a range of other organisms, such as on the surface of corals, and in the region of soil that surrounds plant roots (the rhizosphere).

Significance in Technology and Industry

Extremophile archaea, particularly those resistant either to heat or to extremes of acidity and alkalinity, are a source of enzymes that function under these harsh conditions. These enzymes have found many uses. For example, thermostable DNA polymerases, such as the Pfu DNA polymerase from *Pyrococcus furiosus*, revolutionized molecular biology by allowing the polymerase chain reaction to be used in research as a simple and rapid technique for cloning DNA. In industry, amylases, galactosidases and pullulanases in other species of *Pyrococcus* that function at over 100 °C (212 °F) allow food processing at high temperatures, such as the production of low lactose milk and whey. Enzymes from these thermophilic archaea also tend to be very stable in organic solvents, allowing their use in environmentally friendly processes in green chemistry that synthesize organic compounds. This stability makes them easier to use in structural biology. Consequently, the counterparts of bacterial or eukaryotic enzymes from extremophile archaea are often used in structural studies.

In contrast to the range of applications of archaean enzymes, the use of the organisms themselves in biotechnology is less developed. Methanogenic archaea are a vital part of sewage treatment, since they are part of the community of microorganisms that carry out anaerobic digestion and produce biogas. In mineral processing, acidophilic archaea display promise for the extraction of metals from ores, including gold, cobalt and copper.

Archaea host a new class of potentially useful antibiotics. A few of these archaeocins have been characterized, but hundreds more are believed to exist, especially within *Haloarchaea* and *Sulfolobus*. These compounds differ in structure from bacterial antibiotics, so they may have novel modes of action. In addition, they may allow the creation of new selectable markers for use in archaeal molecular biology.

EUKARYOTE

A **eukaryote** is any organism whose cells contain a nucleus and other organelles enclosed within membranes. Eukaryotes belong to the taxon **Eukarya** or **Eukaryota**. The defining feature that sets eukaryotic cells apart from prokaryotic cells (Bacteria and Archaea) is that they have membrane-bound organelles, especially the nucleus, which contains the genetic material and is enclosed by the nuclear envelope. The presence of a nucleus gives eukaryotes their name, which comes from the Greek ε□ (*eu*, "well" or "true") and κάρυον (*karyon*, "nut" or "kernel"). Eukaryotic cells also contain other membrane-bound organelles such as mitochondria and the Golgi apparatus. In addition, plants and algae contain chloroplasts. Eukaryotic organisms may be unicellular or multicellular. Only eukaryotes form multicellular organisms consisting of many kinds of tissue made up of different cell types.

Eukaryotes can reproduce both asexually through mitosis and sexually through meiosis and gamete fusion. In mitosis, one cell divides to produce two genetically identical cells. In meiosis, DNA replication is followed by two rounds of cell division to produce four daughter cells each with half the number of chromosomes as the original parent cell (haploid cells). These act as sex cells (gametes – each gamete has just one complement of chromosomes, each a unique mix of the corresponding pair of parental chromosomes) resulting from genetic recombination during meiosis.

The domain Eukaryota appears to be monophyletic, and so makes up one of the three domains of life. The two other domains, Bacteria and Archaea, are prokaryotes and have none of the above features. Eukaryotes represent a tiny minority of all living things. However, due to their much larger size, eukaryotes' collective worldwide biomass is estimated at about equal to that of prokaryotes. Eukaryotes first developed approximately 1.6–2.1 billion years ago (during the Proterozoic eon).

Cell Features

Eukaryotic cells are typically much larger than those of prokaryotes. They have a variety of internal membrane-bound structures, called organelles, and a cytoskeleton composed of microtubules, microfilaments, and intermediate filaments, which play an important role in defining the cell's organization and shape. Eukaryotic DNA is divided into several linear bundles called chromosomes, which are separated by a microtubular spindle during nuclear division.

Internal Membrane

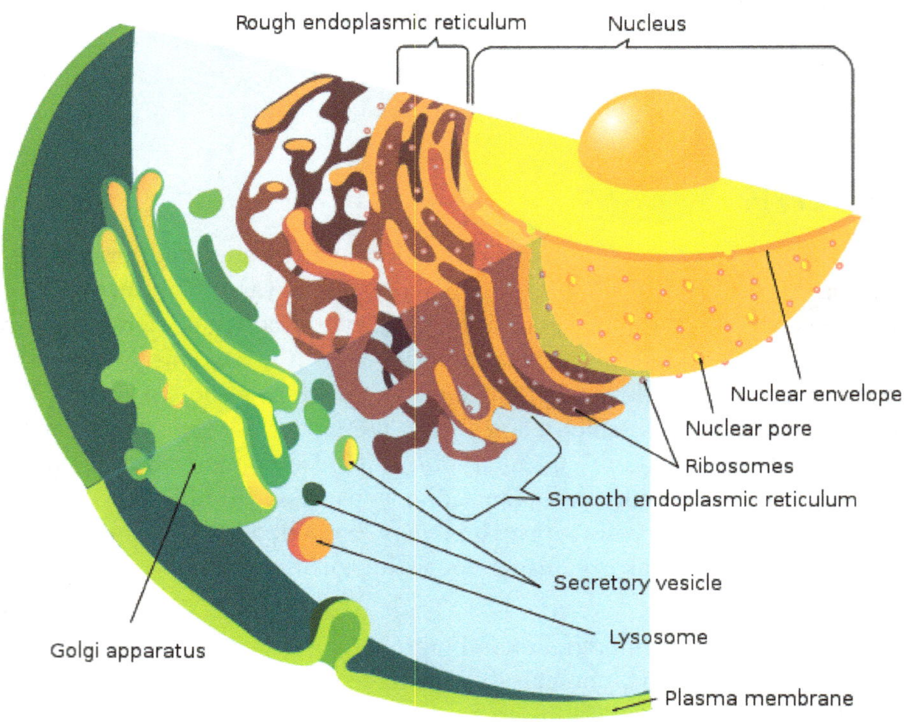

Detail of the endomembrane system and its components

Eukaryote cells include a variety of membrane-bound structures, collectively referred to as the endomembrane system. Simple compartments, called vesicles or vacuoles, can form by budding off other membranes. Many cells ingest food and other materials through a process of endocytosis, where the outer membrane invaginates and then pinches off to form a vesicle. It is probable that most other membrane-bound organelles are ultimately derived from such vesicles. Alternatively some products produced by the cell can leave in a vesicle through exocytosis.

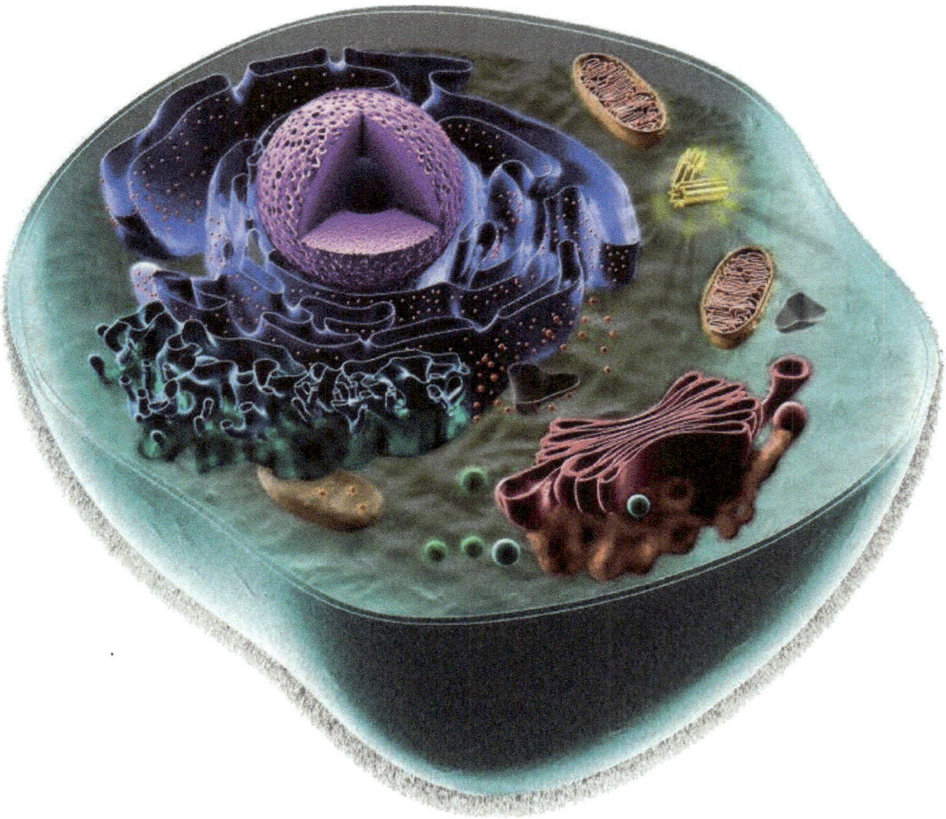

A 3D rendering of an animal cell cut in half.

The nucleus is surrounded by a double membrane (commonly referred to as a nuclear membrane or nuclear envelope), with pores that allow material to move in and out. Various tube- and sheet-like extensions of the nuclear membrane form what is called the endoplasmic reticulum or ER, which is involved in protein transport and maturation. It includes the rough ER where ribosomes are attached to synthesize proteins, which enter the interior space or lumen. Subsequently, they generally enter vesicles, which bud off from the smooth ER. In most eukaryotes, these protein-carrying vesicles are released and further modified in stacks of flattened vesicles, called Golgi bodies or dictyosomes.

Vesicles may be specialized for various purposes. For instance, lysosomes contain digestive enzymes that break down the contents of food vacuoles, and peroxisomes are used to break down peroxide, which is toxic otherwise. Many protozoa have contractile vacuoles, which collect and expel excess water, and extrusomes, which expel material used to deflect predators or capture prey. In higher plants, most of a cell's volume is taken up by a central vacuole, which primarily maintains its osmotic pressure.

Mitochondria and Plastids

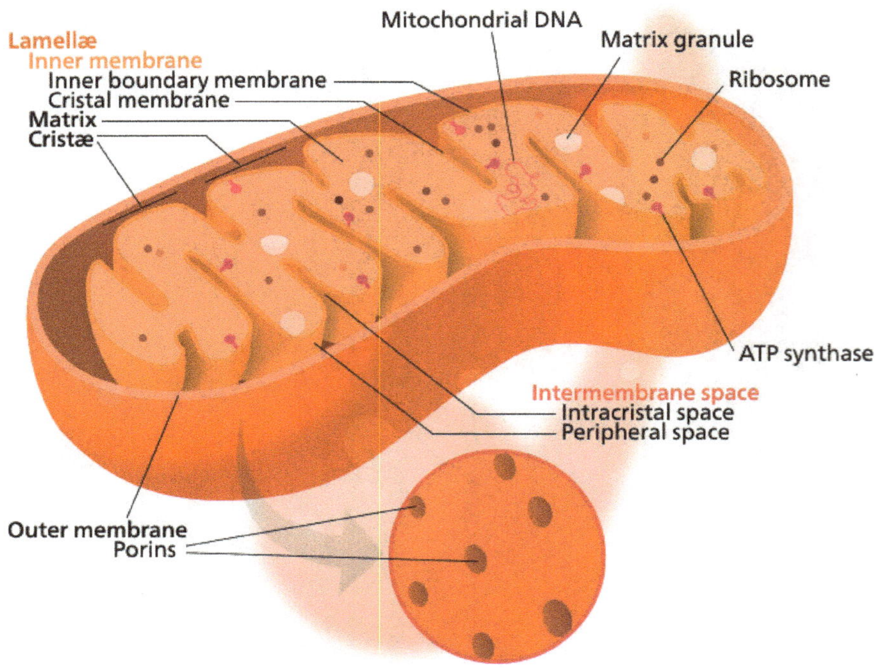

Simplified structure of a mitochondrion

Mitochondria are organelles found in nearly all eukaryotes that provide energy to the cell by converting ingested sugars into ATP. They are surrounded by two membranes (each a phospholipid bi-layer), the inner of which is folded into invaginations called cristae, where aerobic respiration takes place. Mitochondria contain their own DNA. They are now generally held to have developed from endosymbiotic prokaryotes, probably proteobacteria. Protozoa and microbes that lack mitochondria, such as the amoebozoan Pelomyxa and metamonads such as Giardia and Trichomonas, have usually been found to contain mitochondrion-derived organelles, such as hydrogenosomes and mitosomes, and thus probably lost the mitochondria secondarily.

In 2016, *Monocercomonoides*, a metamonad flagellate which resides in the intestines of the chinchilla, has been found to lack mitochondria entirely. *Monocercomonoides* obtains its energy by enzymatic action on nutrients absorbed from the environment. It has also acquired, by lateral gene transfer, a cytosolic sulphur mobilisation system which provides the clusters of iron and sulfur required for protein synthesis. The normal mitochondrial iron-sulphur cluster pathway is considered to have been lost secondarily.

Plants and various groups of algae also have plastids. Plastids have their own DNA and are developed from endosymbionts, in this case cyanobacteria. They usually take the form of chloroplasts, which like cyanobacteria contain chlorophyll and produce organic compounds (such as glucose) through photosynthesis. Others are involved in storing food. Although plastids probably had a single origin, not all plastid-containing groups are closely related. Instead, some eukaryotes have obtained them from others through secondary endosymbiosis or ingestion.

Endosymbiotic origins have also been proposed for the nucleus, for which see below, and for eukaryotic flagella, supposed to have developed from spirochaetes. This is not generally accepted, both from a lack of cytological evidence and difficulty in reconciling this with cellular reproduction.

Cytoskeletal Structures

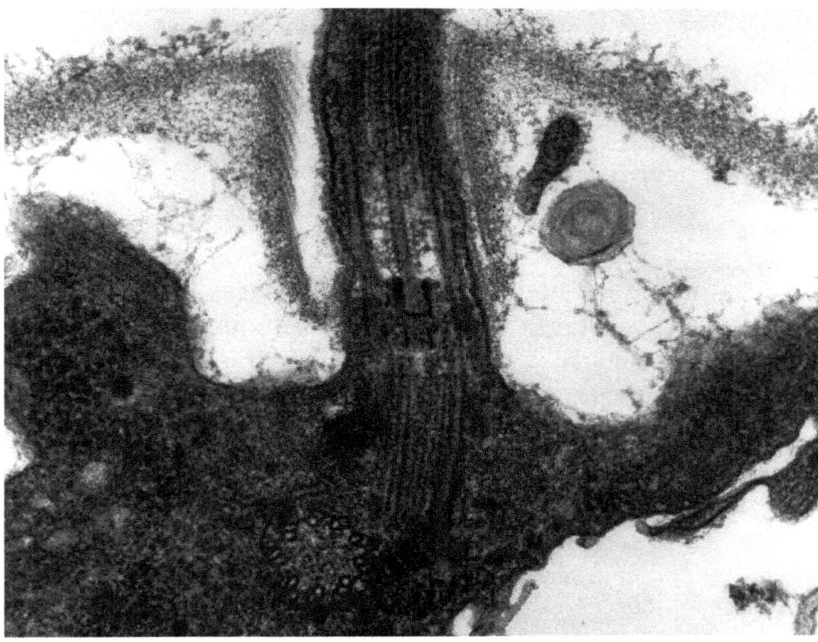

Longitudinal section through the flagellum of *Chlamydomonas reinhardtii*

Many eukaryotes have long slender motile cytoplasmic projections, called flagella, or similar structures called cilia. Flagella and cilia are sometimes referred to as undulipodia, and are variously involved in movement, feeding, and sensation. They are composed mainly of tubulin. These are entirely distinct from prokaryotic flagellae. They are supported by a bundle of microtubules arising from a basal body, also called a kinetosome or centriole, characteristically arranged as nine doublets surrounding two singlets. Flagella also may have hairs, or mastigonemes, and scales connecting membranes and internal rods. Their interior is continuous with the cell's cytoplasm.

Microfilamental structures composed of actin and actin binding proteins, e.g., α-actinin, fimbrin, filamin are present in submembraneous cortical layers and bundles, as well. Motor proteins of microtubules, e.g., dynein or kinesin and actin, e.g., myosins provide dynamic character of the network.

Centrioles are often present even in cells and groups that do not have flagella, but conifers and flowering plants have neither. They generally occur in groups of one or two, called kinetids, that give rise to various microtubular roots. These form a primary component of the cytoskeletal structure, and are often assembled over the course of several cell divisions, with one flagellum retained from the parent and the other derived from it. Centrioles may also be associated in the formation of a spindle during nuclear division.

The significance of cytoskeletal structures is underlined in the determination of shape of the cells, as well as their being essential components of migratory responses like chemotaxis and chemokinesis. Some protists have various other microtubule-supported organelles. These include the radiolaria and heliozoa, which produce axopodia used in flotation or to capture prey, and the haptophytes, which have a peculiar flagellum-like organelle called the haptonema.

Cell Wall

The cells of plants, fungi, and most chromalveolates have a cell wall, a layer outside the cell membrane, providing the cell with structural support, protection, and a filtering mechanism. The cell wall also prevents over-expansion when water enters the cell.

The major polysaccharides making up the primary cell wall of land plants are cellulose, hemicellulose, and pectin. The cellulose microfibrils are linked via hemicellulosic tethers to form the cellulose-hemicellulose network, which is embedded in the pectin matrix. The most common hemicellulose in the primary cell wall is xyloglucan.

Differences among Eukaryotic Cells

There are many different types of eukaryotic cells, though animals and plants are the most familiar eukaryotes, and thus provide an excellent starting point for understanding eukaryotic structure. Fungi and many protists have some substantial differences, however.

Animal Cell

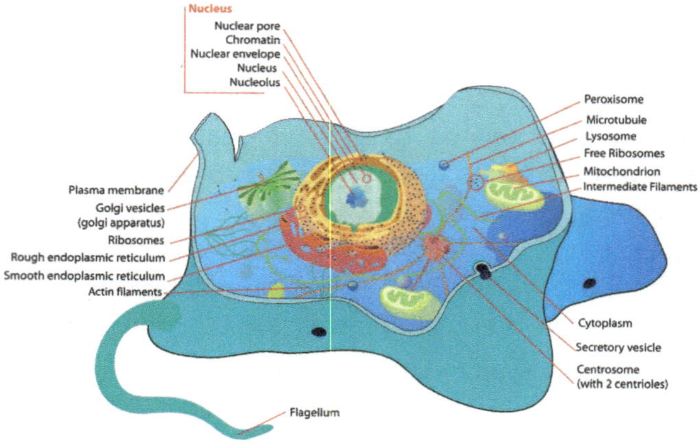

Structure of a typical animal cell

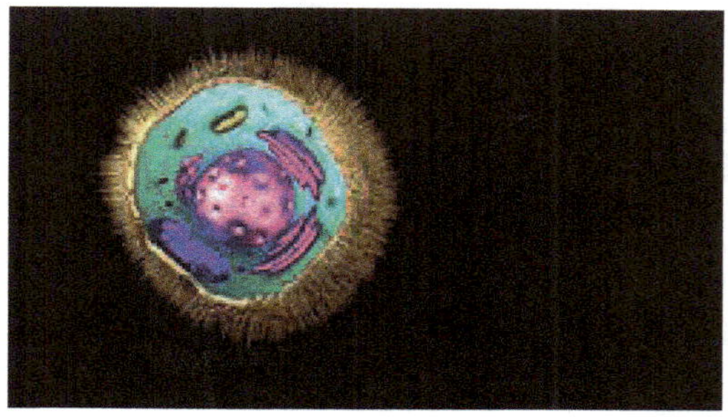

3D Simulation of animal cell

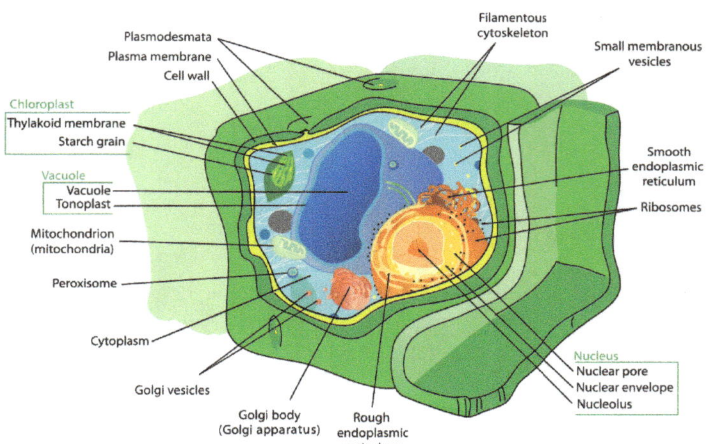

Structure of a typical plant cell

All animals consist of eukaryotic cells. Animal cells are distinct from those of other eukaryotes, most notably plants, as they lack cell walls and chloroplasts and have smaller vacuoles. Due to the lack of a cell wall, animal cells can adopt a variety of shapes. A phagocytic cell can even engulf other structures.

There are many other types of cell. For instance, there are approximately 210 distinct cell types in the adult human body.

Plant Cell

Plant cells are quite different from the cells of the other eukaryotic organisms. Their distinctive features are:

- A large central vacuole (enclosed by a membrane, the tonoplast), which maintains the cell's turgor and controls movement of molecules between the cytosol and sap

- A primary cell wall containing cellulose, hemicellulose and pectin, deposited by the protoplast on the outside of the cell membrane; this contrasts with the cell walls of fungi, which contain chitin, and the cell envelopes of prokaryotes, in which peptidoglycans are the main structural molecules
- The plasmodesmata, linking pores in the cell wall that allow each plant cell to communicate with other adjacent cells; this is different from the functionally analogous system of gap junctions between animal cells.
- Plastids, especially chloroplasts that contain chlorophyll, the pigment that gives plants their green color and allows them to perform photosynthesis
- Bryophytes and seedless vascular plants lack flagellae and centrioles except in the sperm cells. Sperm of cycads and *Ginkgo* are large, complex cells that swim with hundreds to thousands of flagellae.
- Conifers (Pinophyta) and flowering plants (Angiospermae) lack the flagellae and centrioles that are present in animal cells.

Fungal Cell

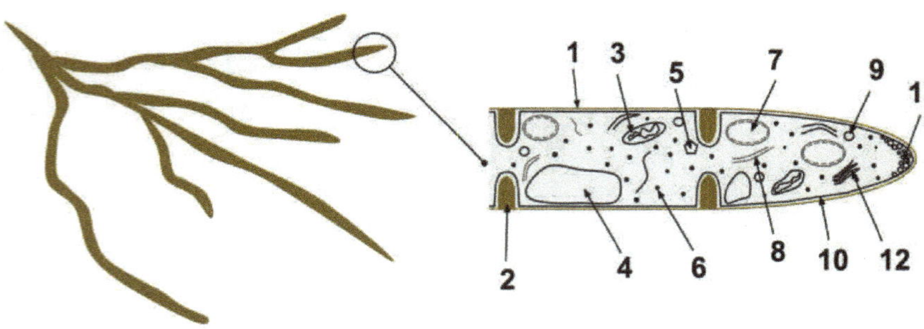

Fungal Hyphae Cells

1- Hyphal wall 2- Septum 3- Mitochondrion 4- Vacuole 5- Ergosterol crystal 6- Ribosome 7- Nucleus 8- Endoplasmic reticulum 9- Lipid body 10- Plasma membrane 11- Spitzenkörper 12- Golgi apparatus

Fungal cells are most similar to animal cells, with the following exceptions:

- A cell wall that contains chitin
- Less definition between cells; the hyphae of higher fungi have porous partitions called septa, which allow the passage of cytoplasm, organelles, and, sometimes, nuclei. Primitive fungi have few or no septa, so each organism is essentially a giant multinucleate supercell; these fungi are described as coenocytic.
- Only the most primitive fungi, chytrids, have flagella.

Other Eukaryotic Cells

Eukaryotes are a very diverse group, and their cell structures are equally diverse. Many have cell walls; many do not. Many have chloroplasts, derived from primary, secondary, or even tertiary endosymbiosis; and many do not. Some groups have unique structures, such as the cyanelles of the glaucophytes, the haptonema of the haptophytes, or the ejectisomes of the cryptomonads. Other structures, such as pseudopods, are found in various eukaryote groups in different forms, such as the lobose amoebozoans or the reticulose foraminiferans.

Reproduction

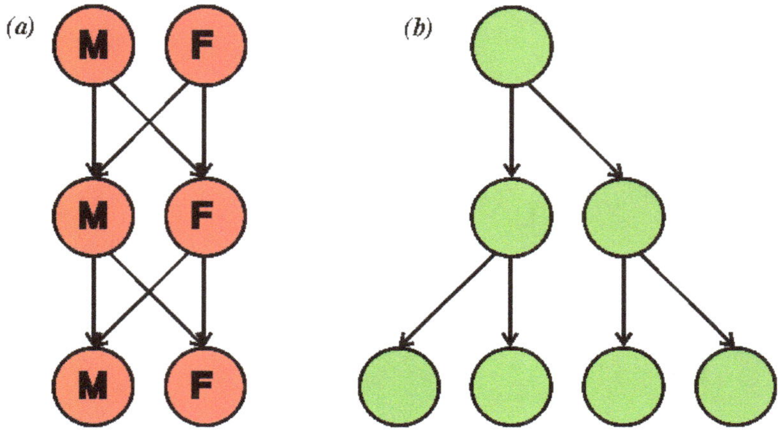

This diagram illustrates the *twofold cost of sex*. If each individual were to contribute to the same number of offspring (two), *(a)* the sexual population remains the same size each generation, where the *(b)* asexual population doubles in size each generation.

Cell division generally takes place asexually by mitosis, a process that allows each daughter nucleus to receive one copy of each chromosome. In most eukaryotes, there is also a process of sexual reproduction, typically involving an alternation between haploid generations, wherein only one copy of each chromosome is present, and diploid generations, wherein two copies of each chromosome are present, occurring through meiosis. There is considerable variation in this pattern.

Eukaryotes have a smaller surface area to volume ratio than prokaryotes, and thus have lower metabolic rates and longer generation times. In some multicellular organisms, cells specialized for metabolism will have enlarged surface areas, such as intestinal vili.

The evolution of sexual reproduction may be a primordial and fundamental characteristic of eukaryotes. Based on a phylogenetic analysis, Dacks and Roger proposed that facultative sex was present in the common ancestor of all eukaryotes. A core set of genes that function in meiosis is present in both *Trichomonas vaginalis* and *Giardia intestinalis*, two organisms previously thought to be asexual. Since these two species are descendants of lineages that diverged early from the eukaryotic evolutionary tree, it was inferred that core meiotic genes, and hence sex, were likely present in a common ancestor of all eukaryotes. Other studies on eukaryotic species once thought to be asexual have revealed evidence for a sexual cycle. For instance, parasitic protozoa of the genus Leishmania have recently been shown to have a sexual cycle. Also, evidence now indicates that amoeba, that were previously regarded as asexual, are anciently sexual and that the majority of present-day asexual groups likely arose recently and independently.

Classification

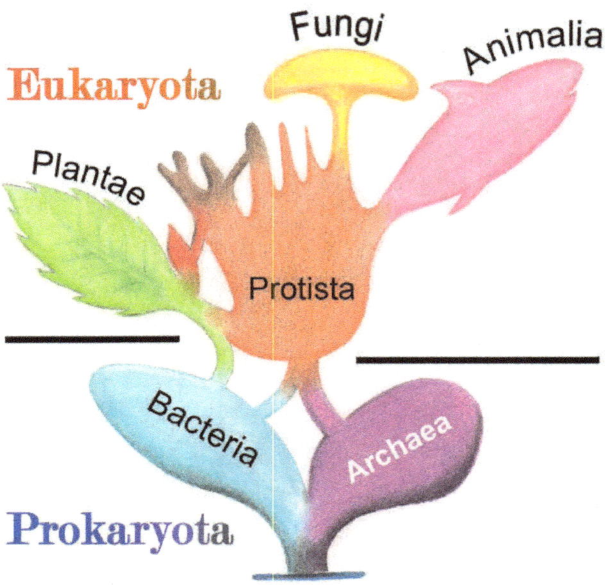

Phylogenetic and symbiogenetic tree of living organisms, showing the origins of eukaryotes & prokaryotes

In antiquity, the two clades of animals and plants were recognized. They were given the taxonomic rank of Kingdom by Linnaeus. Though he included the fungi with plants with some reservations, it was later realized that they are quite distinct and warrant a separate kingdom, the composition of which was not entirely clear until the 1980s. The various single-cell eukaryotes were originally placed with plants or animals when they became known. In 1830, the German biologist Georg A. Goldfuss coined the word *protozoa* to refer to organisms such as ciliates, and this group was expanded until it encompassed all single-celled eukaryotes, and given their own kingdom, the Protista, by Ernst Haeckel in 1866. The eukaryotes thus came to be composed of four kingdoms:

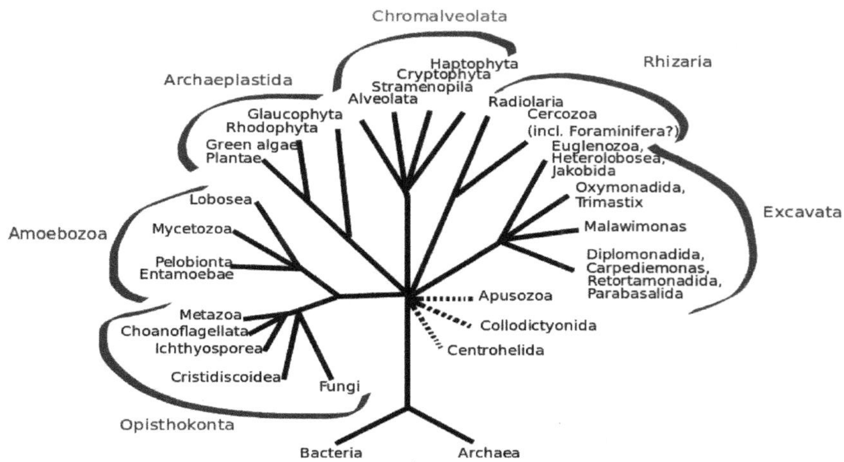

One hypothesis of eukaryotic relationships. The Opisthokonta group includes both animals (Metazoa) and fungi. Plants (Plantae) are placed in Archaeplastida.

- Kingdom Protista
- Kingdom Plantae
- Kingdom Fungi
- Kingdom Animalia

The protists were understood to be "primitive forms", and thus an evolutionary grade, united by their primitive unicellular nature. The disentanglement of the deep splits in the tree of life only really started with DNA sequencing, leading to a system of domains rather than kingdoms as top level rank being put forward by Carl Woese, uniting all the eukaryote kingdoms under the eukaryote domain. At the same time, work on the protist tree intensified, and is still actively going on today. Several alternative classifications have been forwarded, though there is no consensus in the field.

A classification produced in 2005 for the International Society of Protistologists, which reflected the consensus of the time, divided the eukaryotes into six supposedly monophyletic ‹supergroups'. However, in the same year (2005), doubts were expressed as to whether some of these supergroups were monophyletic, particularly the Chromalveolata, and a review in 2006 noted the lack of evidence for several of the supposed six supergroups. A revised classification in 2012 recognizes five supergroups.

Archaeplastida (or Primoplantae)	Land plants, green algae, red algae, and glaucophytes
SAR supergroup	Stramenopiles (brown algae, diatoms, etc.), Alveolata, and Rhizaria (Foraminifera, Radiolaria, and various other amoeboid protozoa).
Excavata	Various flagellate protozoa

Amoebozoa	Most lobose amoeboids and slime molds
Opisthokonta	Animals, fungi, choanoflagellates, etc.

There are also smaller groups of eukaryotes whose position is uncertain or seems to fall outside the major groups. In particular, Haptophyta, Cryptophyta, Centrohelida, Telonemia, Picozoa, Apusomonadida, Ancyromonadida, Breviatea, and the genus *Collodictyon*. Overall, it seems that, although progress has been made, there are still very significant uncertainties in the evolutionary history and classification of eukaryotes. As Roger & Simpson said in 2009 "with the current pace of change in our understanding of the eukaryote tree of life, we should proceed with caution."

In an article published in *Nature Microbiology* in April 2016 the authors, "reinforced once again that the life we see around us – plants, animals, humans and other so-called eukaryotes – represent a tiny percentage of the world's biodiversity." They classified eukaryote "based on the inheritance of their information systems as opposed to lipid or other cellular structures." Jillian F. Banfield of the University of California, Berkeley and fellow scientists used a super computer to generate a diagram of a new tree of life based on DNA from 3000 species including 2,072 known species and 1,011 newly reported microbial organisms, whose DNA they had gathered from diverse environments. As the capacity to sequence DNA became easier, Banfield and team were able to do metagenomic sequencing—"sequencing whole communities of organisms at once and picking out the individual groups based on their genes alone."

Phylogeny

The rRNA trees constructed during the 1980s and 1990s left most eukaryotes in an unresolved "crown" group (not technically a true crown), which was usually divided by the form of the mitochondrial cristae; see crown eukaryotes. The few groups that lack mitochondria branched separately, and so the absence was believed to be primitive; but this is now considered an artifact of long-branch attraction, and they are known to have lost them secondarily.

As of 2011, there is widespread agreement that the Rhizaria belong with the Stramenopiles and the Alveolata, in a clade dubbed the SAR supergroup, so that Rhizaria is not one of the main eukaryote groups; also that the Amoebozoa and Opisthokonta are each monophyletic and form a clade, often called the unikonts. Beyond this, there does not appear to be a consensus.

It has been estimated that there may be 75 distinct lineages of eukaryotes. Most of these lineages are protists.

The known eukaryote genome sizes vary from 8.2 megabases (Mb) in *Babesia bovis* to 112,000–220,050 Mb in the dinoflagellate *Prorocentrum micans*, suggesting that the genome of the ancestral eukaryote has undergone considerable variation during its evolution. The last common ancestor of all eukaryotes is believed to have been a phagotrophic protist with a nucleus, at least one centriole and cilium, facultatively aerobic mitochondria, sex (meiosis and syngamy), a dormant cyst with a cell wall of chitin and/or cellulose and peroxisomes. Later endosymbiosis led to the spread of plastids in some lineages.

Five Supergroups

A global tree of eukaryotes from a consensus of phylogenetic evidence (in particular, phylogenomics), rare genomic signatures, and morphological characteristics is presented in Adl *et al.* 2012 and Burki 2014.

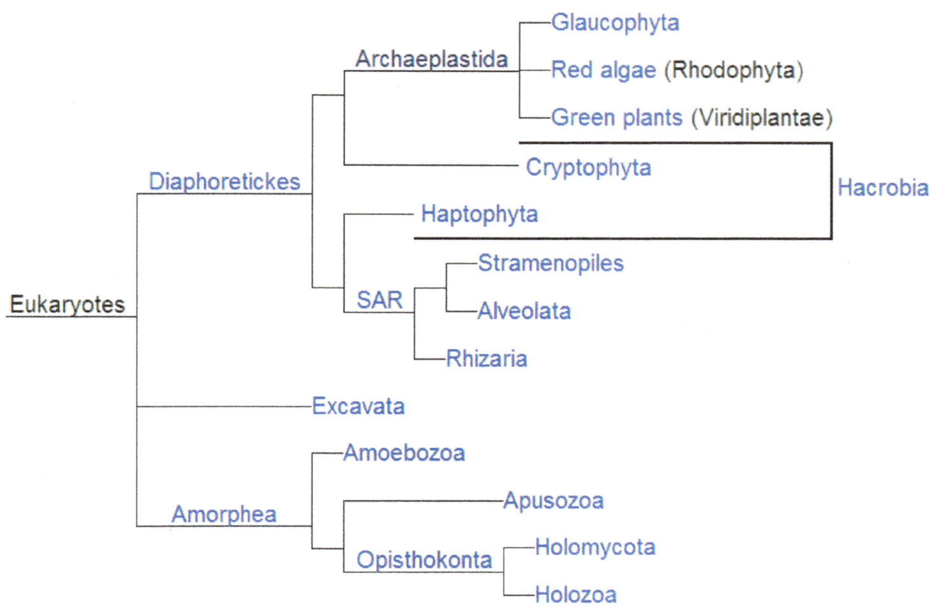

In some analyses, the Hacrobia group (Haptophyta + Cryptophyta) is placed next to Archaeplastida, but in other ones it is nested inside the Archaeplastida.However, several recent studies have concluded that Haptophyta and Cryptophyta do not form a monophyletic group. The former could be a sister group to the SAR group, the latter cluster with the Archaeplastida (plants in the broad sense). As of February 2012, it remains unclear whether the Hacrobia forms a monophyletic group.

The division of the eukaryotes into two primary clades, bikonts (Archaeplastida + SAR + Excavata) and unikonts (Amoebozoa + Opisthokonta), derived from an ancestral biflagellar organism and an ancestral uniflagellar organism, respectively, had been suggested earlier. A 2012 study produced a somewhat similar division, although noting that the terms "unikonts" and "bikonts" were not used in the original sense.

Cavalier-Smith's Tree

Cavalier-Smith 2010, 2013, and 2014 places the eukaryotic tree's root between Excavata (with ventral feeding groove supported by a microtubular root) and the grooveless Euglenozoa:

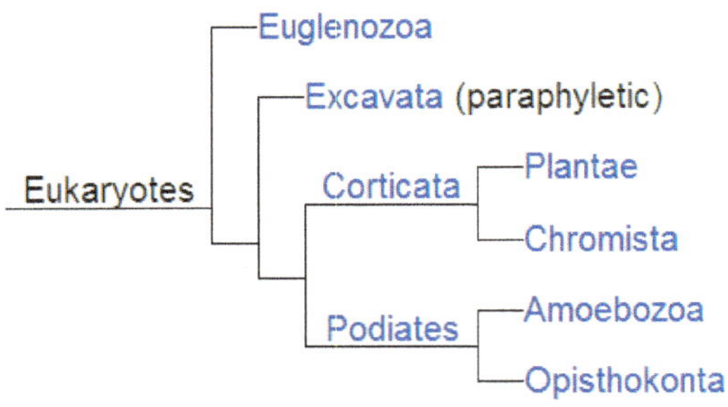

Alternative Views

Other analyses place the SAR supergroup within an expanded Chromalveolata, although they differ on the placement of the resulting five groups. Rogozin *et al.* in 2009 produced the tree shown below, where the primary division is between the Archaeplastida and all other eukaryotes.

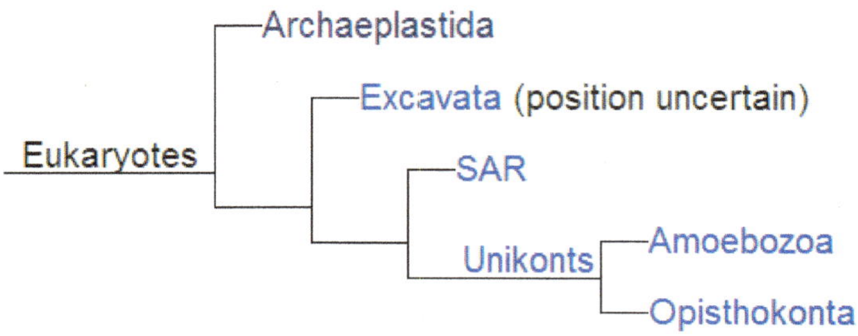

A paper published in 2009, which re-examined the data used in some of the analyses presented above as well as performing new ones, strongly suggested that the Archaeplastida are polyphyletic. The phylogeny finally proposed in the paper is shown below.

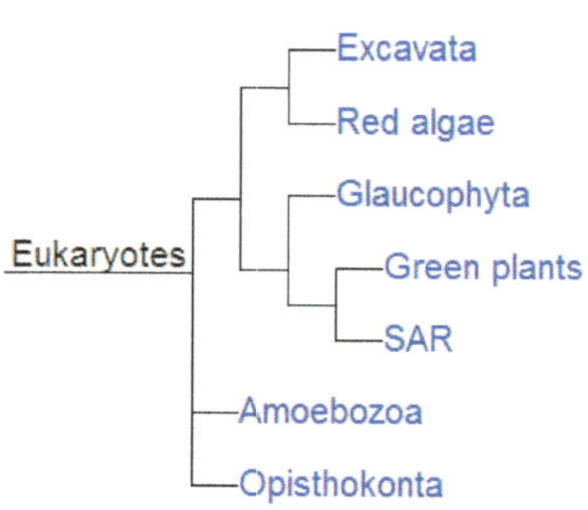

There are also the cladistic analyses of Diana Lipscomb based on classical data which have red algae as basal and Archeoplastida as paraphyletic. In the survey by Parfrey et al. it is recovered in only 42.6% of the molecular analyses that include it, that is, 26 out of 61.

It is not recovered in Goloboff et al.'s combined analysis, and is mostly weakly supported in other molecular analyses. Laura Parfrey et al. point out that Archeoplastida support comes primarily from phylogenomic analyses and these may be picking up misleading endosymbiotic gene transfer signal of genes independently transferred from the plastid to the host nucleus in the 3 archeoplastid clades. And Stiller and Harrell emphasize that the group can be explained by "short-branch exclusion" and "subtle and easily overlooked biases can dominate the overall results of molecular phylogenetic analyses of ancient eukaryotic relationships. Sources of potential phylogenetic artifact should be investigated routinely, not just when obvious ‹long-branch attraction' is encountered."

Red algae as basal is also supported by molecular evidence. *Cyanidioschyzon*, a red alga, is considered basal (sister group to the rest of eukaryotes) by Nagashima et al. and Seckbach. It has the most primitive chloroplast, only 1 mitochondrion, no vacuoles, no trienoic acids, and the smallest eukaryotic genome at 8 Mbp.

Rhizaria are only moderately supported (65.5% of the studies, i.e., 19 of 29), statistical support for them is inconsistent in multigene genealogies with larger taxon sampling and the group is ambiguously supported in Goloboff et al.

Origin of Eukaryotes

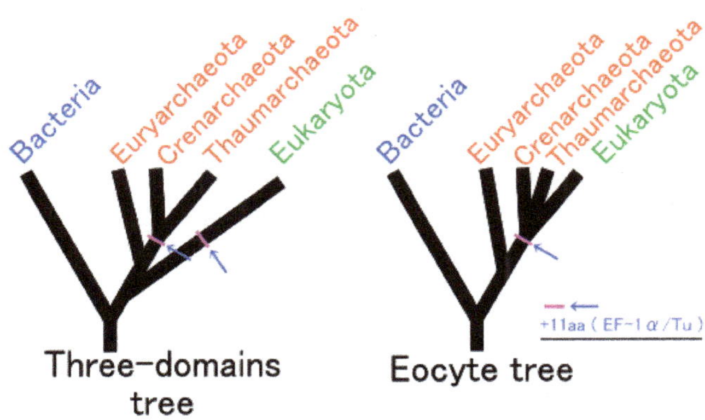

The three-domains tree and the Eocyte hypothesis.

Fossils

The origin of the eukaryotic cell is considered a milestone in the evolution of life, since eukaryotes include all complex cells and almost all multicellular organisms. The timing of this series of events is hard to determine; Knoll (2006) suggests they developed approximately 1.6–2.1 billion years ago. Some acritarchs are known from at least 1.65 billion years ago, and the possible alga *Grypania* has been found as far back as 2.1 billion years ago. The *Geosiphon*-like fossil fungus *Diskagma* has been found in paleosols 2.2 billion years old

Organized living structures have been found in the black shales of the Palaeoproterozoic Francevillian B Formation in Gabon, dated at 2.1 billion years old. Eukaryotic life could have evolved at that time.Fossils that are clearly related to modern groups start appearing an estimated 1.2 billion years ago, in the form of a red alga, though recent work suggests the existence of fossilized filamentous algae in the Vindhya basin dating back perhaps to 1.6 to 1.7 billion years ago.

Biomarkers suggest that at least stem eukaryotes arose even earlier. The presence of steranes in Australian shales indicates that eukaryotes were present in these rocks dated at 2.7 billion years old.

Relationship to Archaea

Eukaryotes are more closely related to Archaea than Bacteria, at least in terms of nuclear DNA and genetic machinery, and one controversial idea is to place them with Archaea in the clade Neomura. However, in other respects, such as membrane composition, eukaryotes are similar to Bacteria. Three main explanations for this have been proposed:

- Eukaryotes resulted from the complete fusion of two or more cells, wherein the cytoplasm formed from a eubacterium, and the nucleus from an archaeon, from a virus, or from a pre-cell.
- Eukaryotes developed from Archaea, and acquired their eubacterial characteristics from the proto-mitochondrion.
- Eukaryotes and Archaea developed separately from a modified eubacterium.

The chronocyte hypothesis for the origin of the eukaryotic cell postulates that a primitive eukaryotic cell was formed by the endosymbiosis of both archaea and bacteria by a third type of cell, termed a chronocyte.

Endomembrane System and Mitochondria

The origins of the endomembrane system and mitochondria are also unclear. The **phagotrophic hypothesis** proposes that eukaryotic-type membranes lacking a cell wall originated first, with the development of endocytosis, whereas mitochondria were acquired by ingestion as endosymbionts. The **syntrophic hypothesis** proposes that the proto-eukaryote relied on the proto-mitochondrion for food, and so ultimately grew to surround it. Here the membranes originated after the engulfment of the mitochondrion, in part thanks to mitochondrial genes (the hydrogen hypothesis is one particular version).

In a study using genomes to construct supertrees, Pisani *et al.* (2007) suggest that, along with evidence that there was never a mitochondrion-less eukaryote, eukaryotes evolved from a syntrophy between an archaea closely related to Thermoplasmatales and an α-proteobacterium, likely a symbiosis driven by sulfur or hydrogen. The mitochondrion and its genome is a remnant of the α-proteobacterial endosymbiont.

Hypotheses for the Origin of Eukaryotes

Different hypotheses have been proposed as to how eukaryotic cells came into existence.

These hypotheses can be classified into two distinct classes – autogenous models and chimeric models.

Autogenous Models

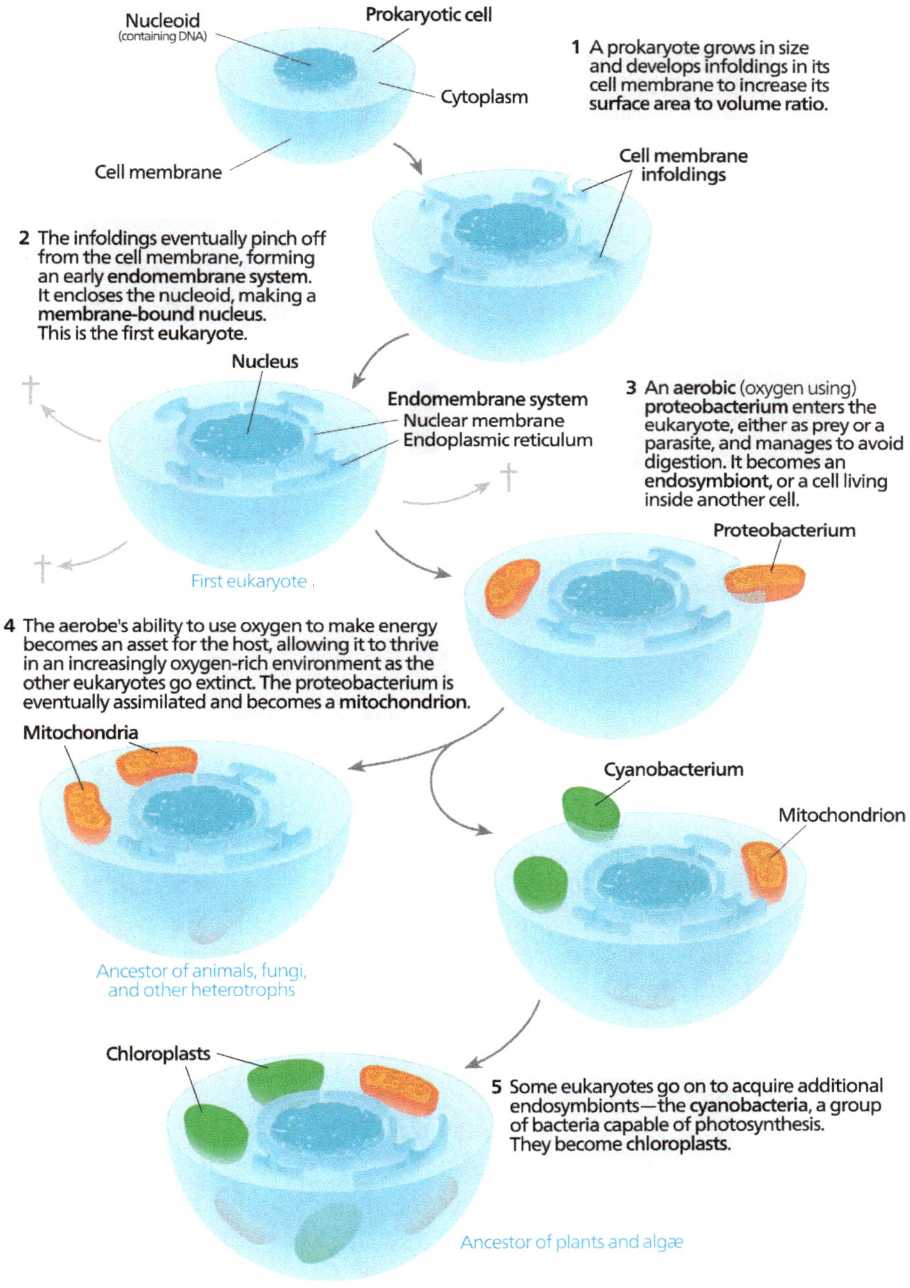

An autogenous model for the origin of eukaryotes.

Autogenous models propose that a proto-eukaryotic cell containing a nucleus existed first, and later acquired mitochondria. According to this model, a large prokaryote developed invaginations in its plasma membrane in order to obtain enough surface area to service its cytoplasmic volume. As the invaginations differentiated in function, some became separate compartments—giving rise to the endomembrane system, including the endoplasmic reticulum, golgi apparatus, nuclear membrane, and single membrane structures such as lysosomes. Mitochondria are proposed to come from the endosymbiosis of an aerobic proteobacterium, and it's assumed that all the eukaryotic lineages that did not acquire mitochondria became extinct. Chloroplasts came about from another endosymbiotic event involving cyanobacteria. Since all eukaryotes have mitochondria, but not all have chloroplasts, mitochondria are thought to have come first. This is the serial endosymbiosis theory.

Some models propose that the origins of double layered organelles, such as mitochondria and chloroplasts, in the proto-eukaryotic cell is due to the compartmentalization of DNA vesicles that were formed from the secondary invaginations or more detailed infoldings of cellular membrane.

Chimeric Models

Chimeric models claim that two prokaryotic cells existed initially – an archaeon and a bacterium. These cells underwent a merging process, either by a physical fusion or by endosymbiosis, thereby leading to the formation of a eukaryotic cell. Within these chimeric models, some studies further claim that mitochondria originated from a bacterial ancestor while others emphasize the role of endosymbiotic processes behind the origin of mitochondria.

Based on the process of mutualistic symbiosis, the hypotheses can be categorized as – the serial endosymbiotic theory (SET), the hydrogen hypothesis (mostly a process of symbiosis where hydrogen transfer takes place among different species), and the syntrophy hypothesis.

According to serial endosymbiotic theory (championed by Dr. Lynn Margulis), a union between a motile anaerobic bacterium (like *Spirochaeta*) and a thermoacidophilic crenarchaeon (like *Thermoplasma* which is sulfidogenic in nature) gave rise to the present day eukaryotes. This union established a motile organism capable of living in the already existing acidic and sulfurous waters. Oxygen is known to cause toxicity to organisms that lack the required metabolic machinery. Thus, the archaeon provided the bacterium with a highly beneficial reduced environment (sulfur and sulfate were reduced to sulfide). In microaerophilic conditions, oxygen was reduced to water thereby creating a mutual benefit platform. The bacterium on the other hand, contributed the necessary fermentation products and electron acceptors along with its motility feature to the archaeon thereby gaining a swimming motility for the organism. From a consortium of bacterial and archaeal DNA originated the nuclear genome of eukaryotic cells. Spirochetes gave rise to the motile features of eukaryotic cells. Endosymbiotic unifications of the ancestors of alpha-proteobacteria and cyanobacteria, led to the origin of mitochondria and plastids respectively. For example, *Thiodendron* has been known to have originated via an ectosymbiotic process based on a similar syntrophy of sulfur existing between the two types of bacteria – *Desulphobacter* and *Spirochaeta*. However, such an association based on motile symbiosis have never been observed practically. Also there is no evidence of archaeans and spirochetes adapting to intense acid-based environments.

In the hydrogen hypothesis, the symbiotic linkage of an anaerobic and autotrophic methanogenic archaeon (host) with an alpha-proteobacterium (the symbiont) gave rise to the eukaryotes. The host utilized hydrogen (H_2) and carbon dioxide (CO_2) to produce methane while the symbiont, capable of aerobic respiration, expelled H_2 and CO_2 as byproducts of anaerobic fermentation process. The host's methanogenic environment worked as a sink for H_2, which resulted in heightened bacterial fermentation. Endosymbiotic gene transfer (EGT) acted as a catalyst for the host to acquire the symbionts' carbohydrate metabolism and turn heterotrophic in nature. Subsequently, the host's methane forming capability was lost. Thus, the origins of the heterotrophic organelle (symbiont) are identical to the origins of the eukaryotic lineage. In this hypothesis, the presence of H_2 represents the selective force that forged eukaryotes out of prokaryotes.

The syntrophy hypothesis was developed in contrast to the hydrogen hypothesis and proposes the existence of two symbiotic events. According to this theory, eukaryogenesis (i.e. origin of eukaryotic cells) occurred based on metabolic symbiosis (syntrophy) between a methanogenic archaeon and a delta-proteobacterium. This syntrophic symbiosis was initially facilitated by H_2 transfer between different species under anaerobic environments. In earlier stages, an alpha-proteobacterium became a member of this integration, and later developed into the mitochondrion. Gene transfer from a delta-proteobacterium to an archaeon led to the methanogenic archaeon developing into a nucleus. The archaeon constituted the genetic apparatus while the delta-proteobacterium contributed towards the cytoplasmic features. This theory incorporates two selective forces that were needed to be considered during the time of nucleus evolution – (a) presence of metabolic partitioning in order to avoid the harmful effects of the co-existence of anabolic and catabolic cellular pathways, and (b) prevention of abnormal biosynthesis of proteins that occur due to a vast spread of introns in the archaeal genes after acquiring the mitochondrion and the loss of methanogenesis.

Thus, the origin of eukaryotes by endosymbiotic processes has been broadly recognized and accepted so far. Mitochondria and plastids have been known to originate from a bacterial ancestor during parallel adaptation to anaerobiosis. However, there still remains a greater need in assessing the question of how much eukaryotic complexity is being originated via an implementation of these symbiogenetic theories.

PROTIST

Protist is an informal term for any eukaryotic organism that is not an animal, plant or fungus. The protists do not form a natural group, or clade, but are often grouped together for convenience, like algae or invertebrates. In some systems of biological classification, such as the popular 5-kingdom scheme proposed by Robert Whittaker in 1969, the protists make up a kingdom called **Protista**, composed of "organisms which are unicellular or unicellular-colonial and which form no tissues."

Besides their relatively simple levels of organization, protists do not necessarily have much in common. When used, the term "protists" is now considered to mean similar-appearing but diverse taxa that are not related through an exclusive common ancestor, and have different life cycles, trophic levels, modes of locomotion, and cellular structures. In the classification system of Lynn Margulis, the term *protist* is reserved for microscopic organisms, while the more inclusive term ***Protoctista*** is applied to a biological kingdom which includes certain large multicellular eukaryotes, such as kelp, red algae and slime molds. Others use the term *protist* more broadly, to encompass both microbial eukaryotes and macroscopic organisms that do not fit into the other traditional kingdoms.

In cladistic systems, there are no equivalents to the taxa Protista or Protoctista, both terms referring to a paraphyletic group which spans the entire eukaryotic tree of life. In cladistic classification, the contents of Protista are distributed among various *supergroups* (SAR, Archaeplastida, Excavata, Opisthokonta, etc.) and "Protista", ''Protoctista" and "Protozoa" are considered obsolete. However, the term "protist" continues to be used informally as a catch-all term for eukaryotic microorganisms. For example, the phrase "protist pathogen" may be used to denote any disease-causing microbe which is not bacteria, virus, viroid or metazoa.

Subdivisions

The term *protista* was first used by Ernst Haeckel in 1866. Protists were traditionally subdivided into several groups based on similarities to the "higher" kingdoms such as:

Protozoa the unicellular "animal-like" (***heterotrophic***/parasitic) protozoa which was further sub-divided based on motility such as (flagellated) *Flagellata*, (ciliated) *Ciliophora*, (phagocytic) *amoeba* and spore-forming *Sporozoans*

Protophyta the "plant-like" (***autotrophic***) protophyta (mostly unicellular algae)

Molds the "fungus-like" (***saprophytic***) slime molds and water molds.

Some protists, sometimes called ambiregnal protists, have been considered to be both protozoa and algae or fungi (e.g., slime molds and flagellated algae), and names for these have been published under either or both of the *ICN* and the *ICZN*. Conflicts, such as these – for example the dual-classification of Euglenids and Dinobryons, which are mixotrophic – is an example of why the kingdom Protista was adopted.

These traditional subdivisions, largely based on superficial commonalities, have been replaced by classifications based on phylogenetics (evolutionary relatedness among organisms). Molecular analyses in modern taxonomy have been used to redistribute former members of this group into diverse and sometimes distantly related phyla. For instance, the water molds are now considered to be closely related to photosynthetic organisms such as Brown algae and Diatoms, the slime molds are grouped mainly under Amoebozoa, and the Amoebozoa itself includes only a subset of "Amoeba" group, and significant number of erstwhile "Amoeboid" genera are distributed among Rhizarians and other Phyla.

However, the older terms are still used as informal names to describe the morphology and ecology of various protists. For example, the term *protozoa* is used to refer to heterotrophic species of protists that do not form filaments.

Classification

Historical Classifications

Among the pioneers in the study of the protists, which were almost ignored by Linnaeus except for some genera (e.g., *Vorticella, Chaos, Volvox, Corallina, Conferva, Ulva, Chara, Fucus*) were Leeuwenhoek, O. F. Müller, C. G. Ehrenberg and Félix Dujardin. The first groups used to classify microscopic organism were the Animalcules and the Infusoria. In 1817, the German naturalist Georg August Goldfuss introduced the word *Protozoa* to refer to organisms such as ciliates and corals. After the cell theory of Schwann and Schleiden (1838–39), this group was modified in 1848 by Carl von Siebold to include only animal-like unicellular organisms, such as foraminifera and amoebae. The formal taxonomic category *Protoctista* was first proposed in the early 1860s by John Hogg, who argued that the protists should include what he saw as primitive unicellular forms of both plants and animals. He defined the Protoctista as a "fourth kingdom of nature", in addition to the then-traditional kingdoms of plants, animals and minerals. The kingdom of minerals was later removed from taxonomy in 1866 by Ernst Haeckel, leaving plants, animals, and the protists (*Protista*), defined as a "kingdom of primitive forms".

In 1938, Herbert Copeland resurrected Hogg's label, arguing that Haeckel's term *Protista* included anucleated microbes such as bacteria, which the term "Protoctista" (literally meaning "first established beings") did not. In contrast, Copeland's term included nucleated eukaryotes such as diatoms, green algae and fungi. This classification was the basis for Whittaker's later definition of Fungi, Animalia, Plantae and Protista as the four kingdoms of life. The kingdom Protista was later modified to separate prokaryotes into the separate kingdom of Monera, leaving the protists as a group of eukaryotic microorganisms. These five kingdoms remained the accepted classification until the development of molecular phylogenetics in the late 20th century, when it became apparent that neither protists nor monera were single groups of related organisms (they were not monophyletic groups).

Modern Classifications

Many systematists today do not treat Protista as a formal taxon, but the term "protist" is still commonly used for convenience in two ways. The most popular contemporary definition is a phylogenetic one, that identifies a paraphyletic group: a protist is any eukaryote that is not an animal, (land) plant, or (true) fungus; this definitionexcludes many unicellular groups, like the Microsporidia (fungi), many Chytridiomycetes (fungi), and yeasts (fungi), and also a non-unicellular group included in Protista in the past, the Myxozoa (animal). Some systematists judge paraphyletic taxa acceptable, and use Protista in this sense as a formal taxon (as found in some secondary textbooks, for pedagogical purpose).

The other definition describes protists primarily by functional or biological criteria: protists are essentially those eukaryotes that are never multicellular, that either exist as independent cells, or if they occur in colonies, do not show differentiation into tissues (but vegetative cell differentiation may occur restricted to sexual reproduction, alternate vegetative morphology, and quiescent or resistant stages, such as cysts); this definition excludes many brown, many red and some green algae, which may have tissues.

The taxonomy of protists is still changing. Newer classifications attempt to present monophyletic groups based on morphological (especially ultrastructural), biochemical (chemotaxonomy) and DNA sequence (molecular research) information. However, there are sometimes discordances between molecular and morphological investigations; these can be categorized as two types: (i) one morphology, multiple lineages (e.g. morphological convergence, cryptic species) and (ii) one lineage, multiple morphologies (e.g. phenotypic plasticity, multiple life-cycle stages).

Because the protists as a whole are paraphyletic, new systems often split up or abandon the kingdom, instead treating the protist groups as separate lines of eukaryotes. The recent scheme by Adl *et al.* (2005) does not recognize formal ranks (phylum, class, etc.) and instead treats groups as clades of phylogenetically related organisms. This is intended to make the classification more stable in the long term and easier to update. Some of the main groups of protists, which may be treated as phyla, are listed in the taxobox, upper right. Many are thought to be monophyletic, though there is still uncertainty. For instance, the excavates are probably not monophyletic and the chromalveolates are probably only monophyletic if the haptophytes and cryptomonads are excluded.

Metabolism

Nutrition can vary according to the type of protist. Most eukaryotic algae are autotrophic, but the pigments were lost in some groups. Other protists are heterotrophic, and may present phagotrophy, osmotrophy, saprotrophy or parasitism. Some are mixotrophic. Some protists that do not have / lost chloroplasts/mitochondria have entered into endosymbiontic relationship with other bacteria/algae to replace the missing functionality. For example *Paramecium bursaria* & *Paulinella* have captured a green algae (*Zoochlorella*) & an cyanobacterium respectively that act as a replacement for chloroplast. Meanwhile, a protist, Mixotricha paradoxa that has lost its mitochondria uses endosymbiontic bacteria as mitochondria and ectosymbiontic hair-like bacteria (*Treponema spirochetes*) for locomotion.

Many protists are flagellate, for example, and filter feeding can take place where the flagella find prey. Other protists can engulf bacteria and other food particles, by extending their cell membrane around them to form a food vacuole and digesting them internally in a process termed phagocytosis.

Nutritional types in protist metabolism

Nutritional type	Source of energy	Source of carbon	Examples
Photoautotrophs	Sunlight	Organic compounds or carbon fixation	Most algae
Chemoheterotrophs	Organic compounds	Organic compounds	Apicomplexa, Trypanosomes or Amoebae

Reproduction

Some protists reproduce sexually using gametes, while others reproduce asexually by binary fission.

Some species, for example *Plasmodium falciparum*, have extremely complex life cycles that involve multiple forms of the organism, some of which reproduce sexually and others asexually. However, it is unclear how frequently sexual reproduction causes genetic exchange between different strains of *Plasmodium* in nature and most populations of parasitic protists may be clonal lines that rarely exchange genes with other members of their species.

Eukaryotes emerged in evolution more than 1.5 billion years ago. The earliest eukaryotes were likely protists. Although sexual reproduction is widespread among extant eukaryotes, it seemed unlikely until recently, that sex could be a primordial and fundamental characteristic of eukaryotes. A principal reason for this view was that sex appeared to be lacking in certain pathogenic protists whose ancestors branched off early from the eukaryotic family tree. However, several of these protists are now known to be capable of, or to recently have had the capability for, meiosis and hence sexual reproduction. For example, the common intestinal parasite *Giardia lamblia* was once considered to be a descendant of a protist lineage that predated the emergence of meiosis and sex. However, *G. lamblia* was recently found to have a core set of genes that function in meiosis and that are widely present among sexual eukaryotes. These results suggested that *G. lamblia* is capable of meiosis and thus sexual reproduction. Furthermore, direct evidence for meiotic recombination, indicative of sex, was also found in *G. lamblia*.

The pathogenic parasitic protists of the genus *Leishmania* have been shown to be capable of a sexual cycle in the invertebrate vector, likened to the meiosis undertaken in the trypanosomes.

Trichomonas vaginalis, a parasitic protist, is not known to undergo meiosis, but when Malik et al. tested for 29 genes that function in meiosis, they found 27 to be present, including 8 of 9 genes specific to meiosis in model eukaryotes. These findings suggest that *T. vaginalis* may be capable of meiosis. Since 21 of the 29 meiotic genes were also present in G. lamblia, it appears that most of these meiotic genes were likely present in a common ancestor of *T. vaginalis* and *G. lamblia*. These two species are descendants of protist lineages that are highly divergent among eukaryotes, leading Malik et al. to suggest that these meiotic genes were likely present in a common ancestor of all eukaryotes.

Based on a phylogenetic analysis, Dacks and Roger proposed that facultative sex was present in the common ancestor of all eukaryotes.

This view was further supported by a study of amoebae by Lahr et al. Amoeba have generally been regarded as asexual protists. However these authors describe evidence that most amoeboid lineages are anciently sexual, and that the majority of asexual groups likely arose recently and independently. It should be noted that early researchers (e.g., Calkins) have interpreted phenomena related to chromidia (chromatin granules free in the cytoplasm) in amoeboid organisms as sexual reproduction.

Protists generally reproduce asexually under favorable environmental conditions, but tend to reproduce sexually under stressful conditions, such as starvation or heat shock.

Oxidative stress, which is associated with the production of reactive oxygen species leading to DNA damage, also appears to be an important factor in the induction of sex in protists.

Ecology

Protists live in almost any environment that contains liquid water. Many protists, such as algae, are photosynthetic and are vital primary producers in ecosystems, particularly in the ocean as part of the plankton. Other protists include pathogenic species such as the kinetoplastid *Trypanosoma brucei*, which causes sleeping sickness and species of the apicomplexan *Plasmodium* which cause malaria.

Parasitism: Role as Pathogens

Some protists are significant parasites of animals (e.g., five species of the parasitic genus *Plasmodium* cause malaria in humans and many others cause similar diseases in other vertebrates), plants (the oomycete *Phytophthora infestans* causes late blight in potatoes) or even of other protists. Protist pathogens share many metabolic pathways with their eukaryotic hosts. This makes therapeutic target development extremely difficult – a drug that harms a protist parasite is also likely to harm its animal/plant host. A more thorough understanding of protist biology may allow these diseases to be treated more efficiently. For example, the apicoplast (a nonphotosynthetic chloroplast but essential to carry out important functions other than photosynthesis) present in apicomplexans provides an attractive target for treating diseases caused by dangerous pathogens such as plasmodium.

Recent papers have proposed the use of viruses to treat infections caused by protozoa.

Researchers from the Agricultural Research Service are taking advantage of protists as pathogens to control red imported fire ant (*Solenopsis invicta*) populations in Argentina. Spore-producing protists such as *Kneallhazia solenopsae* (recognized as a sister clade or the closest relative to the fungus kingdom now) can reduce red fire ant populations by 53–100%. Researchers have also been able to infect phorid fly parasitoids of the ant with the protist without harming the flies. This turns the flies into a vector that can spreads the pathogenic protist between red fire ant colonies.

Fossil Record

Many protists have neither hard parts nor resistant spores, and their fossils are extremely rare or unknown. Examples of such groups include the apicomplexans,most ciliates, some green algae (the Klebsormidiales), choanoflagellates, oomycetes, brown algae, yellow-green algae, excavates (e.g., euglenids). Some of these have been found preserved in amber (fossilized tree resin) or under unusual conditions (e.g., *Paleoleishmania*, a kinetoplastid).

Others are relatively common in the fossil record, as the diatoms, golden algae, haptophytes (coccoliths), silicoflagellates, tintinnids (ciliates), dinoflagellates, green algae, red algae, heliozoans, radiolarians, foraminiferans, ebriids and testate amoebae (euglyphids, arcellaceans). Some are even used as paleoecological indicators to reconstruct ancient environments.

More probable eukaryote fossils begin to appear at about 1.8 billion years ago, the acritarchs, spherical fossils of likely algal protists. Another possible representant of early fossil eukaryotes are the Gabonionta.

FUNGUS

A **fungus** is any member of the group of eukaryotic organisms that includes unicellular microorganisms such as yeasts and molds, as well as multicellular fungi that produce familiar fruiting forms known as mushrooms. These organisms are classified as a kingdom, **Fungi**, which is separate from the other eukaryotic life kingdoms of plants and animals.

A characteristic that places fungi in a different kingdom from plants, bacteria and some protists, is chitin in their cell walls. Similar to animals, fungi are heterotrophs; they acquire their food by absorbing dissolved molecules, typically by secreting digestive enzymes into their environment. Fungi do not photosynthesise. Growth is their means of mobility, except for spores (a few of which are flagellated), which may travel through the air or water. Fungi are the principal decomposers in ecological systems. These and other differences place fungi in a single group of related organisms, named the *Eumycota* (*true fungi* or *Eumycetes*), which share a common ancestor (form a *monophyletic group*), an interpretation that is also strongly supported by molecular phylogenetics. This fungal group is distinct from the structurally similar myxomycetes (slime molds) and oomycetes (water molds). The discipline of biology devoted to the study of fungi is known as mycology (from the Greek μύκης, mukēs, meaning "fungus"). In the past, mycology was regarded as a branch of botany, although it is now known fungi are genetically more closely related to animals than to plants.

Abundant worldwide, most fungi are inconspicuous because of the small size of their structures, and their cryptic lifestyles in soil or on dead matter. Fungi include symbionts of plants, animals, or other fungi and also parasites. They may become noticeable when fruiting, either as mushrooms or as molds. Fungi perform an essential role in the decomposition of organic matter and have fundamental roles in nutrient cycling and exchange in the environment. They have long been used as a direct source of human food, in the form of mushrooms and truffles; as a leavening agent for bread; and in the fermentation of various food products, such as wine, beer, and soy sauce. Since the 1940s, fungi have been used for the production of antibiotics, and, more recently, various enzymes produced by fungi are used industrially and in detergents. Fungi are also used as biological pesticides to control weeds, plant diseases and insect pests. Many species produce bioactive compounds called mycotoxins, such as alkaloids and polyketides, that are toxic to animals including humans. The fruiting structures of a few species contain psychotropic compounds and are consumed recreationally or in traditional spiritual ceremonies. Fungi can break down manufactured materials and buildings, and become significant pathogens of humans and other animals. Losses of crops due to fungal diseases (e.g., rice blast disease) or food spoilage can have a large impact on human food supplies and local economies.

The fungus kingdom encompasses an enormous diversity of taxa with varied ecologies, life cycle strategies, and morphologies ranging from unicellular aquatic chytrids to large mushrooms. However, little is known of the true biodiversity of Kingdom Fungi, which has been estimated at 1.5 million to 5 million species, with about 5% of these having been formally classified. Ever since the pioneering 18th and 19th century taxonomical works of Carl Linnaeus, Christian Hendrik Persoon, and Elias Magnus Fries, fungi have been classified according to their morphology (e.g., characteristics such as spore color or microscopic features) or physiology. Advances in molecular genetics have opened the way for DNA analysis to be incorporated into taxonomy, which has sometimes challenged the historical groupings based on morphology and other traits. Phylogenetic studies published in the last decade have helped reshape the classification within Kingdom Fungi, which is divided into one subkingdom, seven phyla, and ten subphyla.

Etymology

The English word *fungus* is directly adopted from the Latin *fungus* (mushroom), used in the writings of Horace and Pliny. This in turn is derived from the Greek word *sphongos* (σφογγος "sponge"), which refers to the macroscopic structures and morphology of mushrooms and molds; the root is also used in other languages, such as the German *Schwamm* ("sponge") and *Schimmel* ("mold"). The use of the word *mycology*, which is derived from the Greek *mykes* (μύκης "mushroom") and *logos* (λόγος "discourse"), to denote the scientific study of fungi is thought to have originated in 1836 with English naturalist Miles Joseph Berkeley's publication *The English Flora of Sir James Edward Smith, Vol. 5.* A group of all the fungi present in a particular area or geographic region is known as mycobiota (plural noun, no singular), e.g., "the mycobiota of Ireland".

Characteristics

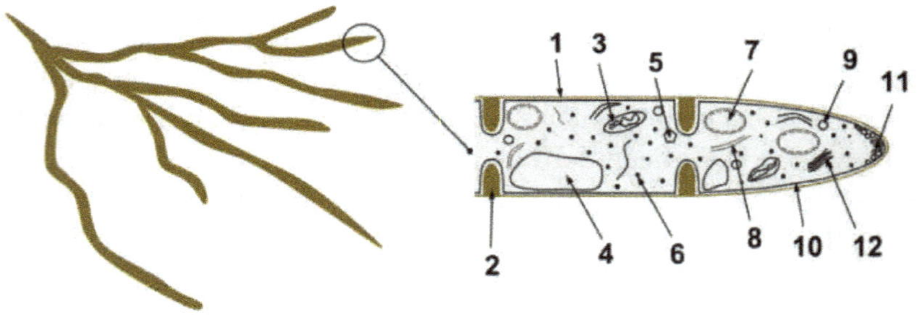

Fungal hyphae cells

- Hyphal wall
- Septum
- Mitochondrion
- Vacuole
- Ergosterol crystal
- Ribosome

- Nucleus
- Endoplasmic reticulum
- Lipid body
- Plasma membrane
- Spitzenkörper
- Golgi apparatus

Before the introduction of molecular methods for phylogenetic analysis, taxonomists considered fungi to be members of the plant kingdom because of similarities in lifestyle: both fungi and plants are mainly immobile, and have similarities in general morphology and growth habitat. Like plants, fungi often grow in soil and, in the case of mushrooms, form conspicuous fruit bodies, which sometimes resemble plants such as mosses. The fungi are now considered a separate kingdom, distinct from both plants and animals, from which they appear to have diverged around one billion years ago. Some morphological, biochemical, and genetic features are shared with other organisms, while others are unique to the fungi, clearly separating them from the other kingdoms:

Shared features:

- With other eukaryotes: Fungal cells contain membrane-bound nuclei with chromosomes that contain DNA with noncoding regions called introns and coding regions called exons. Fungi have membrane-bound cytoplasmic organelles such as mitochondria, sterol-containing membranes, and ribosomes of the 80S type. They have a characteristic range of soluble carbohydrates and storage compounds, including sugar alcohols (e.g., mannitol), disaccharides, (e.g., trehalose), and polysaccharides (e.g., glycogen, which is also found in animals).
- With animals: Fungi lack chloroplasts and are heterotrophic organisms and so require preformed organic compounds as energy sources.
- With plants: Fungi have a cell wall and vacuoles. They reproduce by both sexual and asexual means, and like basal plant groups (such as ferns and mosses) produce spores. Similar to mosses and algae, fungi typically have haploid nuclei.
- With euglenoids and bacteria: Higher fungi, euglenoids, and some bacteria produce the amino acid L-lysine in specific biosynthesis steps, called the α-aminoadipate pathway.
- The cells of most fungi grow as tubular, elongated, and thread-like (filamentous) structures called hyphae, which may contain multiple nuclei and extend by growing at their tips. Each tip contains a set of aggregated vesicles—cellular structures consisting of proteins, lipids, and other organic molecules—called the Spitzenkörper. Both fungi and oomycetes grow as filamentous hyphal cells. In contrast, similar-looking organisms, such as filamentous green algae, grow by repeated cell division within a chain of cells. There are also single-celled fungi (yeasts) that do not form hyphae, and some fungi have both hyphal and yeast forms.
- In common with some plant and animal species, more than 70 fungal species display bioluminescence.

Unique features:

- Some species grow as unicellular yeasts that reproduce by budding or binary fission. Dimorphic fungi can switch between a yeast phase and a hyphal phase in response to environmental conditions.
- The fungal cell wall is composed of glucans and chitin; while glucans are also found in plants and chitin in the exoskeleton of arthropods, fungi are the only organisms that combine these two structural molecules in their cell wall. Unlike those of plants and oomycetes, fungal cell walls do not contain cellulose.

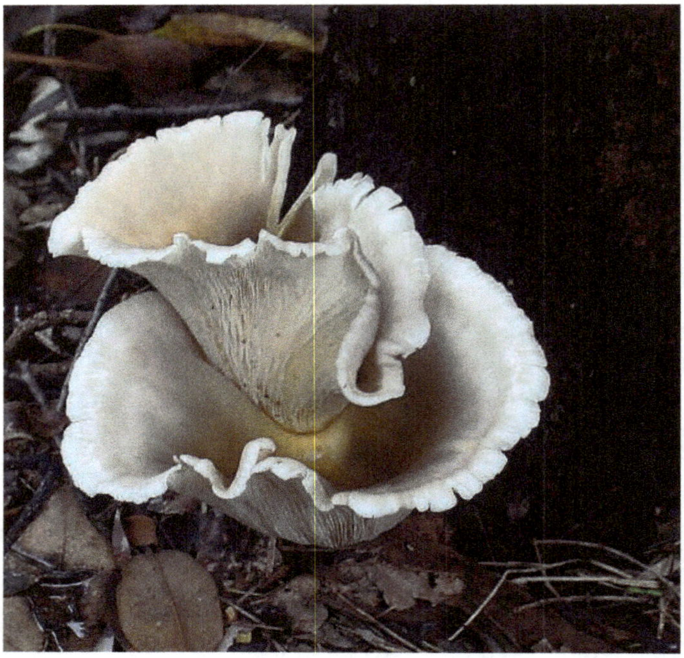

Omphalotus nidiformis, a bioluminescent mushroom

Most fungi lack an efficient system for the long-distance transport of water and nutrients, such as the xylem and phloem in many plants. To overcome this limitation, some fungi, such as *Armillaria*, form rhizomorphs, which resemble and perform functions similar to the roots of plants. As eukaryotes, fungi possess a biosynthetic pathway for producing terpenes that uses mevalonic acid and pyrophosphate as chemical building blocks. Plants and some other organisms have an additional terpene biosynthesis pathway in their chloroplasts, a structure fungi and animals do not have. Fungi produce several secondary metabolites that are similar or identical in structure to those made by plants. Many of the plant and fungal enzymes that make these compounds differ from each other in sequence and other characteristics, which indicates separate origins and convergent evolution of these enzymes in the fungi and plants.

Diversity

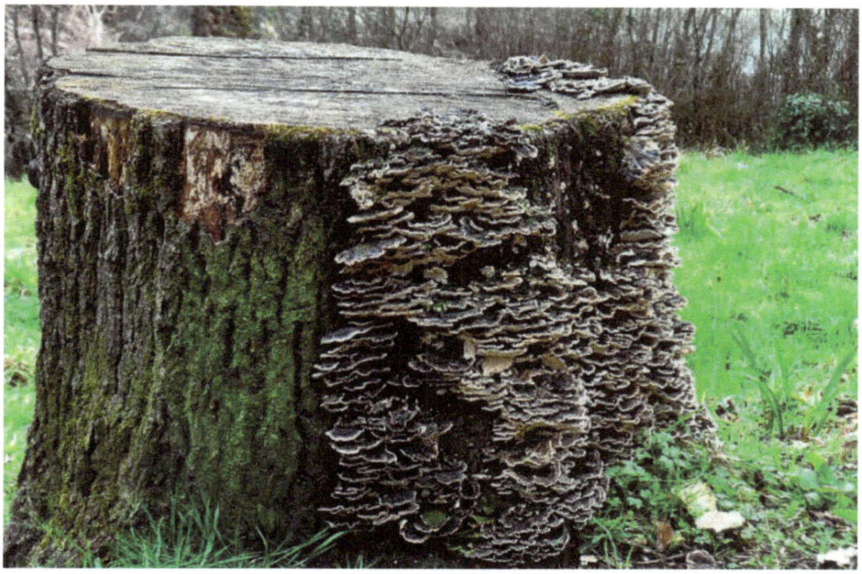

Bracket fungi on a tree stump

Fungi have a worldwide distribution, and grow in a wide range of habitats, including extreme environments such as deserts or areas with high salt concentrations or ionizing radiation, as well as in deep sea sediments. Some can survive the intense UV and cosmic radiation encountered during space travel. Most grow in terrestrial environments, though several species live partly or solely in aquatic habitats, such as the chytrid fungus *Batrachochytrium dendrobatidis*, a parasite that has been responsible for a worldwide decline in amphibian populations. This organism spends part of its life cycle as a motile zoospore, enabling it to propel itself through water and enter its amphibian host. Other examples of aquatic fungi include those living in hydrothermal areas of the ocean.

Around 100,000 species of fungi have been formally described by taxonomists, but the global biodiversity of the fungus kingdom is not fully understood. On the basis of observations of the ratio of the number of fungal species to the number of plant species in selected environments, the fungal kingdom has been estimated to contain about 1.5 million species. A recent (2011) estimate suggests there may be over 5 million species. In mycology, species have historically been distinguished by a variety of methods and concepts. Classification based on morphological characteristics, such as the size and shape of spores or fruiting structures, has traditionally dominated fungal taxonomy. Species may also be distinguished by their biochemical and physiological characteristics, such as their ability to metabolize certain biochemicals, or their reaction to chemical tests. The biological species concept discriminates species based on their ability to mate. The application of molecular tools, such as DNA sequencing and phylogenetic analysis, to study diversity has greatly enhanced the resolution and added robustness to estimates of genetic diversity within various taxonomic groups.

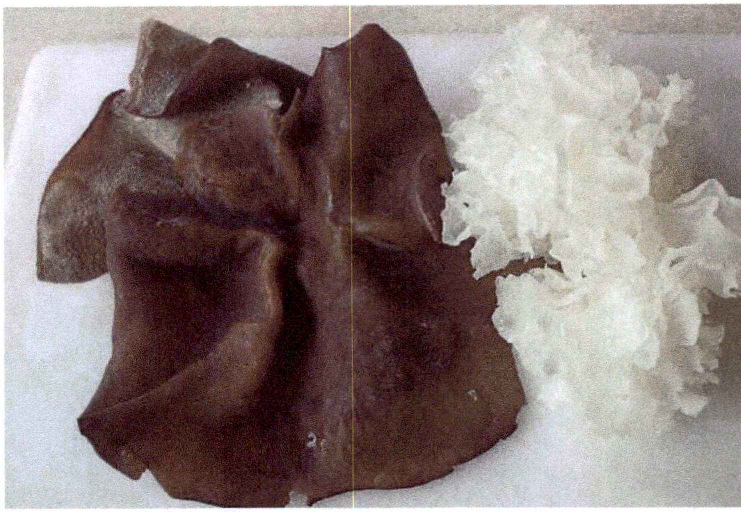

Two types of edible fungi

Mycology

Mycology is the branch of biology concerned with the systematic study of fungi, including their genetic and biochemical properties, their taxonomy, and their use to humans as a source of medicine, food, and psychotropic substances consumed for religious purposes, as well as their dangers, such as poisoning or infection. The field of phytopathology, the study of plant diseases, is closely related because many plant pathogens are fungi.

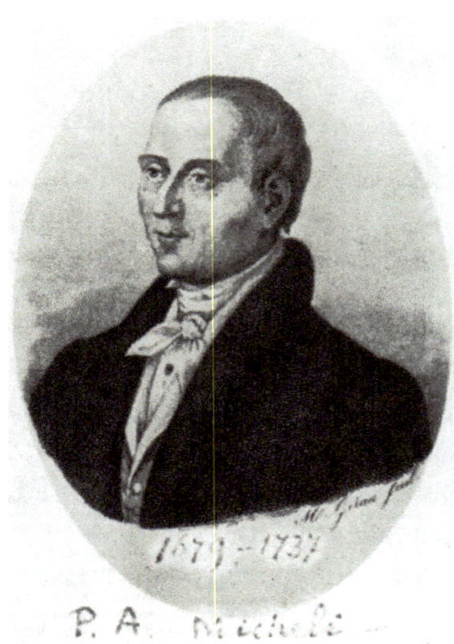

In 1729, Pier A. Micheli first published descriptions of fungi.

The use of fungi by humans dates back to prehistory; Ötzi the Iceman, a well-preserved mummy of a 5,300-year-old Neolithic man found frozen in the Austrian Alps, carried two species of polypore mushrooms that may have been used as tinder (*Fomes fomentarius*), or for medicinal purposes (*Piptoporus betulinus*). Ancient peoples have used fungi as food sources–often unknowingly–for millennia, in the preparation of leavened bread and fermented juices. Some of the oldest written records contain references to the destruction of crops that were probably caused by pathogenic fungi.

Mycology is a relatively new science that became systematic after the development of the microscope in the 17th century. Although fungal spores were first observed by Giambattista della Porta in 1588, the seminal work in the development of mycology is considered to be the publication of Pier Antonio Micheli's 1729 work *Nova plantarum genera*. Micheli not only observed spores but also showed that, under the proper conditions, they could be induced into growing into the same species of fungi from which they originated. Extending the use of the binomial system of nomenclature introduced by Carl Linnaeus in his *Species plantarum* (1753), the Dutch Christian Hendrik Persoon (1761–1836) established the first classification of mushrooms with such skill so as to be considered a founder of modern mycology. Later, Elias Magnus Fries (1794–1878) further elaborated the classification of fungi, using spore color and various microscopic characteristics, methods still used by taxonomists today. Other notable early contributors to mycology in the 17th–19th and early 20th centuries include Miles Joseph Berkeley, August Carl Joseph Corda, Anton de Bary, the brothers Louis René and Charles Tulasne, Arthur H. R. Buller, Curtis G. Lloyd, and Pier Andrea Saccardo. The 20th century has seen a modernization of mycology that has come from advances in biochemistry, genetics, molecular biology, and biotechnology. The use of DNA sequencing technologies and phylogenetic analysis has provided new insights into fungal relationships and biodiversity, and has challenged traditional morphology-based groupings in fungal taxonomy.

Morphology

Microscopic Structures

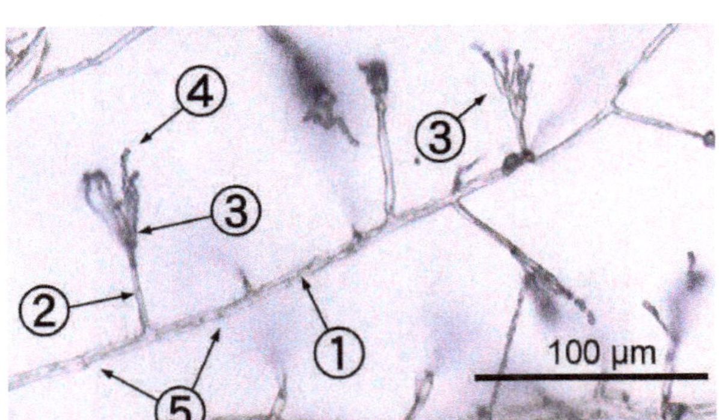

An environmental isolate of *Penicillium*

- hypha
- conidiophore
- phialide
- conidia
- septa

Most fungi grow as hyphae, which are cylindrical, thread-like structures 2–10 μm in diameter and up to several centimeters in length. Hyphae grow at their tips (apices); new hyphae are typically formed by emergence of new tips along existing hyphae by a process called *branching*, or occasionally growing hyphal tips fork, giving rise to two parallel-growing hyphae. Hyphae also sometimes fuse when they come into contact, a process called hyphal fusion (or anastamosis). These growth processes lead to the development of a mycelium, an interconnected network of hyphae. Hyphae can be either septate or coenocytic. Septate hyphae are divided into compartments separated by cross walls (internal cell walls, called septa, that are formed at right angles to the cell wall giving the hypha its shape), with each compartment containing one or more nuclei; coenocytic hyphae are not compartmentalized. Septa have pores that allow cytoplasm, organelles, and sometimes nuclei to pass through; an example is the dolipore septum in fungi of the phylum Basidiomycota. Coenocytic hyphae are in essence multinucleate supercells.

Many species have developed specialized hyphal structures for nutrient uptake from living hosts; examples include haustoria in plant-parasitic species of most fungal phyla, and arbuscules of several mycorrhizal fungi, which penetrate into the host cells to consume nutrients.

Although fungi are opisthokonts—a grouping of evolutionarily related organisms broadly characterized by a single posterior flagellum—all phyla except for the chytrids have lost their posterior flagella. Fungi are unusual among the eukaryotes in having a cell wall that, in addition to glucans (e.g., β-1,3-glucan) and other typical components, also contains the biopolymer chitin.

Macroscopic Structures

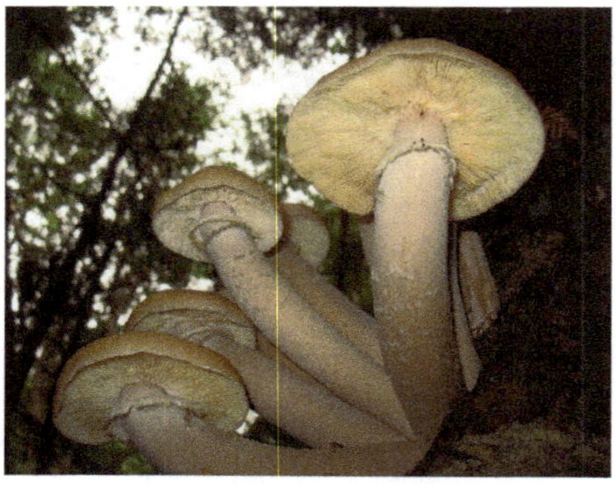

Armillaria solidipes

Fungal mycelia can become visible to the naked eye, for example, on various surfaces and substrates, such as damp walls and spoiled food, where they are commonly called molds. Mycelia grown on solid agar media in laboratory petri dishes are usually referred to as colonies. These colonies can exhibit growth shapes and colors (due to spores or pigmentation) that can be used as diagnostic features in the identification of species or groups. Some individual fungal colonies can reach extraordinary dimensions and ages as in the case of a clonal colony of *Armillaria solidipes*, which extends over an area of more than 900 ha (3.5 square miles), with an estimated age of nearly 9,000 years.

The apothecium—a specialized structure important in sexual reproduction in the ascomycetes—is a cup-shaped fruit body that is often macroscopic and holds the hymenium, a layer of tissue containing the spore-bearing cells. The fruit bodies of the basidiomycetes (basidiocarps) and some ascomycetes can sometimes grow very large, and many are well known as mushrooms.

Growth and Physiology

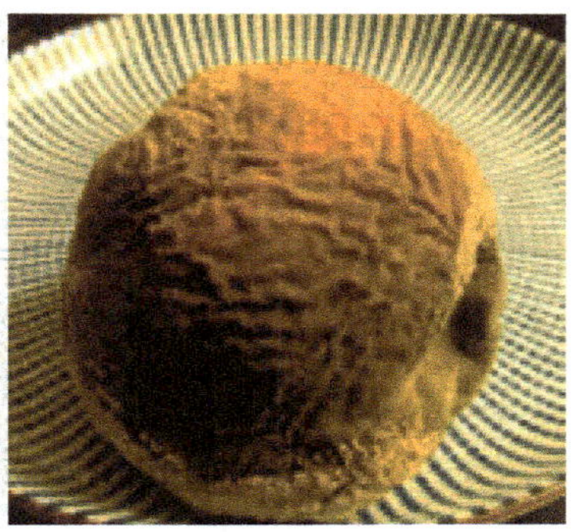

Mold growth covering a decaying peach. The frames were taken approximately 12 hours apart over a period of six days.

The growth of fungi as hyphae on or in solid substrates or as single cells in aquatic environments is adapted for the efficient extraction of nutrients, because these growth forms have high surface area to volume ratios. Hyphae are specifically adapted for growth on solid surfaces, and to invade substrates and tissues. They can exert large penetrative mechanical forces; for example, many plant pathogens, including *Magnaporthe grisea*, form a structure called an appressorium that evolved to puncture plant tissues. The pressure generated by the appressorium, directed against the plant epidermis, can exceed 8 megapascals (1,200 psi). The filamentous fungus *Paecilomyces lilacinus* uses a similar structure to penetrate the eggs of nematodes.

The mechanical pressure exerted by the appressorium is generated from physiological processes that increase intracellular turgor by producing osmolytes such as glycerol. Adaptations such as these are complemented by hydrolytic enzymes secreted into the environment to digest large organic molecules—such as polysaccharides, proteins, and lipids—into smaller molecules that may then be absorbed as nutrients. The vast majority of filamentous fungi grow in a polar fashion (extending in one direction) by elongation at the tip (apex) of the hypha. Other forms of fungal growth include intercalary extension (longitudinal expansion of hyphal compartments that are below the apex) as in the case of some endophytic fungi,or growth by volume expansion during the development of mushroom stipes and other large organs. Growth of fungi as multicellular structures consisting of somatic and reproductive cells—a feature independently evolved in animals and plants—has several functions, including the development of fruit bodies for dissemination of sexual spores (see above) and biofilms for substrate colonization and intercellular communication.

The fungi are traditionally considered heterotrophs, organisms that rely solely on carbon fixed by other organisms for metabolism. Fungi have evolved a high degree of metabolic versatility that allows them to use a diverse range of organic substrates for growth, including simple compounds such as nitrate, ammonia, acetate, or ethanol. In some species the pigment melanin may play a role in extracting energy from ionizing radiation, such as gamma radiation. This form of "radiotrophic" growth has been described for only a few species, the effects on growth rates are small, and the underlying biophysical and biochemical processes are not well known. This process might bear similarity to CO_2 fixation via visible light, but instead uses ionizing radiation as a source of energy.

Reproduction

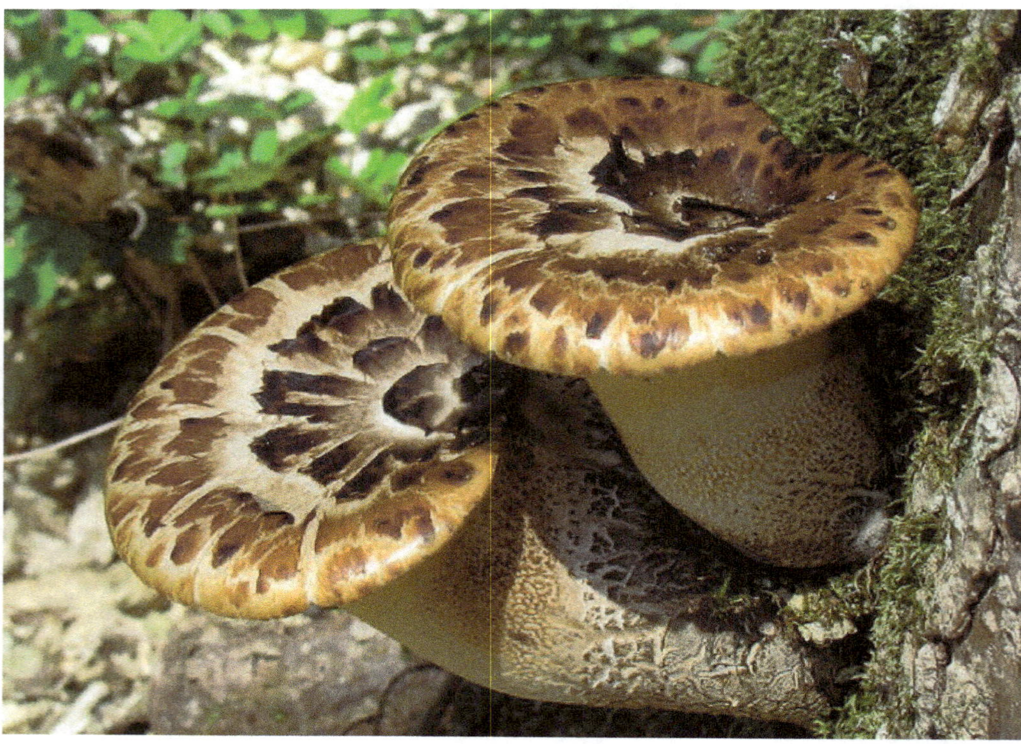

Polyporus squamosus

Fungal reproduction is complex, reflecting the differences in lifestyles and genetic makeup within this diverse kingdom of organisms. It is estimated that a third of all fungi reproduce using more than one method of propagation; for example, reproduction may occur in two well-differentiated stages within the life cycle of a species, the teleomorph and the anamorph. Environmental conditions trigger genetically determined developmental states that lead to the creation of specialized structures for sexual or asexual reproduction. These structures aid reproduction by efficiently dispersing spores or spore-containing propagules.

Asexual Reproduction

Asexual reproduction occurs via vegetative spores (conidia) or through mycelial fragmentation. Mycelial fragmentation occurs when a fungal mycelium separates into pieces, and each component grows into a separate mycelium. Mycelial fragmentation and vegetative spores maintain clonal populations adapted to a specific niche, and allow more rapid dispersal than sexual reproduction. The "Fungi imperfecti" (fungi lacking the perfect or sexual stage) or Deuteromycota comprise all the species that lack an observable sexual cycle. Deuteromycota is not an accepted taxonomic clade, and is now taken to mean simply fungi that lack a known sexual stage.

Sexual Reproduction

Sexual reproduction with meiosis has been directly observed in all fungal phyla except Glomeromycota (genetic analysis suggests meiosis in Glomeromycota as well). It differs in many aspects from sexual reproduction in animals or plants. Differences also exist between fungal groups and can be used to discriminate species by morphological differences in sexual structures and reproductive strategies. Mating experiments between fungal isolates may identify species on the basis of biological species concepts. The major fungal groupings have initially been delineated based on the morphology of their sexual structures and spores; for example, the spore-containing structures, asci and basidia, can be used in the identification of ascomycetes and basidiomycetes, respectively. Some species may allow mating only between individuals of opposite mating type, whereas others can mate and sexually reproduce with any other individual or itself. Species of the former mating system are called heterothallic, and of the latter homothallic.

Most fungi have both a haploid and a diploid stage in their life cycles. In sexually reproducing fungi, compatible individuals may combine by fusing their hyphae together into an interconnected network; this process, anastomosis, is required for the initiation of the sexual cycle. Many ascomycetes and basidiomycetes go through a dikaryotic stage, in which the nuclei inherited from the two parents do not combine immediately after cell fusion, but remain separate in the hyphal cells (see heterokaryosis).

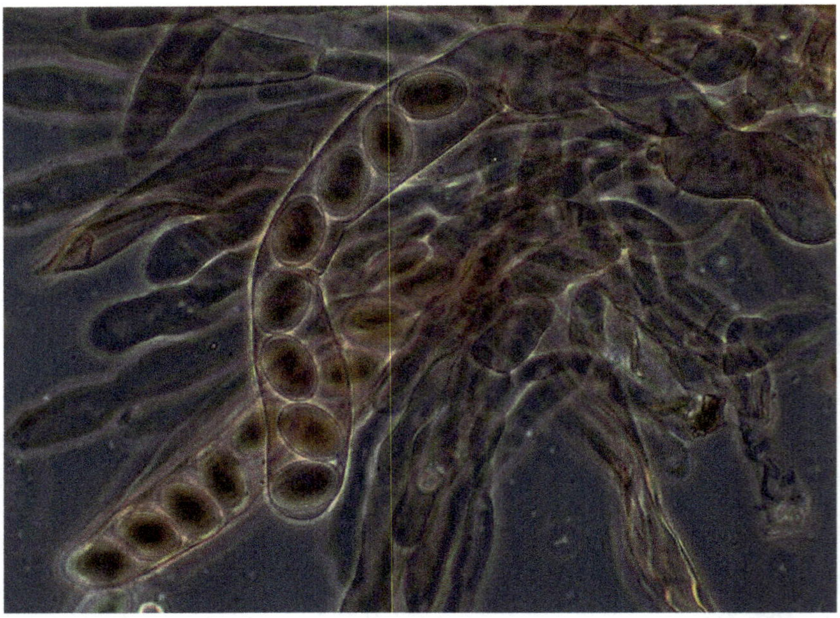

The 8-spore asci of *Morchella elata*, viewed with phase contrast microscopy

In ascomycetes, dikaryotic hyphae of the hymenium (the spore-bearing tissue layer) form a characteristic *hook* at the hyphal septum. During cell division, formation of the hook ensures proper distribution of the newly divided nuclei into the apical and basal hyphal compartments. An ascus (plural *asci*) is then formed, in which karyogamy (nuclear fusion) occurs. Asci are embedded in an ascocarp, or fruiting body. Karyogamy in the asci is followed immediately by meiosis and the production of ascospores. After dispersal, the ascospores may germinate and form a new haploid mycelium.

Sexual reproduction in basidiomycetes is similar to that of the ascomycetes. Compatible haploid hyphae fuse to produce a dikaryotic mycelium. However, the dikaryotic phase is more extensive in the basidiomycetes, often also present in the vegetatively growing mycelium. A specialized anatomical structure, called a clamp connection, is formed at each hyphal septum. As with the structurally similar hook in the ascomycetes, the clamp connection in the basidiomycetes is required for controlled transfer of nuclei during cell division, to maintain the dikaryotic stage with two genetically different nuclei in each hyphal compartment. A basidiocarp is formed in which club-like structures known as basidia generate haploid basidiospores after karyogamy and meiosis. The most commonly known basidiocarps are mushrooms, but they may also take other forms (see Morphology section).

In glomeromycetes (formerly zygomycetes), haploid hyphae of two individuals fuse, forming a gametangium, a specialized cell structure that becomes a fertile gamete-producing cell. The gametangium develops into a zygospore, a thick-walled spore formed by the union of gametes. When the zygospore germinates, it undergoes meiosis, generating new haploid hyphae, which may then form asexual sporangiospores. These sporangiospores allow the fungus to rapidly disperse and germinate into new genetically identical haploid fungal mycelia.

Spore Dispersal

Both asexual and sexual spores or sporangiospores are often actively dispersed by forcible ejection from their reproductive structures. This ejection ensures exit of the spores from the reproductive structures as well as traveling through the air over long distances.

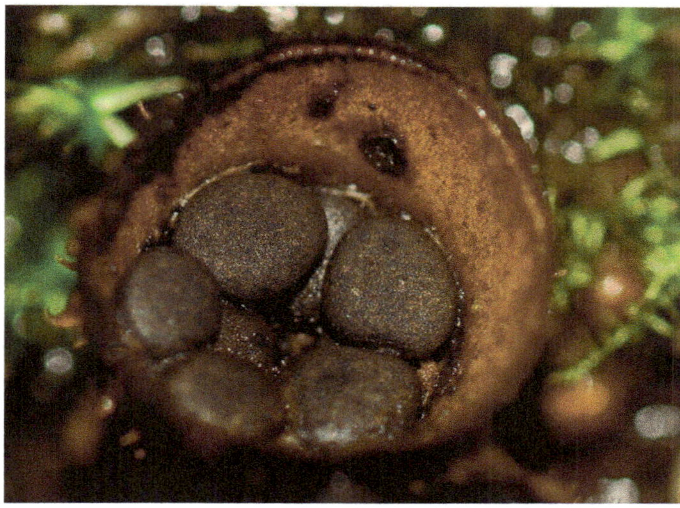

The bird's nest fungus *Cyathus stercoreus*

Specialized mechanical and physiological mechanisms, as well as spore surface structures (such as hydrophobins), enable efficient spore ejection. For example, the structure of the spore-bearing cells in some ascomycete species is such that the buildup of substances affecting cell volume and fluid balance enables the explosive discharge of spores into the air. The forcible discharge of single spores termed *ballistospores* involves formation of a small drop of water (Buller's drop), which upon contact with the spore leads to its projectile release with an initial acceleration of more than 10,000 g; the net result is that the spore is ejected 0.01–0.02 cm, sufficient distance for it to fall through the gills or pores into the air below. Other fungi, like the puffballs, rely on alternative mechanisms for spore release, such as external mechanical forces. The bird's nest fungi use the force of falling water drops to liberate the spores from cup-shaped fruiting bodies. Another strategy is seen in the stinkhorns, a group of fungi with lively colors and putrid odor that attract insects to disperse their spores.

Other Sexual Processes

Besides regular sexual reproduction with meiosis, certain fungi, such as those in the genera *Penicillium* and *Aspergillus*, may exchange genetic material via parasexual processes, initiated by anastomosis between hyphae and plasmogamy of fungal cells. The frequency and relative importance of parasexual events is unclear and may be lower than other sexual processes. It is known to play a role in intraspecific hybridization and is likely required for hybridization between species, which has been associated with major events in fungal evolution.

Evolution

In contrast to plants and animals, the early fossil record of the fungi is meager. Factors that likely contribute to the under-representation of fungal species among fossils include the nature of fungal fruiting bodies, which are soft, fleshy, and easily degradable tissues and the microscopic dimensions of most fungal structures, which therefore are not readily evident. Fungal fossils are difficult to distinguish from those of other microbes, and are most easily identified when they resemble extant fungi. Often recovered from a permineralized plant or animal host, these samples are typically studied by making thin-section preparations that can be examined with light microscopy or transmission electron microscopy. Researchers study compression fossils by dissolving the surrounding matrix with acid and then using light or scanning electron microscopy to examine surface details.

The earliest fossils possessing features typical of fungi date to the Proterozoic eon, some 1,430 million years ago (Ma); these multicellular benthic organisms had filamentous structures with septa, and were capable of anastomosis. More recent studies (2009) estimate the arrival of fungal organisms at about 760–1060 Ma on the basis of comparisons of the rate of evolution in closely related groups. For much of the Paleozoic Era (542–251 Ma), the fungi appear to have been aquatic and consisted of organisms similar to the extant chytrids in having flagellum-bearing spores. The evolutionary adaptation from an aquatic to a terrestrial lifestyle necessitated a diversification of ecological strategies for obtaining nutrients, including parasitism, saprobism, and the development of mutualistic relationships such as mycorrhiza and lichenization. Recent (2009) studies suggest that the ancestral ecological state of the Ascomycota was saprobism, and that independent lichenization events have occurred multiple times.

It is presumed that the fungi colonized the land during the Cambrian (542–488.3 Ma), long before land plants. Fossilized hyphae and spores recovered from the Ordovician of Wisconsin (460 Ma) resemble modern-day Glomerales, and existed at a time when the land flora likely consisted of only non-vascular bryophyte-like plants. Prototaxites, which was probably a fungus or lichen, would have been the tallest organism of the late Silurian. Fungal fossils do not become common and uncontroversial until the early Devonian (416–359.2 Ma), when they occur abundantly in the Rhynie chert, mostly as Zygomycota and Chytridiomycota.At about this same time, approximately 400 Ma, the Ascomycota and Basidiomycota diverged, and all modern classes of fungi were present by the Late Carboniferous (Pennsylvanian, 318.1–299 Ma).

Lichen-like fossils have been found in the Doushantuo Formation in southern China dating back to 635–551 Ma. Lichens formed a component of the early terrestrial ecosystems, and the estimated age of the oldest terrestrial lichen fossil is 400 Ma; this date corresponds to the age of the oldest known sporocarp fossil, a *Paleopyrenomycites* species found in the Rhynie Chert. The oldest fossil with microscopic features resembling modern-day basidiomycetes is *Palaeoancistrus*, found permineralized with a fern from the Pennsylvanian. Rare in the fossil record are the Homobasidiomycetes (a taxon roughly equivalent to the mushroom-producing species of the Agaricomycetes). Two amber-preserved specimens provide evidence that the earliest known mushroom-forming fungi (the extinct species *Archaeomarasmius leggetti*) appeared during the late Cretaceous, 90 Ma.

Some time after the Permian–Triassic extinction event (251.4 Ma), a fungal spike (originally thought to be an extraordinary abundance of fungal spores in sediments) formed, suggesting that fungi were the dominant life form at this time, representing nearly 100% of the available fossil record for this period.However, the relative proportion of fungal spores relative to spores formed by algal species is difficult to assess, the spike did not appear worldwide, and in many places it did not fall on the Permian–Triassic boundary.

Taxonomy

Although commonly included in botany curricula and textbooks, fungi are more closely related to animals than to plants and are placed with the animals in the monophyletic group of opisthokonts. Analyses using molecular phylogenetics support a monophyletic origin of the Fungi. The taxonomy of the Fungi is in a state of constant flux, especially due to recent research based on DNA comparisons. These current phylogenetic analyses often overturn classifications based on older and sometimes less discriminative methods based on morphological features and biological species concepts obtained from experimental matings.

There is no unique generally accepted system at the higher taxonomic levels and there are frequent name changes at every level, from species upwards. Efforts among researchers are now underway to establish and encourage usage of a unified and more consistent nomenclature. Fungal species can also have multiple scientific names depending on their life cycle and mode (sexual or asexual) of reproduction. Web sites such as Index Fungorum and ITIS list current names of fungal species (with cross-references to older synonyms).

The 2007 classification of Kingdom Fungi is the result of a large-scale collaborative research effort involving dozens of mycologists and other scientists working on fungal taxonomy. It recognizes seven phyla, two of which—the Ascomycota and the Basidiomycota—are contained within a branch representing subkingdom Dikarya, the most species rich and familiar group, including all the mushrooms, most food-spoilage molds, most plant pathogenic fungi, and the beer, wine, and bread yeasts. The accompanying cladogram depicts the major fungal taxa and their relationship to opisthokont and unikont organisms, based on the work of Philippe Silar and "The Mycota: A Comprehensive Treatise on Fungi as Experimental Systems for Basic and Applied Research". The lengths of the branches are not proportional to evolutionary distances.

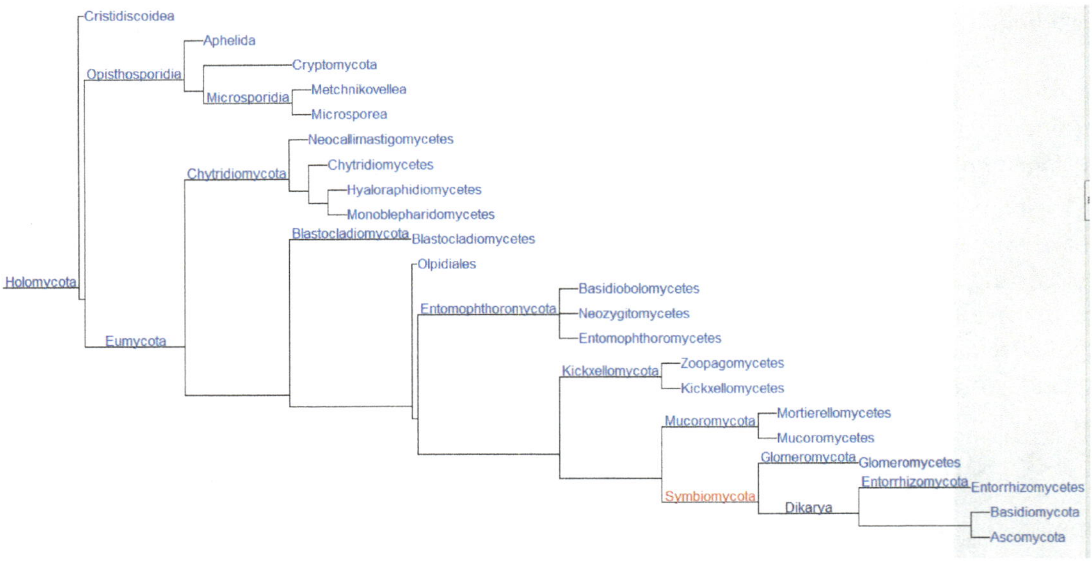
Cristidiscoidea
Aphelida
Cryptomycota
Opisthosporidia
Microsporidia
Metchnikovellea
Microsporea
Neocallimastigomycetes
Chytridiomycota
Chytridiomycetes
Hyaloraphidiomycetes
Monoblepharidomycetes
Blastocladiomycota
Blastocladiomycetes
Olpidiales
Holomycota
Basidiobolomycetes
Entomophthoromycota
Neozygitomycetes
Entomophthoromycetes
Eumycota
Kickxellomycota
Zoopagomycetes
Kickxellomycetes
Mucoromycota
Mortierellomycetes
Mucoromycetes
Glomeromycota
Glomeromycetes
Entorrhizomycota
Entorrhizomycetes
Symbiomycota
Dikarya
Basidiomycota
Ascomycota

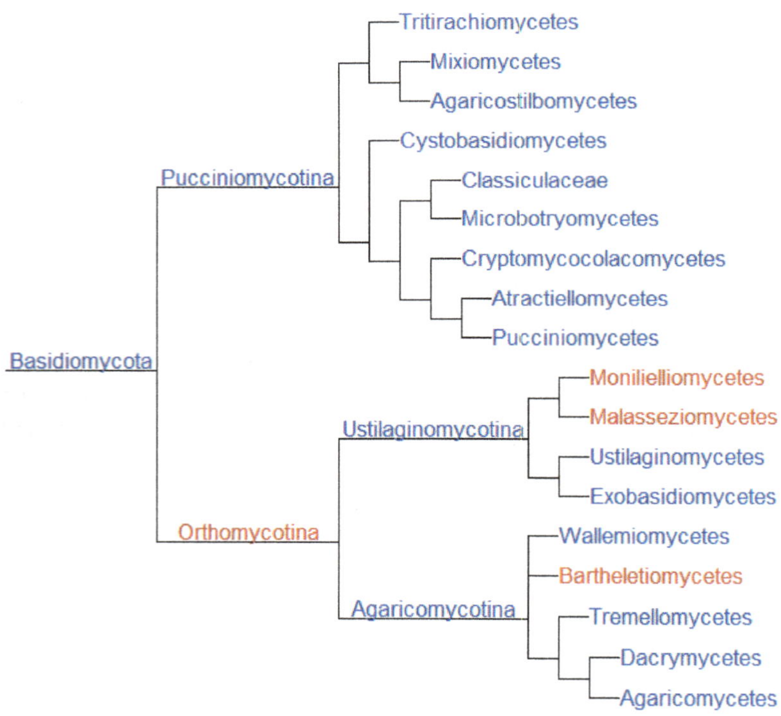
Tritirachiomycetes
Mixiomycetes
Agaricostilbomycetes
Cystobasidiomycetes
Pucciniomycotina
Classiculaceae
Microbotryomycetes
Cryptomycocolacomycetes
Atractiellomycetes
Pucciniomycetes
Basidiomycota
Moniliellomycetes
Malasseziomycetes
Ustilaginomycotina
Ustilaginomycetes
Exobasidiomycetes
Orthomycotina
Wallemiomycetes
Bartheletiomycetes
Agaricomycotina
Tremellomycetes
Dacrymycetes
Agaricomycetes

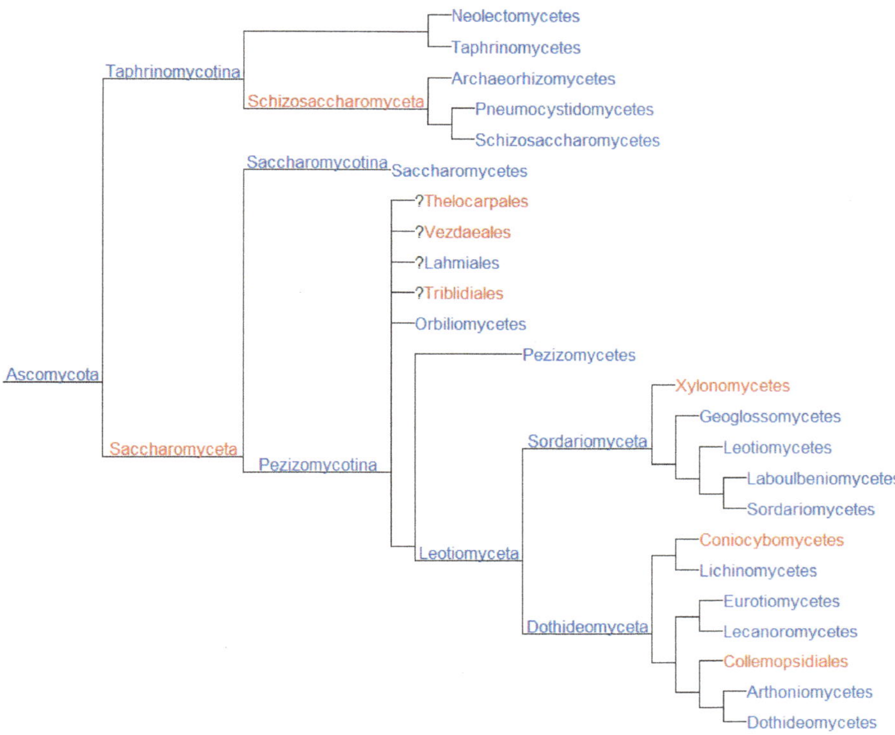

Taxonomic Groups

The major phyla (sometimes called divisions) of fungi have been classified mainly on the basis of characteristics of their sexual reproductive structures. Currently, seven phyla are proposed: Microsporidia, Chytridiomycota, Blastocladiomycota, Neocallimastigomycota, Glomeromycota, Ascomycota, and Basidiomycota.

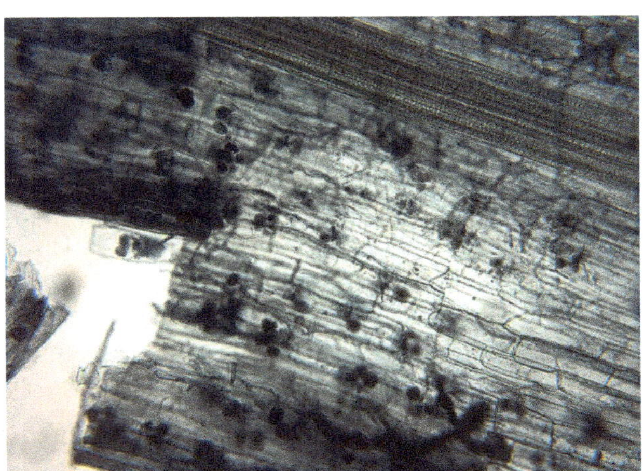

Arbuscular mycorrhiza seen under microscope. Flax root cortical cells containing paired arbuscules.

Phylogenetic analysis has demonstrated that the Microsporidia, unicellular parasites of animals and protists, are fairly recent and highly derived endobiotic fungi (living within the tissue of another species). One 2006 study concludes that the Microsporidia are a sister group to the true fungi; that is, they are each other's closest evolutionary relative. Hibbett and colleagues suggest that this analysis does not clash with their classification of the Fungi, and although the Microsporidia are elevated to phylum status, it is acknowledged that further analysis is required to clarify evolutionary relationships within this group.

The Chytridiomycota are commonly known as chytrids. These fungi are distributed worldwide. Chytrids and their close relatives Neocallimastigomycota and Blastocladiomycota (below) are the only fungi with active motility, producing zoospores that are capable of active movement through aqueous phases with a single flagellum, leading early taxonomists to classify them as protists. Molecular phylogenies, inferred from rRNA sequences in ribosomes, suggest that the Chytrids are a basal group divergent from the other fungal phyla, consisting of four major clades with suggestive evidence for paraphyly or possibly polyphyly.

The Blastocladiomycota were previously considered a taxonomic clade within the Chytridiomycota. Recent molecular data and ultrastructural characteristics, however, place the Blastocladiomycota as a sister clade to the Zygomycota, Glomeromycota, and Dikarya (Ascomycota and Basidiomycota). The blastocladiomycetes are saprotrophs, feeding on decomposing organic matter, and they are parasites of all eukaryotic groups. Unlike their close relatives, the chytrids, most of which exhibit zygotic meiosis, the blastocladiomycetes undergo sporic meiosis.

The Neocallimastigomycota were earlier placed in the phylum Chytridomycota. Members of this small phylum are anaerobic organisms, living in the digestive system of larger herbivorous mammals and in other terrestrial and aquatic environments enriched in cellulose (e.g., domestic waste landfill sites). They lack mitochondria but contain hydrogenosomes of mitochondrial origin. As in the related chrytrids, neocallimastigomycetes form zoospores that are posteriorly uniflagellate or polyflagellate.

Members of the Glomeromycota form arbuscular mycorrhizae, a form of mutualist symbiosis wherein fungal hyphae invade plant root cells and both species benefit from the resulting increased supply of nutrients. All known Glomeromycota species reproduce asexually. The symbiotic association between the Glomeromycota and plants is ancient, with evidence dating to 400 million years ago. Formerly part of the Zygomycota (commonly known as ‹sugar' and ‹pin' molds), the Glomeromycota were elevated to phylum status in 2001 and now replace the older phylum Zygomycota. Fungi that were placed in the Zygomycota are now being reassigned to the Glomeromycota, or the subphyla incertae sedis Mucoromycotina, Kickxellomycotina, the Zoopagomycotina and the Entomophthoromycotina. Some well-known examples of fungi formerly in the Zygomycota include black bread mold (*Rhizopus stolonifer*), and *Pilobolus* species, capable of ejecting spores several meters through the air. Medically relevant genera include *Mucor*, *Rhizomucor*, and *Rhizopus*.

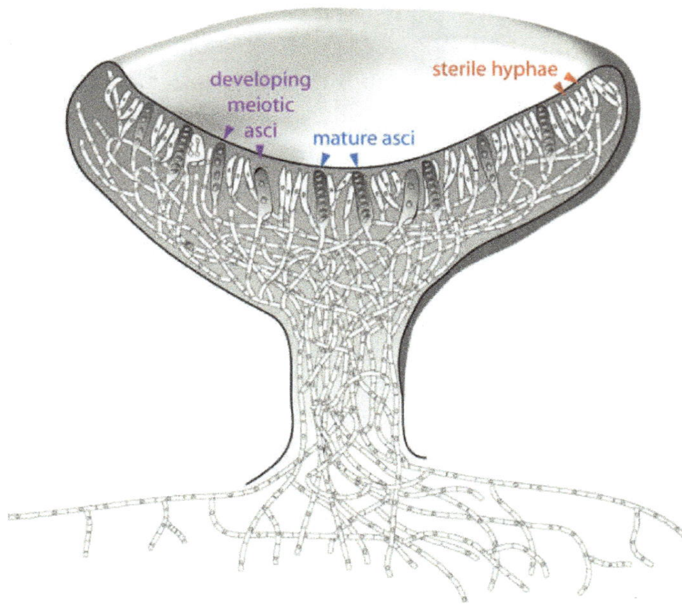

Diagram of an apothecium (the typical cup-like reproductive structure of Ascomycetes) showing sterile tissues as well as developing and mature asci.

The Ascomycota, commonly known as sac fungi or ascomycetes, constitute the largest taxonomic group within the Eumycota. These fungi form meiotic spores called ascospores, which are enclosed in a special sac-like structure called an ascus. This phylum includes morels, a few mushrooms and truffles, unicellular yeasts (e.g., of the genera *Saccharomyces*, *Kluyveromyces*, *Pichia*, and *Candida*), and many filamentous fungi living as saprotrophs, parasites, and mutualistic symbionts (e.g. lichens). Prominent and important genera of filamentous ascomycetes include *Aspergillus*, *Penicillium*, *Fusarium*, and *Claviceps*. Many ascomycete species have only been observed undergoing asexual reproduction (called anamorphic species), but analysis of molecular data has often been able to identify their closest teleomorphs in the Ascomycota. Because the products of meiosis are retained within the sac-like ascus, ascomycetes have been used for elucidating principles of genetics and heredity (e.g., *Neurospora crassa*).

Members of the Basidiomycota, commonly known as the club fungi or basidiomycetes, produce meiospores called basidiospores on club-like stalks called basidia. Most common mushrooms belong to this group, as well as rust and smut fungi, which are major pathogens of grains. Other important basidiomycetes include the maize pathogen *Ustilago maydis*, human commensal species of the genus *Malassezia*, and the opportunistic human pathogen, *Cryptococcus neoformans*.

Fungus-Like Organisms

Because of similarities in morphology and lifestyle, the slime molds (mycetozoans, plasmodiophorids, acrasids, *Fonticula* and labyrinthulids, now in Amoebozoa, Rhizaria, Excavata, Opisthokonta and Stramenopiles, respectively), water molds (oomycetes) and hyphochytrids (both Stramenopiles) were formerly classified in the kingdom Fungi, in groups like Mastigomycotina, Gymnomycota and Phycomycetes. The slime molds were studied also as protozoans, leading to a ambiregnal, duplicated taxonomy.

Unlike true fungi, the cell walls of oomycetes contain cellulose and lack chitin. Hyphochytrids have both chitin and cellulose. Slime molds lack a cell wall during the assimilative phase (except labyrinthulids, which have a wall of scales), and ingest nutrients by ingestion (phagocytosis, except labyrinthulids) rather than absorption (osmotrophy, as fungi, labyrinthulids, oomycetes and hyphochytrids). Neither water molds nor slime molds are closely related to the true fungi, and, therefore, taxonomists no longer group them in the kingdom Fungi. Nonetheless, studies of the oomycetes and myxomycetes are still often included in mycology textbooks and primary research literature.

The Eccrinales and Amoebidiales are opisthokont protists, previously thought to be zygomycete fungi. Other groups now in Opisthokonta (e.g., *Corallochytrium*, Ichthyosporea) were also at given time classified as fungi. The genus *Blastocystis*, now in Stramenopiles, was originally classified as a yeast. *Ellobiopsis*, now in Alveolata, was considered a chytrid. The bacteria were also included in fungi in some classifications, as the group Schizomycetes.

The Rozellida clade, including the "ex-chytrid" *Rozella*, is a genetically disparate group known mostly from environmental DNA sequences that is a sister group to fungi. Members of the group that have been isolated lack the chitinous cell wall that is characteristic of fungi.

The nucleariids, protists currently grouped in the Choanozoa (Opisthokonta), may be the next sister group to the eumycete clade, and as such could be included in an expanded fungal kingdom.

Many Actinomycetales (Actinobacteria), a group with many filamentous bacteria, were also long believed to be fungi.

Ecology

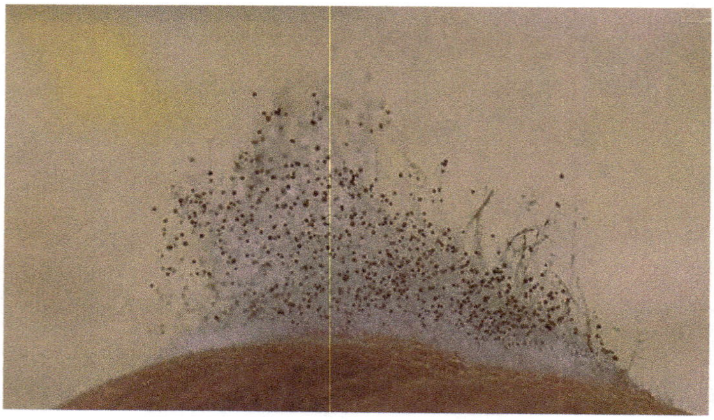

A pin mold decomposing a peach

Although often inconspicuous, fungi occur in every environment on Earth and play very important roles in most ecosystems. Along with bacteria, fungi are the major decomposers in most terrestrial (and some aquatic) ecosystems, and therefore play a critical role in biogeochemical cyclesand in many food webs. As decomposers, they play an essential role in nutrient cycling, especially as saprotrophs and symbionts, degrading organic matter to inorganic molecules, which can then re-enter anabolic metabolic pathways in plants or other organisms.

Symbiosis

Many fungi have important symbiotic relationships with organisms from most if not all Kingdoms. These interactions can be mutualistic or antagonistic in nature, or in the case of commensal fungi are of no apparent benefit or detriment to the host.

With Plants

Mycorrhizal symbiosis between plants and fungi is one of the most well-known plant–fungus associations and is of significant importance for plant growth and persistence in many ecosystems; over 90% of all plant species engage in mycorrhizal relationships with fungi and are dependent upon this relationship for survival.

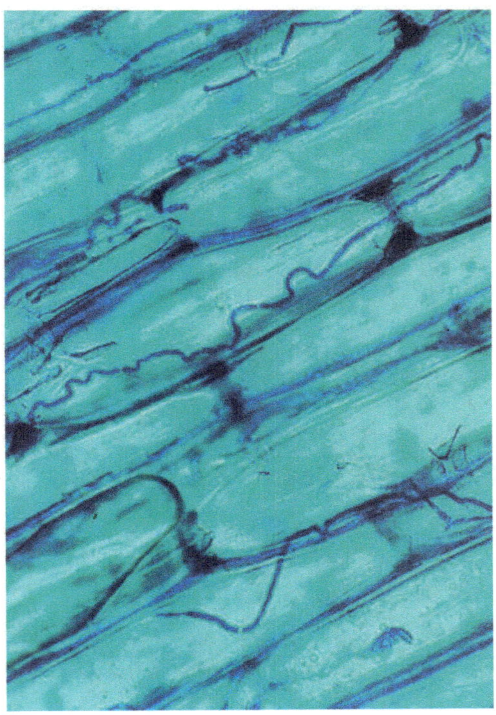

The dark filaments are hyphae of the endophytic fungus *Neotyphodium coenophialum* in the intercellular spaces of tall fescue leaf sheath tissue

The mycorrhizal symbiosis is ancient, dating to at least 400 million years ago. It often increases the plant's uptake of inorganic compounds, such as nitrate and phosphate from soils having low concentrations of these key plant nutrients. The fungal partners may also mediate plant-to-plant transfer of carbohydrates and other nutrients. Such mycorrhizal communities are called "common mycorrhizal networks". A special case of mycorrhiza is myco-heterotrophy, whereby the plant parasitizes the fungus, obtaining all of its nutrients from its fungal symbiont. Some fungal species inhabit the tissues inside roots, stems, and leaves, in which case they are called endophytes. Similar to mycorrhiza, endophytic colonization by fungi may benefit both symbionts; for example, endophytes of grasses impart to their host increased resistance to herbivores and other environmental stresses and receive food and shelter from the plant in return.

With Algae and Cyanobacteria

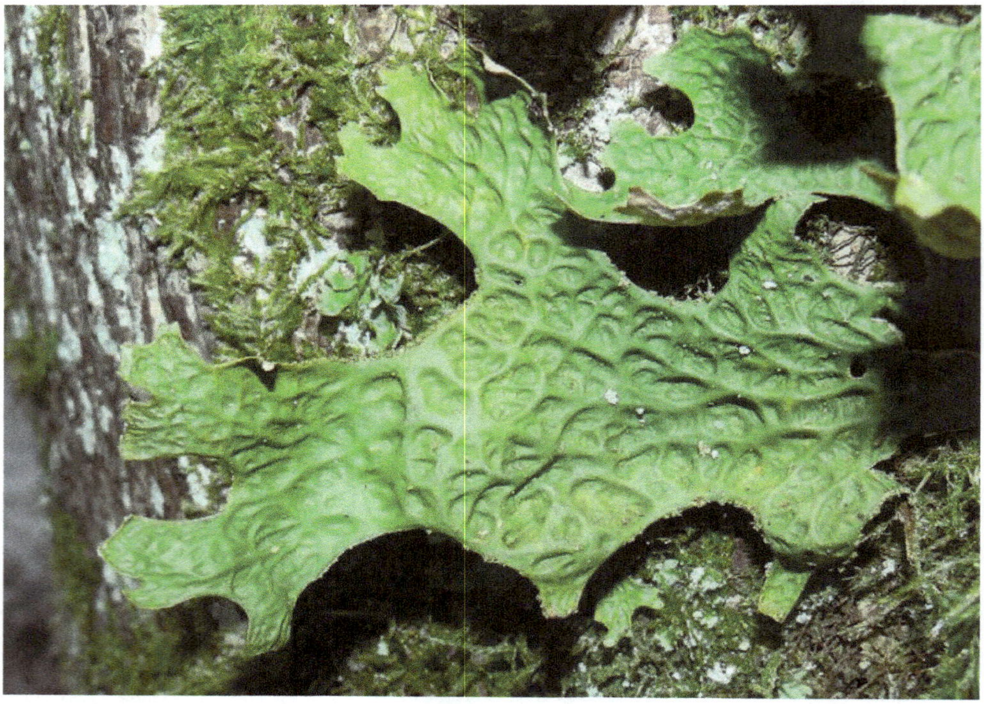

The lichen *Lobaria pulmonaria*, a symbiosis of fungal, algal, and cyanobacterial species

Lichens are a symbiotic relationship between fungi and photosynthetic algae or cyanobacteria. The photosynthetic partner in the relationship is referred to in lichen terminology as a "photobiont". The fungal part of the relationship is composed mostly of various species of ascomycetes and a few basidiomycetes. Lichens occur in every ecosystem on all continents, play a key role in soil formation and the initiation of biological succession, and are prominent in some extreme environments, including polar, alpine, and semiarid desert regions. They are able to grow on inhospitable surfaces, including bare soil, rocks, tree bark, wood, shells, barnacles and leaves. As in mycorrhizas, the photobiont provides sugars and other carbohydrates via photosynthesis to the fungus, while the fungus provides minerals and water to the photobiont. The functions of both symbiotic organisms are so closely intertwined that they function almost as a single organism; in most cases the resulting organism differs greatly from the individual components. Lichenization is a common mode of nutrition for fungi; around 20% of fungi—between 17,500 and 20,000 described species—are lichenized. Characteristics common to most lichens include obtaining organic carbon by photosynthesis, slow growth, small size, long life, long-lasting (seasonal) vegetative reproductive structures, mineral nutrition obtained largely from airborne sources, and greater tolerance of desiccation than most other photosynthetic organisms in the same habitat.

With Insects

Many insects also engage in mutualistic relationships with fungi. Several groups of ants cultivate fungi in the order Agaricales as their primary food source, while ambrosia beetles cultivate various species of fungi in the bark of trees that they infest. Likewise, females of several wood wasp species (genus *Sirex*) inject their eggs together with spores of the wood-rotting fungus *Amylostereum areolatum* into the sapwood of pine trees; the growth of the fungus provides ideal nutritional conditions for the development of the wasp larvae. At least one species of stingless bee has a relationship with a fungus in the genus *Monascus*, where the larvae consume and depend on fungus transferred from old to new nests. Termites on the African savannah are also known to cultivate fungi, and yeasts of the genera *Candida* and *Lachancea* inhabit the gut of a wide range of insects, including neuropterans, beetles, and cockroaches; it is not known whether these fungi benefit their hosts. Fungi ingrowing dead wood are essential for xylophagous insects (e.g. woodboring beetles). They deliver nutrients needed by xylophages to nutritionally scarce dead wood. Thanks to this nutritional enrichment the larvae of woodboring insect is able to grow and develop to adulthood. The larvae of many families of fungicolous flies, particularly those within the superfamily Sciaroidea such as the Mycetophilidae and some Keroplatidae feed on fungal fruiting bodies and sterile mycorrhizae.

As Pathogens and Parasites

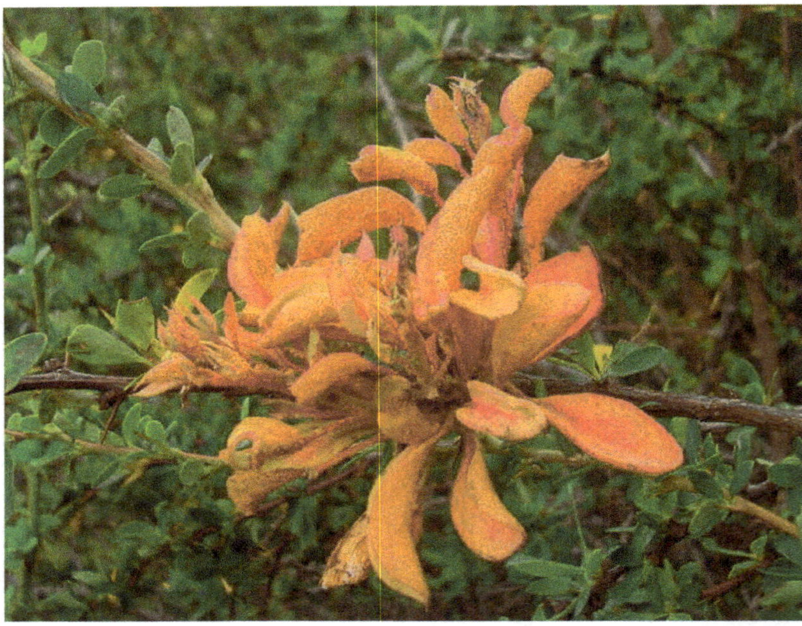

The plant pathogen *Aecidium magellanicum* causes calafate rust, seen here on a *Berberis* shrub in Chile.

Many fungi are parasites on plants, animals (including humans), and other fungi. Serious pathogens of many cultivated plants causing extensive damage and losses to agriculture and forestry include the rice blast fungus *Magnaporthe oryzae*, tree pathogens such as *Ophiostoma ulmi* and *Ophiostoma novo-ulmi* causing Dutch elm disease and *Cryphonectria parasitica* responsible for chestnut blight, and plant pathogens in the genera *Fusarium*, *Ustilago*, *Alternaria*, and *Cochliobolus*. Some carnivorous fungi, like *Paecilomyces lilacinus*, are predators of nematodes, which they capture using an array of specialized structures such as constricting rings or adhesive nets.

Some fungi can cause serious diseases in humans, several of which may be fatal if untreated. These include aspergillosis, candidiasis, coccidioidomycosis, cryptococcosis, histoplasmosis, mycetomas, and paracoccidioidomycosis. Furthermore, persons with immuno-deficiencies are particularly susceptible to disease by genera such as *Aspergillus*, *Candida*, *Cryptoccocus*, *Histoplasma*, and *Pneumocystis*.Other fungi can attack eyes, nails, hair, and especially skin, the so-called dermatophytic and keratinophilic fungi, and cause local infections such as ringworm and athlete's foot. Fungal spores are also a cause of allergies, and fungi from different taxonomic groups can evoke allergic reactions.

As Targets of Mycoparasites

The organisms which parasitize fungi are known as mycoparasitic organisms. Certain species of the *Pythium* genus, which are oomycetes, have potential as biocontrol agents against certain fungi. Fungi can also act as mycoparasites or antagonists of other fungi, such as *Hypomyces chrysospermus*, which grows on bolete mushrooms.

Fungi can become the target of infection by mycoviruses.

Mycotoxins

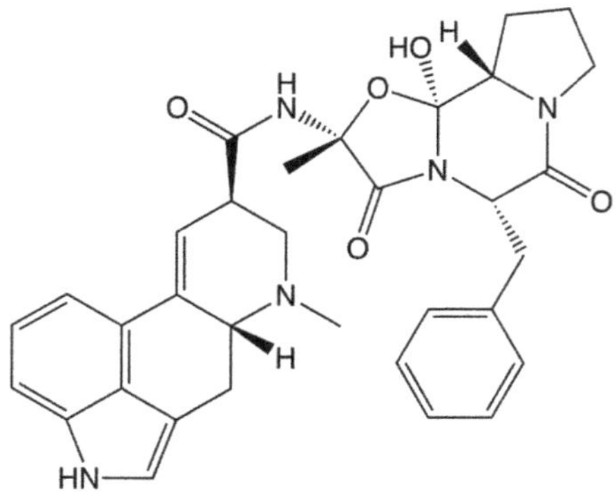

Ergotamine, a major mycotoxin produced by *Claviceps* species, which if ingested can cause gangrene, convulsions, and hallucinations

Many fungi produce biologically active compounds, several of which are toxic to animals or plants and are therefore called mycotoxins. Of particular relevance to humans are mycotoxins produced by molds causing food spoilage, and poisonous mushrooms (see above). Particularly infamous are the lethal amatoxins in some *Amanita* mushrooms, and ergot alkaloids, which have a long history of causing serious epidemics of ergotism (St Anthony's Fire) in people consuming rye or related cereals contaminated with sclerotia of the ergot fungus, *Claviceps purpurea*. Other notable mycotoxins include the aflatoxins, which are insidious liver toxins and highly carcinogenic metabolites produced by certain *Aspergillus* species often growing in or on grains and nuts consumed by humans, ochratoxins, patulin, and trichothecenes (e.g., T-2 mycotoxin) and fumonisins, which have significant impact on human food supplies or animal livestock.

Mycotoxins are secondary metabolites (or natural products), and research has established the existence of biochemical pathways solely for the purpose of producing mycotoxins and other natural products in fungi. Mycotoxins may provide fitness benefits in terms of physiological adaptation, competition with other microbes and fungi, and protection from consumption (fungivory). Many fungal secondary metabolites (or derivatives) are used medically, as described under Human Use below.

Pathogenic Mechanisms

Ustilago maydis is a pathogenic plant fungus that causes smut disease in maize and teosinte. Plants have evolved efficient defense systems against pathogenic microbes such as *U. maydis*. A rapid defense reaction after pathogen attack is the oxidative burst where the plant produces reactive oxygen species at the site of the attempted invasion. *U. maydis* can respond to the oxidative burst with an oxidative stress response, regulated by the gene *YAP1*. The response protects *U. maydis* from the host defense, and is necessary for the pathogen's virulence. Furthermore, *U. maydis* has a well-established recombinational DNA repair system which acts during mitosis and meiosis. The system may assist the pathogen in surviving DNA damage arising from the host plant's oxidative defensive response to infection.

Cryptococcus neoformans is an encapsulated yeast that can live in both plants and animals. *C. neoformans* usually infects the lungs, where it is phagocytosed by alveolar macrophages. Some *C. neoformans* can survive inside macrophages, which appears to be the basis for latency, disseminated disease, and resistance to antifungal agents. One mechanism by which *C. neoformans* survives the hostile macrophage environment is by up-regulating the expression of genes involved in the oxidative stress response. Another mechanism involves meiosis. The majority of *C. neoformans* are mating "type a". Filaments of mating "type a" ordinarily have haploid nuclei, but they can become diploid (perhaps by endoduplication or by stimulated nuclear fusion) to form blastospores. The diploid nuclei of blastospores can undergo meiosis, including recombination, to form haploid basidiospores that can be dispersed. This process is referred to as monokaryotic fruiting. this process requires a gene called *DMC1*, which is a conserved homologue of genes *recA* in bacteria and *RAD51* in eukaryotes, that mediates homologous chromosome pairing during meiosis and repair of DNA double-strand breaks. Thus, *C. neoformans* can undergo a meiosis, monokaryotic fruiting, that promotes recombinational repair in the oxidative, DNA damaging environment of the host macrophage, and the repair capability may contribute to its virulence.

Human Use

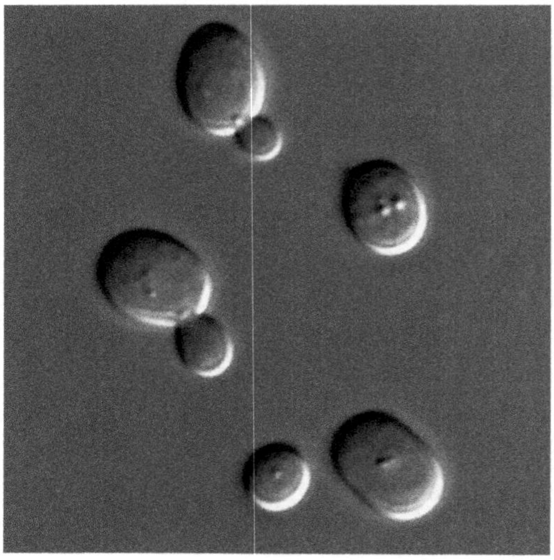

Saccharomyces cerevisiae cells shown with DIC microscopy

The human use of fungi for food preparation or preservation and other purposes is extensive and has a long history. Mushroom farming and mushroom gathering are large industries in many countries. The study of the historical uses and sociological impact of fungi is known as ethnomycology. Because of the capacity of this group to produce an enormous range of natural products with antimicrobial or other biological activities, many species have long been used or are being developed for industrial production of antibiotics, vitamins, and anti-cancer and cholesterol-lowering drugs. More recently, methods have been developed for genetic engineering of fungi, enabling metabolic engineering of fungal species. For example, genetic modification of yeast species—which are easy to grow at fast rates in large fermentation vessels—has opened up ways of pharmaceutical production that are potentially more efficient than production by the original source organisms.

Therapeutic Uses

Modern Chemotherapeutics

Many species produce metabolites that are major sources of pharmacologically active drugs. Particularly important are the antibiotics, including the penicillins, a structurally related group of β-lactam antibiotics that are synthesized from small peptides. Although naturally occurring penicillins such as penicillin G (produced by *Penicillium chrysogenum*) have a relatively narrow spectrum of biological activity, a wide range of other penicillins can be produced by chemical modification of the natural penicillins. Modern penicillins are semisynthetic compounds, obtained initially from fermentation cultures, but then structurally altered for specific desirable properties. Other antibiotics produced by fungi include: ciclosporin, commonly used as an immunosuppressant during transplant surgery; and fusidic acid, used to help control infection from methicillin-resistant *Staphylococcus aureus* bacteria. Widespread use of antibiotics for the treatment of bacterial diseases, such as tuberculosis, syphilis, leprosy, and others began in the early 20th century and continues to date. In nature, antibiotics of fungal or bacterial origin appear to play a dual role: at high concentrations they act as chemical defense against competition with other microorganisms in species-rich environments, such as the rhizosphere, and at low concentrations as quorum-sensing molecules for intra- or interspecies signaling. Other drugs produced by fungi include griseofulvin isolated from *Penicillium griseofulvum*, used to treat fungal infections, and statins (HMG-CoA reductase inhibitors), used to inhibit cholesterol synthesis. Examples of statins found in fungi include mevastatin from *Penicillium citrinum* and lovastatin from *Aspergillus terreus* and the oyster mushroom.

Traditional and Folk Medicine

Certain mushrooms enjoy usage as therapeutics in folk medicines, such as Traditional Chinese medicine. Notable medicinal mushrooms with a well-documented history of use include *Agaricus subrufescens*, *Ganoderma lucidum*, and *Ophiocordyceps sinensis*. Research has identified compounds produced by these and other fungi that have inhibitory biological effects against viruses and cancer cells.Specific metabolites, such as polysaccharide-K, ergotamine, and β-lactam antibiotics, are routinely used in clinical medicine. The shiitake mushroom is a source of lentinan, a clinical drug approved for use in cancer treatments in several countries, including Japan. In Europe and Japan, polysaccharide-K (brand name Krestin), a chemical derived from *Trametes versicolor*, is an approved adjuvant for cancer therapy.

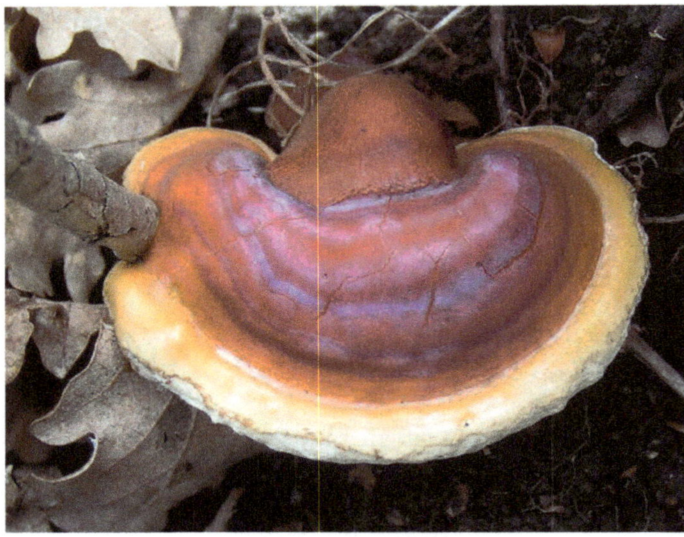

The medicinal fungi *Ganoderma lucidum* (left) and *Ophiocordyceps sinensis* (right)

Cultured Foods

Baker's yeast or *Saccharomyces cerevisiae*, a unicellular fungus, is used to make bread and other wheat-based products, such as pizza dough and dumplings. Yeast species of the genus *Saccharomyces* are also used to produce alcoholic beverages through fermentation. Shoyu koji mold (*Aspergillus oryzae*) is an essential ingredient in brewing Shoyu (soy sauce) and sake, and the preparation of miso, while *Rhizopus* species are used for making tempeh. Several of these fungi are domesticated species that were bred or selected according to their capacity to ferment food without producing harmful mycotoxins (see below), which are produced by very closely related *Aspergilli*. Quorn, a meat substitute, is made from *Fusarium venenatum*.

Edible and Poisonous species

Edible mushrooms are well-known examples of fungi. Many are commercially raised, but others must be harvested from the wild. *Agaricus bisporus*, sold as button mushrooms when small or Portobello mushrooms when larger, is a commonly eaten species, used in salads, soups, and many other dishes. Many Asian fungi are commercially grown and have increased in popularity in the West. They are often available fresh in grocery stores and markets, including straw mushrooms (*Volvariella volvacea*), oyster mushrooms (*Pleurotus ostreatus*), shiitakes (*Lentinula edodes*), and enokitake (*Flammulina* spp.).

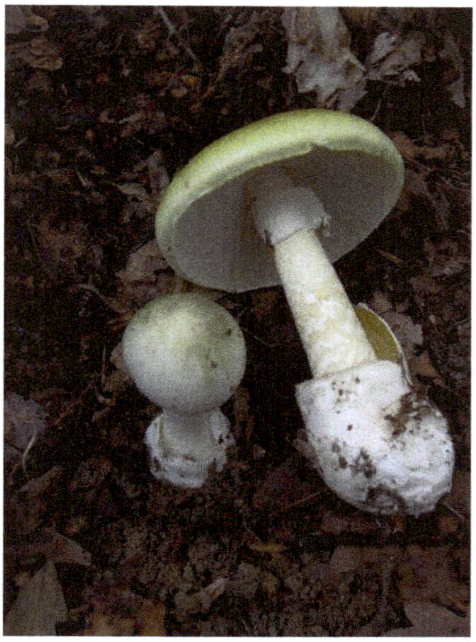

Amanita phalloides accounts for the majority of fatal mushroom poisonings worldwide.

There are many more mushroom species that are harvested from the wild for personal consumption or commercial sale. Milk mushrooms, morels, chanterelles, truffles, black trumpets, and *porcini* mushrooms (*Boletus edulis*) (also known as king boletes) demand a high price on the market. They are often used in gourmet dishes.

Certain types of cheeses require inoculation of milk curds with fungal species that impart a unique flavor and texture to the cheese. Examples include the blue color in cheeses such as Stilton or Roquefort, which are made by inoculation with *Penicillium roqueforti*. Molds used in cheese production are non-toxic and are thus safe for human consumption; however, mycotoxins (e.g., aflatoxins, roquefortine C, patulin, or others) may accumulate because of growth of other fungi during cheese ripening or storage.

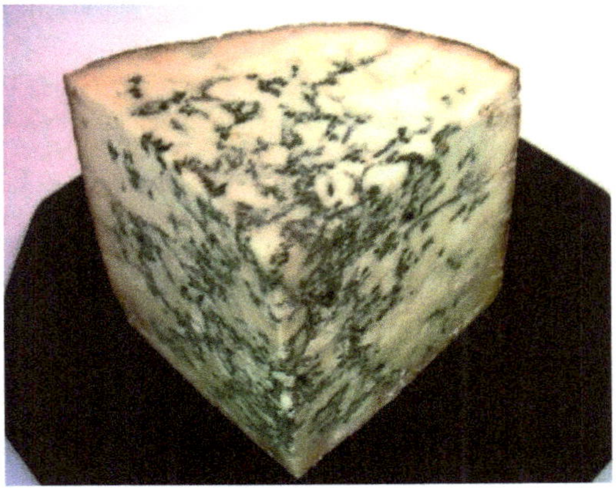

Stilton cheese veined with *Penicillium roqueforti*

Many mushroom species are poisonous to humans, with toxicities ranging from slight digestive problems or allergic reactions as well as hallucinations to severe organ failures and death. Genera with mushrooms containing deadly toxins include *Conocybe*, *Galerina*, *Lepiota*, and, the most infamous, *Amanita*. The latter genus includes the destroying angel *(A. virosa)* and the death cap *(A. phalloides)*, the most common cause of deadly mushroom poisoning. The false morel (*Gyromitra esculenta*) is occasionally considered a delicacy when cooked, yet can be highly toxic when eaten raw. *Tricholoma equestre* was considered edible until it was implicated in serious poisonings causing rhabdomyolysis. Fly agaric mushrooms (*Amanita muscaria*) also cause occasional non-fatal poisonings, mostly as a result of ingestion for its hallucinogenic properties. Historically, fly agaric was used by different peoples in Europe and Asia and its present usage for religious or shamanic purposes is reported from some ethnic groups such as the Koryak people of north-eastern Siberia.

As it is difficult to accurately identify a safe mushroom without proper training and knowledge, it is often advised to assume that a wild mushroom is poisonous and not to consume it.

Pest Control

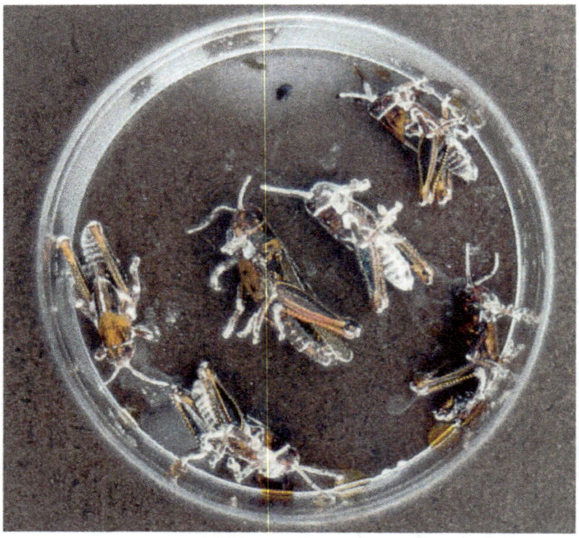

Grasshoppers killed by *Beauveria bassiana*

In agriculture, fungi may be useful if they actively compete for nutrients and space with pathogenic microorganisms such as bacteria or other fungi via the competitive exclusion principle, or if they are parasites of these pathogens. For example, certain species may be used to eliminate or suppress the growth of harmful plant pathogens, such as insects, mites, weeds, nematodes, and other fungi that cause diseases of important crop plants. This has generated strong interest in practical applications that use these fungi in the biological control of these agricultural pests. Entomopathogenic fungi can be used as biopesticides, as they actively kill insects. Examples that have been used as biological insecticides are *Beauveria bassiana*, *Metarhizium* spp, *Hirsutella* spp, *Paecilomyces* (*Isaria*) spp, and *Lecanicillium lecanii*. Endophytic fungi of grasses of the genus *Neotyphodium*, such as *N. coenophialum*, produce alkaloids that are toxic to a range of invertebrate and vertebrate herbivores. These alkaloids protect grass plants from herbivory, but several endophyte alkaloids can poison grazing animals, such as cattle and sheep. Infecting cultivars of pasture or forage grasses with *Neotyphodium* endophytes is one approach being used in grass breeding programs; the fungal strains are selected for producing only alkaloids that increase resistance to herbivores such as insects, while being non-toxic to livestock.

Bioremediation

Certain fungi, in particular "white rot" fungi, can degrade insecticides, herbicides, pentachlorophenol, creosote, coal tars, and heavy fuels and turn them into carbon dioxide, water, and basic elements. Fungi have been shown to biomineralize uranium oxides, suggesting they may have application in the bioremediation of radioactively polluted sites.

Model Organisms

Several pivotal discoveries in biology were made by researchers using fungi as model organisms, that is, fungi that grow and sexually reproduce rapidly in the laboratory. For example, the one gene-one enzyme hypothesis was formulated by scientists using the bread mold *Neurospora crassa* to test their biochemical theories. Other important model fungi are *Aspergillus nidulans* and the yeasts *Saccaromyces cerevisiae* and *Schizosaccharomyces pombe*, each of which with a long history of use to investigate issues in eukaryotic cell biology and genetics, such as cell cycle regulation, chromatin structure, and gene regulation. Other fungal models have more recently emerged that address specific biological questions relevant to medicine, plant pathology, and industrial uses; examples include *Candida albicans*, a dimorphic, opportunistic human pathogen, *Magnaporthe grisea*, a plant pathogen, and *Pichia pastoris*, a yeast widely used for eukaryotic protein production.

Others

Fungi are used extensively to produce industrial chemicals like citric, gluconic, lactic, and malic acids, and industrial enzymes, such as lipases used in biological detergents,cellulases used in making cellulosic ethanol and stonewashed jeans, and amylases, invertases, proteases and xylanases. Several species, most notably *Psilocybin mushrooms* (colloquially known as *magic mushrooms*), are ingested for their psychedelic properties, both recreationally and religiously.

Habitats and Ecology

Microorganisms are found in almost every habitat present in nature. Even in hostile environments such as the poles, deserts, geysers, rocks, and the deep sea. Some types of microorganisms have adapted to the extreme conditions and sustained colonies; these organisms are known as extremophiles. Extremophiles have been isolated from rocks as much as 7 kilometres below the Earth's surface, and it has been suggested that the amount of living organisms below the Earth's surface is comparable with the amount of life on or above the surface. Extremophiles have been known to survive for a prolonged time in a vacuum, and can be highly resistant to radiation, which may even allow them to survive in space. Many types of microorganisms have intimate symbiotic relationships with other larger organisms; some of which are mutually beneficial (mutualism), while others can be damaging to the host organism (parasitism). If microorganisms can cause disease in a host they are known as pathogens and then they are sometimes referred to as microbes.

Extremophiles

Extremophiles are microorganisms that have adapted so that they can survive and even thrive in conditions that are normally fatal to most life-forms. For example, some species have been found in the following extreme environments:

- Temperature: as high as 130 °C (266 °F), as low as −17 °C (1 °F)
- Acidity/alkalinity: less than pH 0, up to pH 11.5
- Salinity: up to saturation
- Pressure: up to 1,000-2,000 atm, down to 0 atm (e.g. vacuum of space)
- Radiation: up to 5kGy

Extremophiles are significant in different ways. They extend terrestrial life into much of the Earth's hydrosphere, crust and atmosphere, their specific evolutionary adaptation mechanisms to their extreme environment can be exploited in bio-technology, and their very existence under such extreme conditions increases the potential for extraterrestrial life.

Soil Microorganisms

The nitrogen cycle in soils depends on the fixation of atmospheric nitrogen. One way this can occur is in the nodules in the roots of legumes that contain symbiotic bacteria of the genera *Rhizobium*, *Mesorhizobium*, *Sinorhizobium*, *Bradyrhizobium*, and *Azorhizobium*.

Symbiotic Microorganisms

Symbiotic microorganisms such as fungi and algae form an association in lichen. Certain fungi form mycorrhizal symbioses with trees that increase the supply of nutrients to the tree.

Applications

Microorganisms are vital to humans and the environment, as they participate in the carbon and nitrogen cycles, as well as fulfilling other vital roles in virtually all ecosystems, such as recycling other organisms' dead remains and waste products through decomposition. Microorganisms also have an important place in most higher-order multicellular organisms as symbionts. Many blame the failure of Biosphere 2 on an improper balance of microorganisms.

Food Production

Microorganisms are used to make yoghurt, cheese and curd. They are used to leaven bread, and to convert sugars to alcohol in wine and beer.

Soil

Microbes can make nutrients and minerals in the soil available to plants, produce hormones that spur growth, stimulate the plant immune system and trigger or dampen stress responses. In general a more diverse soil microbiome results in fewer plant diseases and higher yield.

Fermentation

Microorganisms are used in brewing, wine making, baking, pickling and other food-making processes.

They are also used to control the fermentation process in the production of cultured dairy products such as yogurt and cheese. The cultures also provide flavor and aroma, and inhibit undesirable organisms.

Hygiene

Hygiene is the avoidance of infection or food spoiling by eliminating microorganisms from the surroundings. As microorganisms, in particular bacteria, are found virtually everywhere, the levels of harmful microorganisms can be reduced to acceptable levels. However, in some cases, it is required that an object or substance be completely sterile, i.e. devoid of all living entities and viruses. A good example of this is a hypodermic needle.

In food preparation microorganisms are reduced by preservation methods (such as the addition of vinegar), clean utensils used in preparation, short storage periods, or by cool temperatures. If complete sterility is needed, the two most common methods are irradiation and the use of an autoclave, which resembles a pressure cooker.

There are several methods for investigating the level of hygiene in a sample of food, drinking water, equipment, etc. Water samples can be filtrated through an extremely fine filter. This filter is then placed in a nutrient medium. Microorganisms on the filter then grow to form a visible colony. Harmful microorganisms can be detected in food by placing a sample in a nutrient broth designed to enrich the organisms in question. Various methods, such as selective media or polymerase chain reaction, can then be used for detection. The hygiene of hard surfaces, such as cooking pots, can be tested by touching them with a solid piece of nutrient medium and then allowing the microorganisms to grow on it.

There are no conditions where all microorganisms would grow, and therefore often several methods are needed. For example, a food sample might be analyzed on three different nutrient mediums designed to indicate the presence of "total" bacteria (conditions where many, but not all, bacteria grow), molds (conditions where the growth of bacteria is prevented by, e.g., antibiotics) and coliform bacteria (these indicate a sewage contamination).

Water Treatment

The majority of all oxidative sewage treatment processes rely on a large range of microorganisms to oxidise organic constituents which are not amenable to sedimentation or flotation. Anaerobic microorganisms are also used to reduce sludge solids producing methane gas (amongst other gases) and a sterile mineralised residue. In potable water treatment, one method, the slow sand filter, employs a complex gelatinous layer composed of a wide range of microorganisms to remove both dissolved and particulate material from raw water.

Energy

Microorganisms are used in fermentation to produce ethanol, and in biogas reactors to produce methane. Scientists are researching the use of algae to produce liquid fuels, and bacteria to convert various forms of agricultural and urban waste into usable fuels.

Chemicals, Enzymes

Microorganisms are used for many commercial and industrial production of chemicals, enzymes and other bioactive molecules. Examples of organic acid produced include

- **Acetic acid**: Produced by the bacterium *Acetobacter aceti* and other acetic acid bacteria (AAB)
- **Butyric acid** (butanoic acid): Produced by the bacterium *Clostridium butyricum*
- **Lactic acid**: *Lactobacillus* and others commonly called as lactic acid bacteria (LAB)
- **Citric acid**: Produced by the fungus *Aspergillus niger*

Microorganisms are used for preparation of bioactive molecules and enzymes.

- Streptokinase produced by the bacterium *Streptococcus* and modified by genetic engineering is used as a clot buster for removing clots from the blood vessels of patients who have undergone myocardial infarctions leading to heart attack.
- Cyclosporin A is a bioactive molecule used as an immunosuppressive agent in organ transplantation
- Statins produced by the yeast *Monascus purpureus* are commercialised as blood cholesterol lowering agents which act by competitively inhibiting the enzyme responsible for synthesis of cholesterol.

Science

Microorganisms are essential tools in biotechnology, biochemistry, genetics, and molecular biology. The yeasts (*Saccharomyces cerevisiae*) and fission yeast (*Schizosaccharomyces pombe*) are important model organisms in science, since they are simple eukaryotes that can be grown rapidly in large numbers and are easily manipulated. They are particularly valuable in genetics, genomics and proteomics. Microorganisms can be harnessed for uses such as creating steroids and treating skin diseases. Scientists are also considering using microorganisms for living fuel cells, and as a solution for pollution.

Warfare

In the Middle Ages, diseased corpses were thrown into castles during sieges using catapults or other siege engines. Individuals near the corpses were exposed to the pathogen and were likely to spread that pathogen to others.

Human Health

Human Digestion

Microorganisms can form an endosymbiotic relationship with other, larger organisms. For example, the bacteria that live within the human digestive system contribute to gut immunity, synthesise vitamins such as folic acid and biotin, and ferment complex indigestible carbohydrates.

Disease

Microorganisms are the causative agents (pathogens) in many infectious diseases. The organisms involved include pathogenic bacteria, causing diseases such as plague, tuberculosis and anthrax; protozoa, causing diseases such as malaria, sleeping sickness, dysentery and toxoplasmosis; and also fungi causing diseases such as ringworm, candidiasis or histoplasmosis. However, other diseases such as influenza, yellow fever or AIDS are caused by pathogenic viruses, which are not usually classified as living organisms and are not, therefore, microorganisms by the strict definition. No clear examples of archaean pathogens are known, although a relationship has been proposed between the presence of some archaean methanogens and human periodontal disease.

Ecology

Microorganisms play critical roles in Earth's biogeochemical cycles as they are responsible for decomposition and play vital parts in carbon and nitrogen fixation, as well as oxygen production.

Etymology and Pronunciation

The word *microorganism* uses combining forms of *micro-* (from the Greek: μικρός, *mikros*, "small") and *organism* from the Greek: ργανισμός, *organismós*, "organism"). It is usually styled solid but is sometimes hyphenated (*micro-organism*), especially in older texts. The word *microbe* comes from μικρός, mikrós, "small" and βίος, bíos, "life".

MICROORGANISMS USED IN FOOD AND BEVERAGE PREPARATION

This is an incomplete list of bacteria and fungi that are used in preparing food.

List of microorganisms used in food and beverage preparation

Microorganism	Type Of Microorganism	Food or Beverage	Reference(s)
Acetobacter aceti	bacterium	chocolate	
Acetobacter aceti	bacterium	vinegar	
Acetobacter cerevisiae	bacterium	Beer	
Acetobacter fabarum	bacterium	chocolate	
Acetobacter fabarum	bacterium	coffee	
Acetobacter lovaniensis	bacterium	vegetables	
Acetobacter malorum	bacterium	vinegar	
Acetobacter orientalis	bacterium	vegetables	
Acetobacter pasteurianus	bacterium	chocolate	
Acetobacter pasteurianus	bacterium	vinegar	
Acetobacter pomorum	bacterium	vinegar	
Acetobacter syzygii	bacterium	chocolate	
Acetobacter syzygii	bacterium	vinegar	
Acetobacter tropicalis	bacterium	chocolate	
Acetobacter tropicalis	bacterium	coffee	
Arthrobacter arilaitensis	bacterium	smear-ripened cheese	
Arthrobacter bergerei	bacterium	smear-ripened cheese	
Arthrobacter globiformis	bacterium	smear-ripened cheese	
Arthrobacter nicotianae	bacterium	surface-ripened cheese	
Arthrobacter nicotianae	bacterium	Tilsit cheese	
Arthrobacter variabilis	bacterium	smear-ripened cheese	
Aspergillus acidus	fungus	tea	
Aspergillus niger	fungus	awamori	
Aspergillus fumigatus	fungus	chocolate	
Aspergillus oryzae	fungus	miso	
Aspergillus oryzae	fungus	sake	
Aspergillus oryzae	fungus	soy sauce	
Aspergillus sojae	fungus	miso	
Aspergillus sojae	fungus	soy sauce	
Bacillus cereus	bacterium	chocolate	
Bacillus coagulans	bacterium	chocolate	
Bacillus licheniformis	bacterium	chocolate	
Bacillus pumilus	bacterium	chocolate	
Bacillus sphaericus	bacterium	stinky tofu	
Bacillus stearothermophilus	bacterium	chocolate	
Bacillus subtilis	bacterium	chocolate	
Bacillus subtilis	bacterium	natto	
Bifidobacterium adolescentis	bacterium	yogurt	
Bifidobacterium animalis	bacterium	daisy	
Bifidobacterium bifidum	bacterium	daisy	
Bifidobacterium breve	bacterium	daisy	
Bifidobacterium breve	bacterium	soy	

Microorganism	Type Of Microorganism	Food or Beverage	Reference(s)
Bifidobacterium infantis	bacterium	daisy	
Bifidobacterium lactis	bacterium	daisy	
Bifidobacterium longum	bacterium	daisy	
Bifidobacterium pseudolongum	bacterium	daisy	
Bifidobacterium thermophilum	bacterium	daisy	
Brachybacterium alimentarium	bacterium	Beaufort cheese	
Brachybacterium alimentarium	bacterium	Gruyère cheese	
Brachybacterium tyrofermentans	bacterium	Beaufort cheese	
Brachybacterium tyrofermentans	bacterium	Gruyère cheese	
Brevibacterium aurantiacum	bacterium	cheese	
Brevibacterium casei	bacterium	smear-ripened cheese	
Brevibacterium linens	bacterium	smear-ripened cheese	
Candida colliculosa	fungus	cheese	
Candida colliculosa	fungus	kefir	
Candida exiguus	fungus	sourdough bread	
Candida humicola	fungus	chocolate	
Candida kefyr	fungus	surface-ripened cheese	
Candida krusei	fungus	surface-ripened cheese	
Candida milleri	fungus	sourdough bread	
Candida mycoderma	fungus	Limburger cheese	
Candida pelliculosa	fungus	chocolate	
Candida rugosa	fungus	chocolate	
Candida tropicalis	fungus	chocolate	
Candida utilis	fungus	cheese	
Candida valida	fungus	sourdough	
Candida vini	fungus	Reblochon cheese, wine	
Candida zeylanoides	fungus	Reblochon cheese	
Carnobacterium divergens	bacterium	cheese	
Carnobacterium divergens	bacterium	fish	
Carnobacterium divergens	bacterium	meat	
Carnobacterium maltaromaticum	bacterium	dairy	
Carnobacterium piscicola	bacterium	meat	
Corynebacterium ammoniagenes	bacterium	cheese	
Corynebacterium casei	bacterium	smear-ripened cheese	
Corynebacterium flavescens	bacterium	cheese	
Corynebacterium mooreparkense	bacterium	smear-ripened cheese	
Corynebacterium variabile	bacterium	cheese	
Cyberlindnera mrakii	fungus	wine	
Cystofilobasidium infirmominiatum	fungus	cheese	
Debaryomyces hansenii	fungus	smear-ripened cheese	

Microorganism	Type Of Microorganism	Food or Beverage	Reference(s)
Debaryomyces hansenii	fungus	Reblochon cheese	
Debaryomyces kloeckeri	fungus	Limburger cheese	
Enterococcus faecalis	bacterium	cheese	
Enterococcus faecalis	bacterium	cream	
Enterococcus faecalis	bacterium	ham	
Enterococcus faecalis	bacterium	miso	
Enterococcus faecalis	bacterium	pickle	
Enterococcus faecalis	bacterium	sausage	
Enterococcus faecalis	bacterium	soy sauce	
Enterococcus faecium	bacterium	Manchego cheese	
Enterococcus faecium	bacterium	ham	
Enterococcus faecium	bacterium	miso	
Enterococcus faecium	bacterium	pickle	
Enterococcus faecium	bacterium	soy sauce	
Fusarium domesticum	fungus	cheese	
Geotrichum candidum	fungus	cheese	
Gluconacetobacter azotocaptans	bacterium	chocolate	
Gluconacetobacter azotocaptans	bacterium	coffee	
Gluconacetobacter diazotrophicus	bacterium	chocolate	
Gluconacetobacter diazotrophicus	bacterium	coffee	
Gluconacetobacter entanii	bacterium	vinegar	
Gluconacetobacter europaeus	bacterium	vinegar	
Gluconacetobacter hansenii	bacterium	vinegar	
Gluconacetobacter johannae	bacterium	chocolate	
Gluconacetobacter johannae	bacterium	coffee	
Gluconacetobacter oboediens	bacterium	vinegar	
Gluconacetobacter xylinus	bacterium	vinegar	
Gluconobacter oxydans	bacterium	chocolate	
Hafnia alvei	bacterium	cheese	
Halomonas elongata	bacterium	meat	
Issatchenkia orientalis	fungus	kefir	
Kazachstania exigua	fungus	kefir	
Kazachstania unispora	fungus	kefir	
Kloeckera africana	fungus	chocolate	
Kloeckera apis	fungus	chocolate	.
Kloeckera javanica	fungus	chocolate	
Kluyveromyces lactis	fungus	cheese	
Kluyveromyces marxianus	fungus	cheese	
Kluyveromyces marxianus	fungus	chocolate	
Kocuria rhizophila	bacterium	cheese	
Kocuria rhizophila	bacterium	meat	
Kocuria varians	bacterium	dairy	
Kocuria varians	bacterium	sausage	
Lactobacillus acetotolerans	bacterium	fruit	
Lactobacillus acetotolerans	bacterium	sourdough bread	

Microorganism	Type Of Microorganism	Food or Beverage	Reference(s)
Lactobacillus acetotolerans	bacterium	vegetables	
Lactobacillus acidifarinae	bacterium	sourdough bread	
Lactobacillus acidipiscis	bacterium	dairy	
Lactobacillus acidipiscis	bacterium	fish	
Lactobacillus acidophilus	bacterium	vegetables	
Lactobacillus acidophilus	bacterium	yogurt	
Lactobacillus alimentarius	bacterium	fish	
Lactobacillus alimentarius	bacterium	meat	
Lactobacillus brevis	bacterium	Canestrato Pugliese cheese	
Lactobacillus brevis	bacterium	vegetables	
Lactobacillus brevis ssp. *linens*	bacterium	kefir	
Lactobacillus bucheri	bacterium	bread	
Lactobacillus bucheri	bacterium	wine	
Lactobacillus cacaonum	bacterium	chocolate	
Lactobacillus casei	bacterium	Idiazabal cheese	
Lactobacillus casei	bacterium	Manchego cheese	
Lactobacillus casei	bacterium	Roncal cheese	
Lactobacillus casei	bacterium	yogurt	
Lactobacillus casei ssp. *pseudoplantarum*	bacterium	Grana Padano cheese	
Lactobacillus casei ssp. *pseudoplantarum*	bacterium	Parmigiano-Reggiano cheese	
Lactobacillus cellobiosus	bacterium	chocolate	
Lactobacillus collinoides	bacterium	cider	
Lactobacillus composti	bacterium	*sh ch*	
Lactobacillus coryniformis	bacterium	cheese	
Lactobacillus crispatus	bacterium	sourdough bread	
Lactobacillus curvatus	bacterium	Cacio di Fossa cheese	
Lactobacillus curvatus	bacterium	Canestrato Pugliese cheese	
Lactobacillus curvatus	bacterium	Pecorino Romano cheese	
Lactobacillus curvatus	bacterium	Pecorino Sardo cheese	
Lactobacillus curvatus	bacterium	sausage	
Lactobacillus delbrueckii	bacterium	vegetables	
Lactobacillus delbrueckii ssp. *bulgaricus*	bacterium	cheese	
Lactobacillus delbrueckii ssp. *bulgaricus*	bacterium	yogurt	
Lactobacillus delbrueckii ssp. *lactis*	bacterium	Pecorino Romano cheese	
Lactobacillus dextrinicus	bacterium	meat	
Lactobacillus diolivorans	bacterium	chicha	
Lactobacillus fabifermentans	bacterium	chocolate	
Lactobacillus farciminis	bacterium	fish	
Lactobacillus farciminis	bacterium	soy	
Lactobacillus fermentum	bacterium	chocolate	

Microorganism	Type Of Microorganism	Food or Beverage	Reference(s)
Lactobacillus fermentum	bacterium	Pecorino Romano cheese	
Lactobacillus fermentum	bacterium	sourdough bread	
Lactobacillus gasseri	bacterium	dairy	
Lactobacillus gasseri	bacterium	sourdough bread	
Lactobacillus ghanensis	bacterium	chocolate	
Lactobacillus hammesii	bacterium	sourdough bread	
Lactobacillus harbinensis	bacterium	vegetables	
Lactobacillus helveticus	bacterium	cheese	
Lactobacillus helveticus	bacterium	vegetables	
Lactobacillus hilgardii	bacterium	chocolate	
Lactobacillus hilgardii	bacterium	wine	
Lactobacillus homohiochii	bacterium	sake	
Lactobacillus homohiochii	bacterium	sourdough bread	
Lactobacillus jensenii	bacterium	bread	
Lactobacillus johnsonii	bacterium	dairy	
Lactobacillus johnsonii	bacterium	sourdough bread	
Lactobacillus kefiranofaciens	bacterium	kefir	
Lactobacillus kefiri	bacterium	kefir	
Lactobacillus kimchii	bacterium	kimchi	
Lactobacillus kisonensis	bacterium	pickle	
Lactobacillus kunkeei	bacterium	wine	
Lactobacillus mali	bacterium	cider	
Lactobacillus mali	bacterium	rum	
Lactobacillus mali	bacterium	wine	
Lactobacillus manihotivorans	bacterium	cassava	
Lactobacillus mindensis	bacterium	sourdough bread	
Lactobacillus mucosae	bacterium	sourdough bread	
Lactobacillus nagelii	bacterium	wine	
Lactobacillus namuresis	bacterium	sourdough bread	
Lactobacillus nantesis	bacterium	sourdough bread	
Lactobacillus nodensis	bacterium	dairy	
Lactobacillus oeni	bacterium	wine	
Lactobacillus otakiensis	bacterium	pickle	
Lactobacillus panis	bacterium	sourdough bread	
Lactobacillus parabrevis	bacterium	cheese	
Lactobacillus parabrevis	bacterium	kefir	
Lactobacillus parabrevis	bacterium	vegetables	
Lactobacillus parabuchneri	bacterium	sourdough bread	
Lactobacillus paracasei	bacterium	dairy	
Lactobacillus paracasei	bacterium	meat	
Lactobacillus paracasei ssp. *paracasei*	bacterium	Cacio di Fossa cheese	
Lactobacillus paracasei ssp. *paracasei*	bacterium	Canestrato Pugliese cheese	
Lactobacillus paracasei ssp. *paracasei*	bacterium	Pecorino Sardo cheese	
Lactobacillus parakefiri	bacterium	kefir	
Lactobacillus paralimentarius	bacterium	sourdough bread	

Microorganism	Type Of Microorganism	Food or Beverage	Reference(s)
Lactobacillus paraplantarum	bacterium	cheese	
Lactobacillus paraplantarum	bacterium	vegetables	
Lactobacillus pentosus	bacterium	Canestrato Pugliese cheese	
Lactobacillus pentosus	bacterium	fish	
Lactobacillus pentosus	bacterium	fruit	
Lactobacillus pentosus	bacterium	wine	
Lactobacillus perolens	bacterium	cheese	
Lactobacillus perolens	bacterium	vegetables	
Lactobacillus plantarum	bacterium	Cacio di Fossa cheese	
Lactobacillus plantarum	bacterium	Canestrato Pugliese cheese	
Lactobacillus plantarum	bacterium	chocolate	
Lactobacillus plantarum	bacterium	Idiazabal cheese	
Lactobacillus plantarum	bacterium	Manchego cheese	
Lactobacillus plantarum	bacterium	Pecorino Romano cheese	
Lactobacillus plantarum	bacterium	Roncal cheese	
Lactobacillus plantarum	bacterium	sausage	
Lactobacillus plantarum	bacterium	vegetables	
Lactobacillus pobuzihii	bacterium	fruit	
Lactobacillus pontis	bacterium	sourdough bread	
Lactobacillus rapi	bacterium	pickle	
Lactobacillus rapi	bacterium	vegetables	
Lactobacillus reuteri	bacterium	sourdough bread	
Lactobacillus rhamnosus	bacterium	Grana Padano cheese	
Lactobacillus rhamnosus	bacterium	Parmigiano-Reggiano cheese	
Lactobacillus rhamnosus	bacterium	meat	
Lactobacillus rhamnosus	bacterium	vegetables	
Lactobacillus rossiae	bacterium	sourdough bread	
Lactobacillus sakei	bacterium	sake	
Lactobacillus sakei	bacterium	sausage	
Lactobacillus salivarius	bacterium	dairy	
Lactobacillus sanfranciscensis	bacterium	sourdough bread	
Lactobacillus satsumensis	bacterium	*sh ch*	
Lactobacillus secaliphilus	bacterium	sourdough bread	
Lactobacillus senmaizukei	bacterium	pickles	
Lactobacillus siliginis	bacterium	sourdough bread	
Lactobacillus similis	bacterium	rum	
Lactobacillus spicheri	bacterium	sourdough bread	
Lactobacillus suebicus	bacterium	fruit	
Lactobacillus spp.	bacterium	butter	
Lactobacillus spp.	bacterium	olive	
Lactobacillus sunkii	bacterium	pickle	
Lactobacillus tucceti	bacterium	dairy	
Lactobacillus tucceti	bacterium	sausage	
Lactobacillus vaccinostercus	bacterium	fruit	
Lactobacillus vaccinostercus	bacterium	vegetables	

Microorganism	Type Of Microorganism	Food or Beverage	Reference(s)
Lactobacillus versmoldesis	bacterium	sausage	
Lactobacillus yamanashiensis	bacterium	cider	
Lactobacillus yamanashiensis	bacterium	wine	
Lactococcus lactis	bacterium	buttermilk	
Lactococcus lactis	bacterium	chocolate	
Lactococcus lactis ssp. *cremoris*	bacterium	Cheddar cheese	
Lactococcus lactis ssp. *lactis*	bacterium	cheese	
Lactococcus raffinolactis	bacterium	cheese	
Lactococcus spp.	bacterium	butter	
Lecanicillium lecanii	fungus	cheese	
Leuconostoc carnosum	bacterium	meat	
Leuconostoc citreum	bacterium	cheese	
Leuconostoc citreum	bacterium	fish	
Leuconostoc fallax	bacterium	sauerkraut	
Leuconostoc holzapfelii	bacterium	coffee	
Leuconostoc inhae	bacterium	kimchi	
Leuconostoc kimchii	bacterium	kimchi	
Leuconostoc lactis	bacterium	cheese	
Leuconostoc mesenteroides	bacterium	chocolate	
Leuconostoc mesenteroides	bacterium	vegetables	
Leuconostoc mesenteroides ssp. *cremoris*	bacterium	cheese	
Leuconostoc mesenteroides ssp. *cremoris*	bacterium	vegetables	
Leuconostoc mesenteroides ssp. *dextranicum*	bacterium	butter	
Leuconostoc mesenteroides ssp. *dextranicum*	bacterium	Idiazabal cheese	
Leuconostoc mesenteroides ssp. *dextranicum*	bacterium	pickle	
Leuconostoc mesenteroides ssp. *dextranicum*	bacterium	Roncal cheese	
Leuconostoc mesenteroides ssp. *mesenteroides*	bacterium	Idiazabal cheese	
Leuconostoc mesenteroides ssp. *mesenteroides*	bacterium	Roncal cheese	
Leuconostoc palmae	bacterium	palm wine	
Leuconostoc pseudomesenteroides	bacterium	butter	
Leuconostoc pseudomesenteroides	bacterium	buttermilk	
Leuconostoc pseudomesenteroides	bacterium	sour cream	
Leuconostoc spp.	bacterium	butter	
Leuconostoc spp.	bacterium	olive	
Leuconostoc spp.	bacterium	wine	
Macrococcus caseolyticus	bacterium	cheese	
Macrococcus caseolyticus	bacterium	sausage	
Microbacterium foliorum	bacterium	surface-ripened cheese	

Microorganism	Type Of Microorganism	Food or Beverage	Reference(s)
Microbacterium gubbeenense	bacterium	Limburger cheese	
Microbacterium gubbeenense	bacterium	smear-ripened cheese	
Microbacterium gubbeenense	bacterium	Tilsit cheese	
Micrococcus luteus	bacterium	cheese	
Micrococcus lylae	bacterium	sausage	
Mucor hiemalis	fungus	soy bean curd	
Mucor plumbeus	fungus	cheese	
Mucor racemosus	fungus	cheese	
Mucor racemosus	fungus	chocolate	
Neurospora intermedia	fungus	oncom	
Oenococcus oeni	bacterium	wine	
Pediococcus acidilactici	bacterium	sausage	
Pediococcus acidilactici	bacterium	vegetables	
Pediococcus pentosaceus	bacterium	sausage	
Penicillium album	fungus	farmhouse cheeses	
Penicillium camemberti	fungus	cheese	v
Penicillium caseifulvum	fungus	cheese	
Penicillium chrysogenum	fungus	cheese	
Penicillium chrysogenum	fungus	sausage	
Penicillium commune	fungus	surface-ripened cheese	
Penicillium nalgiovense	fungus	cheese	
Penicillium nalgiovense	fungus	ham	
Penicillium nalgiovense	fungus	sausage	
Penicillium roqueforti	fungus	cheese	
Penicillium solitum	fungus	meat	
Pichia fermentans	fungus	dairy	
Pichia fermentans	fungus	kefir	
Pichia fermentans	fungus	wine	
Propionibacterium acidipropionici	bacterium	cheese	
Propionibacterium freudenreichii ssp. *freudenreichii*	bacterium	dairy	
Propionibacterium freudenreichii ssp. *shermanii*	bacterium	Emmental cheese	
Propionibacterium jensenii	bacterium	cheese	
Propionibacterium thoenii	bacterium	cheese	
Proteus vulgaris	bacterium	surface-ripened cheese	
Pseudomonas fluorescens	bacterium	yogurt	
Psychrobacter celer	bacterium	cheese	
Rhizopus microsporus ssp. *oligosporus*	fungus	oncom	
Rhizopus microsporus ssp. *oligosporus*	fungus	tempeh	
Rhodosporidium infirmominiatum	fungus	cheese	
Rhodotorula glutinis	fungus	chocolate	
Rhodotorula minuta	fungus	smear-ripened cheese	
Rhodotorula rubra	fungus	chocolate	

Microorganism	Type Of Microorganism	Food or Beverage	Reference(s)
Saccharomyces bayanus	fungus	beer	
Saccharomyces bayanus	fungus	cider	
Saccharomyces bayanus	fungus	wine	
Saccharomyces carlsbergensis	fungus	lager beer	
Saccharomyces cerevisiae	fungus	ale beer	
Saccharomyces cerevisiae	fungus	bread	
Saccharomyces cerevisiae	fungus	cider	
Saccharomyces cerevisiae	fungus	cheese	
Saccharomyces cerevisiae	fungus	chocolate	
Saccharomyces cerevisiae	fungus	wine	
Saccharomyces pastorianus	fungus	lager beer	
Saccharomyces rouzii	fungus	miso	
Saccharomyces uvarum	fungus	lager beer	
Staphylococcus carnosus	bacterium	cheese	
Staphylococcus carnosus ssp. *carnosus*	bacterium	sausage	
Staphylococcus condimenti	bacterium	soy	
Staphylococcus equorum	bacterium	meat	
Staphylococcus equorum ssp. *linens*	bacterium	cheese	
Staphylococcus fleurettii	bacterium	cheese	
Staphylococcus piscifermentans	bacterium	fish	
Staphylococcus saphrophyticus	bacterium	Harzer cheese	
Staphylococcus sciuri ssp. *carnaticus*	bacterium	cheese	
Staphylococcus simulans	bacterium	sausage	
Staphylococcus succinus	bacterium	dairy	
Staphylococcus succinus	bacterium	meat	
Staphylococcus vitulinus	bacterium	cheese	
Staphylococcus vitulinus	bacterium	meat	
Staphylococcus warneri	bacterium	meat	
Staphylococcus xylosus	bacterium	cheese	
Staphylococcus xylosus	bacterium	sausage	
Streptococcus gallolyticus	bacterium	dairy	
Streptococcus salivarius	bacterium	yogurt	
Streptococcus thermophilus	bacterium	cheese	
Streptococcus thermophilus	bacterium	yogurt	
Streptomyces griseus	bacterium	meat	
Tetragenococcus halophilus	bacterium	miso	
Tetragenococcus halophilus	bacterium	soy sauce	
Tetragenococcus koreensis	bacterium	kimchi	
Torulaspora delbrueckii	fungus	smear-ripened cheese	
Torulopsis versatilis	fungus	miso	
Thrichosporon beigelii	fungus	smear-ripened cheese	
Verticillium lecanii	fungus	Tomme cheese	
Weissella beninensis	bacterium	cassava	
Weissella cibaria	bacterium	kimchi	

Microorganism	Type Of Microorganism	Food or Beverage	Reference(s)
Weissella fabaria	bacterium	chocolate	
Weissella ghanesis	bacterium	chocolate	
Weissella koreensis	bacterium	kimchi	
Weissella paramesenteroides	bacterium	sausage	
Weissella thailandensis	bacterium	fish	
Yarrowia lipolytica	fungus	Raclette cheese	
Yarrowia lipolytica	fungus	smear-ripened cheese	
Yarrowia lipolytica	fungus	dairy	
Zygotorulaspora florentina	fungus	kefir	
Zymomonas mobilis	bacterium	palm wine	
Zymomonas mobilis	bacterium	pulque	

REFERENCES

1. Madigan M; Martinko J, eds. (2006). Brock Biology of Microorganisms (13th ed.). Pearson Education. p. 1096. ISBN 0-321-73551-X.
2. Rybicki EP (1990). “The classification of organisms at the edge of life, or problems with virus systematics”. S Aft J Sci. 86: 182–6. ISSN 0038-2353.
3. Lwoff A (1956). “The concept of virus”. J. Gen. Microbiol. 17 (2): 239–53. doi:10.1099/00221287-17-2-239. PMID 13481308.
4. Wade, Nicholas (25 July 2016). “Meet Luca, the Ancestor of All Living Things”. New York Times. Retrieved 25 July 2016.
5. University of Georgia (25 August 1998). “First-Ever Scientific Estimate Of Total Bacteria On Earth Shows Far Greater Numbers Than Ever Known Before”. Science Daily. Retrieved 10 November 2014.
6. Dose, K; Bieger-Dose, A.; Dillmann, R.; Gill, M.; Kerz, O.; Klein, A.; Meinert, H.; Nawroth, T.; Risi, S.; Stridde, C. (1995). “ERA-experiment “space biochemistry””. Advances in Space Research. 16 (8): 119–129. doi:10.1016/0273-1177(95)00280-R. PMID 11542696.
7. Vaisberg, Horneck G.; Eschweiler, U.; Reitz, G.; Wehner, J.; Willimek, R.; Strauch, K. (1995). “Biological responses to space: results of the experiment “Exobiological Unit” of ERA on EURECA I”. Adv Space Res. 16 (8): 105–18. Bibcode:1995AdSpR..16..105V. doi:10.1016/0273-1177(95)00279-N. PMID 11542695.
8. Staff (2012). “The JTM Effect”. jtmnutrients.com. Archived from the original on 2012-11-14. Retrieved 10 November 2014.
9. Staff (2014). “The Biosphere”. Aspen Global Change Institute. Retrieved 10 November 2014.
10. Choi, Charles Q. (17 March 2013). “Microbes Thrive in Deepest Spot on Earth”. LiveScience. Retrieved 17 March 2013.
11. Glud, Ronnie; Wenzhöfer, Frank; Middelboe, Mathias; Oguri, Kazumasa; Turnewitsch, Robert; Canfield, Donald E.; Kitazato, Hiroshi (17 March 2013).

"High rates of microbial carbon turnover in sediments in the deepest oceanic trench on Earth". Nature Geoscience. 6 (4): 284–288. Bibcode:2013NatGe...6..284G. doi:10.1038/ngeo1773. Retrieved 17 March 2013.

12. Oskin, Becky (14 March 2013). "Intraterrestrials: Life Thrives in Ocean Floor". LiveScience. Retrieved 17 March 2013.
13. Morelle, Rebecca (15 December 2014). "Microbes discovered by deepest marine drill analysed". BBC News. Retrieved 15 December 2014.
14. Fox, Douglas (20 August 2014). "Lakes under the ice: Antarctica's secret garden". Nature. 512 (7514): 244–246. Bibcode:2014Natur.512..244F. doi:10.1038/512244a. Retrieved 21 August 2014.
15. Mack, Eric (20 August 2014). "Life Confirmed Under Antarctic Ice; Is Space Next?". Forbes. Retrieved 21 August 2014.
16. Christner BC, Morris CE, Foreman CM, Cai R, Sands DC (2008). "Ubiquity of biological ice nucleators in snowfall". Science. 319 (5867): 1214. Bibcode:2008Sci...319.1214C. doi:10.1126/science.1149757. PMID 18309078.
17. 2002 WHO mortality data Accessed 20 January 2007
18. Schopf J (2006). "Fossil evidence of Archaean life". Philos Trans R Soc Lond B Biol Sci. 361 (1470): 869–85. doi:10.1098/rstb.2006.1834. PMC 1578735 . PMID 16754604.
19. Altermann W, Kazmierczak J (2003). "Archean microfossils: a reappraisal of early life on Earth". Res Microbiol. 154 (9): 611–7. doi:10.1016/j.resmic.2003.08.006. PMID 14596897.
20. Cavalier-Smith T (2006). "Cell evolution and Earth history: stasis and revolution". Philos Trans R Soc Lond B Biol Sci. 361 (1470): 969–1006. doi:10.1098/rstb.2006.1842. PMC 1578732 . PMID 16754610.
21. Schopf J (1994). "Disparate rates, differing fates: tempo and mode of evolution changed from the Precambrian to the Phanerozoic". Proc Natl Acad Sci USA. 91 (15): 6735–42. Bibcode:1994PNAS...91.6735S. doi:10.1073/pnas.91.15.6735. PMC 44277 . PMID 8041691.
22. Stanley S (May 1973). "An Ecological Theory for the Sudden Origin of Multicellular Life in the Late Precambrian". Proc Natl Acad Sci USA. 70 (5): 1486–9. Bibcode:1973PNAS...70.1486S. doi:10.1073/pnas.70.5.1486. PMC 433525 . PMID 16592084.
23. DeLong E, Pace N (2001). "Environmental diversity of bacteria and archaea". Syst Biol. 50 (4): 470–8. doi:10.1080/106351501750435040. PMID 12116647.
24. Schmidt A, Ragazzi E, Coppellotti O, Roghi G (2006). "A microworld in Triassic amber". Nature. 444 (7121): 835. Bibcode:2006Natur.444..835S. doi:10.1038/444835a. PMID 17167469.
25. Schirber, Michael (July 27, 2014). "Microbe's Innovation May Have Started Largest Extinction Event on Earth". Space.com. Astrobiology Magazine. .... That spike in nickel allowed methanogens to take off.
26. Wolska K (2003). "Horizontal DNA transfer between bacteria in the environment".

Acta Microbiol Pol. 52 (3): 233–43. PMID 14743976.

27. Enright M, Robinson D, Randle G, Feil E, Grundmann H, Spratt B (May 2002). "The evolutionary history of methicillin-resistant Staphylococcus aureus (MRSA)". Proc Natl Acad Sci USA. 99 (11): 7687–92. Bibcode:2002PNAS...99.7687E. doi:10.1073/pnas.122108599. PMC 124322 . PMID 12032344.
28. Mahavira is dated 599 BCE - 527 BCE. See. Dundas, Paul; John Hinnels, eds. (2002). The Jains. London: Routledge. ISBN 0-415-26606-8. p. 24
29. Dundas, Paul (2002) p. 88
30. Jaini, Padmanabh (1998). The Jaina Path of Purification. New Delhi: Motilal Banarsidass. ISBN 81-208-1578-5. p. 109
31. Varro On Agriculture 1,xii Loeb
32. Tschanz, David W. "Arab Roots of European Medicine". Heart Views. 4 (2). Archived from the original on 3 May 2011.
33. Colgan, Richard (2009). Advice to the Young Physician: On the Art of Medicine. Springer. p. 33. ISBN 978-1-4419-1033-2.
34. Payne, A.S. The Cleere Observer: A Biography of Antoni Van Leeuwenhoek, p. 13, Macmillan, 1970
35. Leeuwenhoek A (1753). "Part of a Letter from Mr Antony van Leeuwenhoek, concerning the Worms in Sheeps Livers, Gnats, and Animalcula in the Excrements of Frogs". Philosophical Transactions (1683–1775). 22 (260–276): 509–18. doi:10.1098/rstl.1700.0013.
36. Leeuwenhoek A (1753). "Part of a Letter from Mr Antony van Leeuwenhoek, F. R. S. concerning Green Weeds Growing in Water, and Some Animalcula Found about Them". Philosophical Transactions (1683–1775). 23 (277–288): 1304–11. doi:10.1098/rstl.1702.0042.
37. The Nobel Prize in Physiology or Medicine 1905Nobelprize.org Accessed 22 November 2006.
38. O'Brien S, Goedert J (1996). "HIV causes AIDS: Koch's postulates fulfilled". Curr Opin Immunol. 8 (5): 613–18. doi:10.1016/S0952-7915(96)80075-6. PMID 8902385.
39. Borenstein, Seth (13 November 2013). "Oldest fossil found: Meet your microbial mom". Associated Press. Retrieved 15 November 2013.
40. Noffke, Nora; Christian, Christian; Wacey, David; Hazen, Robert M. (8 November 2013). "Microbially Induced Sedimentary Structures Recording an Ancient Ecosystem in the ca. 3.48 Billion-Year-Old Dresser Formation, Pilbara, Western Australia". Astrobiology (journal). 13 (12): 1103–24. doi:10.1089/ast.2013.1030. PMC 3870916 . PMID 24205812. Retrieved 15 November 2013.
41. Ciccarelli FD, Doerks T, von Mering C, Creevey CJ, Snel B, Bork P (2006). "Toward automatic reconstruction of a highly resolved tree of life". Science. 311 (5765): 1283–7. Bibcode:2006Sci...311.1283C. doi:10.1126/science.1123061. PMID 16513982.
42. Gold T (1992). "The deep, hot biosphere". Proc. Natl. Acad. Sci. U.S.A. 89

(13): 6045–9. Bibcode:1992PNAS...89.6045G. doi:10.1073/pnas.89.13.6045. PMC 49434 . PMID 1631089.

43. Whitman W, Coleman D, Wiebe W (1998). "Prokaryotes: The unseen majority". Proc Natl Acad Sci USA. 95 (12): 6578–83. Bibcode:1998PNAS...95.6578W. doi:10.1073/pnas.95.12.6578. PMC 33863 . PMID 9618454.
44. Staff (2 May 2016). "Researchers find that Earth may be home to 1 trillion species". National Science Foundation. Retrieved 6 May 2016.
45. Schulz H, Jorgensen B (2001). "Big bacteria". Annu Rev Microbiol. 55: 105–37. doi:10.1146/annurev.micro.55.1.105. PMID 11544351.
46. Shapiro JA (1998). "Thinking about bacterial populations as multicellular organisms" (PDF). Annu. Rev. Microbiol. 52: 81–104. doi:10.1146/annurev.micro.52.1.81. PMID 9891794. Archived from the original (PDF) on 17 July 2011.
47. Johnsborg O, Eldholm V, Håvarstein LS (December 2007). "Natural genetic transformation: prevalence, mechanisms and function". Res. Microbiol. 158 (10): 767–78. doi:10.1016/j.resmic.2007.09.004. PMID 17997281.
48. Transformation (genetics)
49. Eagon R (1962). "PSEUDOMONAS NATRIEGENS, A MARINE BACTERIUM WITH A GENERATION TIME OF LESS THAN 10 MINUTES". J Bacteriol. 83 (4): 736–7. PMC 279347 . PMID 13888946.
50. Woese C, Kandler O, Wheelis M (1990). "Towards a natural system of organisms: proposal for the domains Archaea, Bacteria, and Eucarya". Proc Natl Acad Sci USA. 87 (12): 4576–9. Bibcode:1990PNAS...87.4576W. doi:10.1073/pnas.87.12.4576. PMC 54159 . PMID 2112744.
51. De Rosa M, Gambacorta A, Gliozzi A (1 March 1986). "Structure, biosynthesis, and physicochemical properties of archaebacterial lipids". Microbiol. Rev. 50 (1): 70–80. PMC 373054 . PMID 3083222.
52. Robertson C, Harris J, Spear J, Pace N (2005). "Phylogenetic diversity and ecology of environmental Archaea". Curr Opin Microbiol. 8 (6): 638–42. doi:10.1016/j.mib.2005.10.003. PMID 16236543.
53. Karner MB, DeLong EF, Karl DM (2001). "Archaeal dominance in the mesopelagic zone of the Pacific Ocean". Nature. 409 (6819): 507–10. doi:10.1038/35054051. PMID 11206545.
54. Sinninghe Damsté JS, Rijpstra WI, Hopmans EC, Prahl FG, Wakeham SG, Schouten S (June 2002). "Distribution of Membrane Lipids of Planktonic Crenarchaeota in the Arabian Sea". Appl. Environ. Microbiol. 68 (6): 2997–3002. doi:10.1128/AEM.68.6.2997-3002.2002. PMC 123986 . PMID 12039760.
55. Leininger, S.; Urich, T.; Schloter, M.; Schwark, L.; Qi, J.; Nicol, G. W.; Prosser, J. I.; Schuster, S. C.; Schleper, C. (2006). "Archaea predominate among ammonia-oxidizing prokaryotes in soils". Nature. 442 (7104): 806–809. Bibcode:2006Natur.442..806L. doi:10.1038/nature04983. PMID 16915287.
56. Eukaryota: More on Morphology. (Retrieved 10 October 2006)
57. Dyall S, Brown M, Johnson P (2004). "Ancient invasions: from endosymbionts

to organelles". Science. 304 (5668): 253–7. Bibcode:2004Sci...304..253D. doi:10.1126/science.1094884. PMID 15073369.

58. See coenocyte.
59. Bernstein, H; Bernstein, C; Michod, RE (2012). "Chapter 1". In Kimura, Sakura; Shimizu, Sora. DNA repair as the primary adaptive function of sex in bacteria and eukaryotes. DNA Repair: New Research. Hauppauge, N.Y.: Nova Sci. Publ. pp. 1–49. ISBN 978-1-62100-808-8.
60. Cavalier-Smith T (1 December 1993). "Kingdom protozoa and its 18 phyla". Microbiol. Rev. 57 (4): 953–94. PMC 372943 . PMID 8302218.
61. Corliss JO (1992). "Should there be a separate code of nomenclature for the protists?". BioSystems. 28 (1–3): 1–14. doi:10.1016/0303-2647(92)90003-H. PMID 1292654.
62. Devreotes P (1989). "Dictyostelium discoideum: a model system for cell-cell interactions in development". Science. 245 (4922): 1054–8. Bibcode:1989Sci...245.1054D. doi:10.1126/science.2672337. PMID 2672337.
63. Slapeta J, Moreira D, López-García P (2005). "The extent of protist diversity: insights from molecular ecology of freshwater eukaryotes". Proc. Biol. Sci. 272 (1576): 2073–81. doi:10.1098/rspb.2005.3195. PMC 1559898 . PMID 16191619.
64. Moreira D, López-García P (2002). "The molecular ecology of microbial eukaryotes unveils a hidden world" (PDF). Trends Microbiol. 10 (1): 31–8. doi:10.1016/S0966-842X(01)02257-0. PMID 11755083.
65. Lapinski J, Tunnacliffe A (2003). "Anhydrobiosis without trehalose in bdelloid rotifers". FEBS Lett. 553 (3): 387–90. doi:10.1016/S0014-5793(03)01062-7. PMID 14572656.
66. Kumamoto CA, Vinces MD (2005). "Contributions of hyphae and hypha-co-regulated genes to Candida albicans virulence". Cell. Microbiol. 7 (11): 1546–54. doi:10.1111/j.1462-5822.2005.00616.x. PMID 16207242.
67. Thomas, David C. (2002). Seaweeds. London: Natural History Museum. ISBN 0-565-09175-1.
68. Szewzyk U, Szewzyk R, Stenström T (1994). "Thermophilic, anaerobic bacteria isolated from a deep borehole in granite in Sweden". Proc Natl Acad Sci USA. 91 (5): 1810–3. Bibcode:1994PNAS...91.1810S. doi:10.1073/pnas.91.5.1810. PMC 43253 . PMID 11607462.
69. Horneck G (1981). "Survival of microorganisms in space: a review". Adv Space Res. 1 (14): 39–48. doi:10.1016/0273-1177(81)90241-6. PMID 11541716.
70. Strain 121, a hyperthermophilic archaea, has been shown to reproduce at 121 °C (250 °F), and survive at 130 °C (266 °F).
71. Some Psychrophilic bacteria can grow at −17 °C (1 °F), and can survive near absolute zero.
72. Picrophilus can grow at pH -0.06.
73. The alkaliphilic bacteria Bacillus alcalophilus can grow at up to pH 11.5.

74. Dyall-Smith, Mike, HALOARCHAEA, University of Melbourne. Haloarchaea.

75. The piezophilic bacteria Halomonas salaria requires a pressure of 1,000 atm; nanobes, a speculative organism, have been reportedly found in the earth's crust at 2,000 atm.

76. See Deinococcus radiodurans

77. Cavicchioli R (2002). "Extremophiles and the search for extraterrestrial life". Astrobiology. 2 (3): 281–92. Bibcode:2002AsBio...2..281C. doi:10.1089/153110702762027862. PMID 12530238.

78. Barea J, Pozo M, Azcón R, Azcón-Aguilar C (2005). "Microbial co-operation in the rhizosphere". J Exp Bot. 56 (417): 1761–78. doi:10.1093/jxb/eri197. PMID 15911555.

79. Gillen, Alan L. (2007). The Genesis of Germs: The Origin of Diseases and the Coming Plagues. New Leaf Publishing Group. p. 10. ISBN 0-89051-493-3.

80. Vrieze, Jop de (2015-08-14). "The littlest farmhands". Science. 349 (6249): 680–683. doi:10.1126/science.349.6249.680. ISSN 0036-8075. PMID 26273035.

81. "Dairy Microbiology". University of Guelph. Retrieved 9 October 2006.

82. Gray, N.F. (2004). Biology of Wastewater Treatment. Imperial College Press. p. 1164. ISBN 1-86094-332-2.

83. Kitani, Osumu; Carl W. Hall (1989). Biomass Handbook. Taylor & Francis US. p. 256. ISBN 2-88124-269-3.

84. Pimental, David (2007). Food, Energy, and Society. CRC Press. p. 289. ISBN 1-4200-4667-5.

85. Tickell, Joshua; et al. (2000). From the Fryer to the Fuel Tank: The Complete Guide to Using Vegetable Oil as an Alternative Fuel. Biodiesel America. p. 53. ISBN 0-9707227-0-2.

86. Inslee, Jay; et al. (2008). Apollo's Fire: Igniting America's Clean Energy Economy. Island Press. p. 157. ISBN 1-59726-175-0.

87. Biology textbook for class XII. National council of educational research and training. p. 183. ISBN 81-7450-639-X.

88. Castrillo JI, Oliver SG (2004). "Yeast as a touchstone in post-genomic research: strategies for integrative analysis in functional genomics". J. Biochem. Mol. Biol. 37 (1): 93–106. doi:10.5483/BMBRep.2004.37.1.093. PMID 14761307.

89. Suter B, Auerbach D, Stagljar I (2006). "Yeast-based functional genomics and proteomics technologies: the first 15 years and beyond". BioTechniques. 40 (5): 625–44. doi:10.2144/000112151. PMID 16708762.

90. Sunnerhagen P (2002). "Prospects for functional genomics in Schizosaccharomyces pombe". Curr. Genet. 42 (2): 73–84. doi:10.1007/s00294-002-0335-6. PMID 12478386.

91. Soni, S.K. (2007). Microbes: A Source of Energy for 21st Century. New India Publishing. ISBN 81-89422-14-6.

92. Moses, Vivian; et al. (1999). Biotechnology: The Science and the Business. CRC Press. p. 563. ISBN 90-5702-407-1.
93. Langford, Roland E. (2004). Introduction to Weapons of Mass Destruction: Radiological, Chemical, and Biological. Wiley-IEEE. p. 140. ISBN 0-471-46560-7.
94. O'Hara A, Shanahan F (2006). "The gut flora as a forgotten organ". EMBO Rep. 7 (7): 688–93. doi:10.1038/sj.embor.7400731. PMC 1500832 . PMID 16819463.
95. Eckburg P, Lepp P, Relman D (2003). "Archaea and Their Potential Role in Human Disease". Infect Immun. 71 (2): 591–6. doi:10.1128/IAI.71.2.591-596.2003. PMC 145348 . PMID 12540534.
96. Lepp P, Brinig M, Ouverney C, Palm K, Armitage G, Relman D (2004). "Methanogenic Archaea and human periodontal disease". Proc Natl Acad Sci USA. 101 (16): 6176–81. Bibcode:2004PNAS..101.6176L. doi:10.1073/pnas.0308766101. PMC 395942 . PMID 15067114.

CHAPTER 3

The Microbiology of Food Preservation

Chapter Contents

- **Introduction**
- **Traditional Techniques**
- **Smoking**
- **Curing**
- **ssssIndustrial/Modern Techniques**

Food preservation is the science of extending the shelf life of food while maintaining as much as possible of its nutritional quality and avoiding the growth of unwanted micro-organisms. There are a number of different ways of preserving foods. Some involve storage methods, some involve packaging, and some involve treating the food in particular ways prior to or during storage, either cooking it in whole or part or combining it with other foods or substances. This science has been practiced in a variety of ways for hundreds of years.

INTRODUCTION

Food preservation involves preventing the growth of bacteria, fungi (such as yeasts), or other micro-organisms (although some methods work by introducing benign bacteria or fungi to the food), as well as slowing the oxidation of fats that cause rancidity. Food preservation may also include processes that inhibit visual deterioration, such as the enzymatic browning reaction in apples after they are cut during food preparation.

Many processes designed to preserve food will involve a number of food preservation methods. Preserving fruit by turning it into jam, for example, involves boiling (to reduce the fruit's moisture content and to kill bacteria, etc.), sugaring (to prevent their re-growth) and sealing within an airtight jar (to prevent recontamination). Some traditional methods of preserving food have been shown to have a lower energy input and carbon footprint, when compared to modern methods.

Some methods of food preservation are known to create carcinogens. In 2015, the International Agency for Research on Cancer of the World Health Organization (WHO) classified processed meat, i.e. meat that has undergone salting, curing, fermenting, and smoking, as "carcinogenic to humans".

Maintaining or creating nutritional value, texture and flavor is an important aspect of food preservation, although, historically, some methods drastically altered the character of the food being preserved. In many cases these changes have come to be seen as desirable qualities – cheese, yogurt and pickled onions being common examples.

TRADITIONAL TECHNIQUES

New techniques of food preservation became available to the home chef from the dawn of agriculture until the Industrial Revolution.

Drying

Drying is one of the oldest techniques used to hamper the decomposition of food products. As early as 12,000 B.C., Middle Eastern and Oriental cultures were drying foods using the power of the sun. Vegetables and fruits are naturally dried by the sun and wind, but "still houses" were built in areas that did not have enough sunlight to dry things. A fire would be built inside the building to provide the heat to dry the various fruits, vegetables, and herbs.

Cooling

Cooling preserves food by slowing down the growth and reproduction of microorganisms and the action of enzymes that cause food to rot. The introduction of commercial and domestic refrigerators drastically improved the diets of many in the Western world by allowing foods such as fresh fruit, salads and dairy products to be stored safely for longer periods, particularly during warm weather.

Before the era of mechanical refrigeration, cooling for food storage occurred in the forms of root cellars and iceboxes. Rural people often did their own ice cutting, whereas town and city dwellers often relied on the ice trade. Today, root cellaring remains popular among people who value various goals, including local food, heirloom crops, traditional home cooking techniques, family farming, frugality, self-sufficiency, organic farming, and others.

Freezing

Freezing is also one of the most commonly used processes, both commercially and domestically, for preserving a very wide range of foods, including prepared foods that would not have required freezing in their unprepared state. For example, potato waffles are stored in the freezer, but potatoes themselves require only a cool dark place to ensure many months' storage. Cold stores provide large-volume, long-term storage for strategic food stocks held in case of national emergency in many countries.

Boiling

Boiling liquid food items can kill any existing microbes. Milk and water are often boiled to kill any harmful microbes that may be present in them.

Heating

Heating to temperatures which are sufficient to kill microorganisms inside the food is a method used with perpetual stews. Milk is also boiled before storing to kill many microorganisms.

Salting

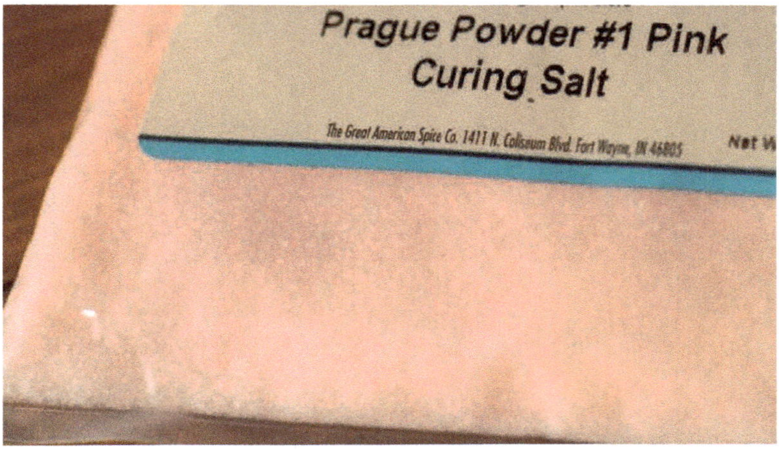

Bag of Prague powder #1, also known as "curing salt" or "pink salt". It is typically a combination of salt and sodium nitrite, with the pink color added to distinguish it from ordinary salt.

Salting or curing draws moisture from a substance through a process of osmosis. substances are cured with salt or sugar, or a combination of the two. Nitrates and nitrites are also often used to cure meat and contribute the characteristic pink colour. It was a main method of preservation in medieval times and around the 1700s.

Sugaring

The earliest cultures have used sugar as a preservative, and it was commonplace to store fruit in honey. Similar to pickled foods, sugar cane was brought to Europe through the trade routes. In northern climates without sufficient sun to dry foods, preserves are made by heating the fruit with sugar. "Sugar tends to draw water from the microbes (plasmolysis). This process leaves the microbial cells dehydrated, thus killing them. In this way, the food will remain safe from microbial spoilage." Sugar is used to preserve fruits, either in an anti-microbial syrup with fruit such as apples, pears, peaches, apricots and plums, or in crystallized form where the preserved material is cooked in sugar to the point of crystallization and the resultant product is then stored dry. This method is used for the skins of citrus fruit (candied peel), angelica and ginger. Also sugaring can be used in jam jellies.

SMOKING

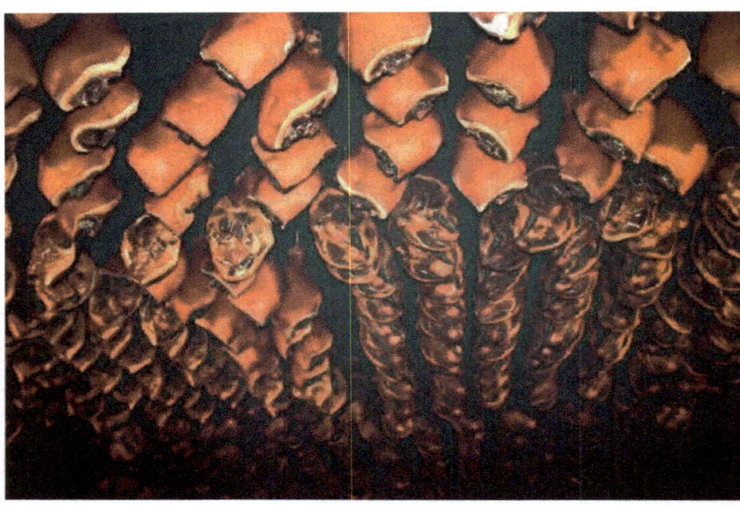

Smoked ham in a smokehouse in Schleswig-Holstein, Germany

Smoking is used to lengthen the shelf life of perishable food items. This effect is achieved by exposing the food to smoke from burning plant materials such as wood. Smoke deposits a number of pyrolysis products onto the food, including the phenols syringol, guaiacol and catechol.These compounds aid in the drying and preservation of meats and other foods. Most commonly subjected to this method of food preservation are meats and fish that have undergone curing. Fruits and vegetables like paprika, cheeses, spices, and ingredients for making drinks such as malt and tea leaves are also smoked, but mainly for cooking or flavoring them. It is one of the oldest food preservation methods, which probably arose after the development of cooking with fire.

Pickling

Pickling is a method of preserving food in an edible anti-microbial liquid. Pickling can be broadly classified into two categories: chemical pickling and fermentation pickling.

In chemical pickling, the food is placed in an edible liquid that inhibits or kills bacteria and other micro-organisms. Typical pickling agents include brine (high in salt), vinegar, alcohol, and vegetable oil, especially olive oil but also many other oils. Many chemical pickling processes also involve heating or boiling so that the food being preserved becomes saturated with the pickling agent. Common chemically pickled foods include cucumbers, peppers, corned beef, herring, and eggs, as well as mixed vegetables such as piccalilli.

In fermentation pickling, the food itself produces the preservation agent, typically by a process that produces lactic acid. Fermented pickles include sauerkraut, nukazuke, kimchi, surströmming,

Lye

Sodium hydroxide (lye) makes food too alkaline for bacterial growth. Lye will saponify fats in the food, which will change its flavor and texture. Lutefisk uses lye in its preparation, as do some olive recipes. Modern recipes for century eggs also call for lye.

Canning

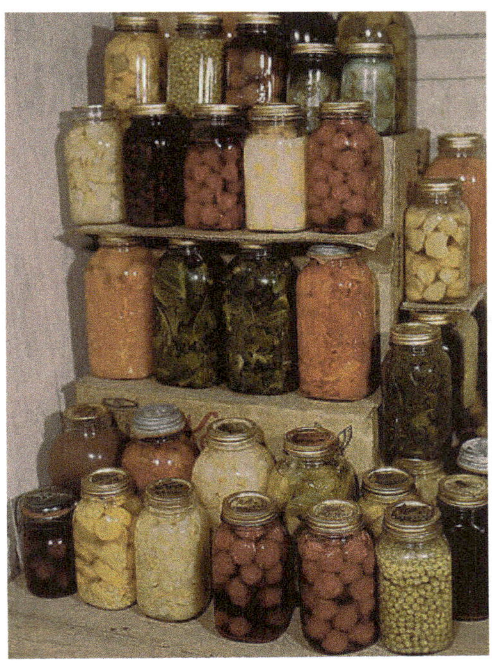

Preserved Food

Canning involves cooking food, sealing it in sterile cans or jars, and boiling the containers to kill or weaken any remaining bacteria as a form of sterilization. It was invented by the French confectioner Nicolas Appert. By 1806, this process was used by the French Navy to preserve meat, fruit, vegetables, and even milk. Although Appert had discovered a new way of preservation, it wasn't understood until 1864 when Louis Pasteur found the relationship between microorganisms, food spoilage, and illness.

Foods have varying degrees of natural protection against spoilage and may require that the final step occur in a pressure cooker. High-acid fruits like strawberries require no preservatives to can and only a short boiling cycle, whereas marginal vegetables such as carrots require longer boiling and addition of other acidic elements. Low-acid foods, such as vegetables and meats, require pressure canning. Food preserved by canning or bottling is at immediate risk of spoilage once the can or bottle has been opened.

Lack of quality control in the canning process may allow ingress of water or micro-organisms. Most such failures are rapidly detected as decomposition within the can causes gas production and the can will swell or burst. However, there have been examples of poor manufacture (underprocessing) and poor hygiene allowing contamination of canned food by the obligate anaerobe *Clostridium botulinum*, which produces an acute toxin within the food, leading to severe illness or death. This organism produces no gas or obvious taste and remains undetected by taste or smell. Its toxin is denatured by cooking, however. Cooked mushrooms, handled poorly and then canned, can support the growth of Staphylococcus aureus, which produces a toxin that is not destroyed by canning or subsequent reheating.

Jellying

Food may be preserved by cooking in a material that solidifies to form a gel. Such materials include gelatin, agar, maize flour, and arrowroot flour. Some foods naturally form a protein gel when cooked, such as eels and elvers, and sipunculid worms, which are a delicacy in Xiamen, in the Fujian province of the People's Republic of China. Jellied eels are a delicacy in the East End of London, where they are eaten with mashed potatoes. Potted meats in aspic (a gel made from gelatine and clarified meat broth) were a common way of serving meat off-cuts in the UK until the 1950s. Many jugged meats are also jellied.

A traditional British way of preserving meat (particularly shrimp) is by setting it in a pot and sealing it with a layer of fat. Also common is potted chicken liver; compare pâté.

Jugging

Meat can be preserved by jugging. Jugging is the process of stewing the meat (commonly game or fish) in a covered earthenware jug or casserole. The animal to be jugged is usually cut into pieces, placed into a tightly-sealed jug with brine or gravy, and stewed. Red wine and/or the animal's own blood is sometimes added to the cooking liquid. Jugging was a popular method of preserving meat up until the middle of the 20th century.

Burial

Burial of food can preserve it due to a variety of factors: lack of light, lack of oxygen, cool temperatures, pH level, or desiccants in the soil. Burial may be combined with other methods such as salting or fermentation. Most foods can be preserved in soil that is very dry and salty (thus a desiccant) such as sand, or soil that is frozen.

Many root vegetables are very resistant to spoilage and require no other preservation than storage in cool dark conditions, for example by burial in the ground, such as in a storage clamp. Century eggs are created by placing eggs in alkaline mud (or other alkaline substance), resulting in their "inorganic" fermentation through raised pH instead of spoiling. The fermentation preserves them and breaks down some of the complex, less flavorful proteins and fats into simpler, more flavorful ones. Cabbage was traditionally buried in the fall in northern farms in the U.S. for preservation. Some methods keep it crispy while other methods produce sauerkraut. A similar process is used in the traditional production of kimchi. Sometimes meat is buried under conditions that cause preservation. If buried on hot coals or ashes, the heat can kill pathogens, the dry ash can desiccate, and the earth can block oxygen and further contamination. If buried where the earth is very cold, the earth acts like a refrigerator.

In Orissa, India, it is practical to store rice by burying it underground. This method helps to store for three to six months during the dry season.

CURING

The earliest form of curing was dehydration. To accelerate this process, salt is usually added. In the culinary world, it was common to choose raw salts from various sources (rock salt, sea salt, etc.). More modern "examples of salts that are used as preservatives include sodium chloride (NaCl), sodium nitrate ($NaNO_3$) and sodium nitrite ($NaNO_2$). Even at mild concentrations (up to 2%), sodium chloride, found in many food products, is capable of neutralizing the antimicrobial character of natural compounds."

Fermentation

Some foods, such as many cheeses, wines, and beers, use specific micro-organisms that combat spoilage from other less-benign organisms. These micro-organisms keep pathogens in check by creating an environment toxic for themselves and other micro-organisms by producing acid or alcohol. Methods of fermentation include, but are not limited to, starter micro-organisms, salt, hops, controlled (usually cool) temperatures and controlled (usually low) levels of oxygen. These methods are used to create the specific controlled conditions that will support the desirable organisms that produce food fit for human consumption.

Fermentation is the microbial conversion of starch and sugars into alcohol. Not only can fermentation produce alcohol, but it can also be a valuable preservation technique. Fermentation can also make foods more nutritious and palatable. For example, drinking water in the Middle Ages was dangerous because it often contained pathogens that could spread disease. When the water is made into beer, the boiling during the brewing process kills any bacteria in the water that could make people sick. Additionally, the water now has the nutrients from the barley and other ingredients, and the microorganisms can also produce vitamins as they ferment.

INDUSTRIAL/MODERN TECHNIQUES

Techniques of food preservation were developed in research laboratories for commercial applications.

Pasteurization

Pasteurization is a process for preservation of liquid food. It was originally applied to combat the souring of young local wines. Today, the process is mainly applied to daily products. In this method, milk is heated at about 70 °C for 15 to 30 seconds to kill the bacteria present in it and cooling it quickly to 10 °C to prevent the remaining bacteria from growing. The milk is then stored in sterilized bottles or pouches in cold places. This method was invented by Louis Pasteur, a French chemist, in 1862.

Vacuum Packing

Vacuum-packing stores food in a vacuum environment, usually in an air-tight bag or bottle. The vacuum environment strips bacteria of oxygen needed for survival. Vacuum-packing is commonly used for storing nuts to reduce loss of flavor from oxidization. A major drawback to vacuum packaging, at the consumer level, is that vacuum sealing can deform contents and rob certain foods, such as cheese, of its flavor.

Artificial Food Additives

Preservative food additives can be *antimicrobial*, which inhibit the growth of bacteria or fungi, including mold, or *antioxidant*, such as oxygen absorbers, which inhibit the oxidation of food constituents. Common antimicrobial preservatives include calcium propionate, sodium nitrate, sodium nitrite, sulfites (sulfur dioxide, sodium bisulfite, potassium hydrogen sulfite, etc.) and disodium EDTA. Antioxidants include BHA and BHT. Other preservatives include formaldehyde (usually in solution), glutaraldehyde (kills insects), ethanol, and methylchloroisothiazolinone.

Radiation

Irradiation of food is the exposure of food to ionizing radiation. The two types of ionizing radiation used are beta particles (high-energy electrons) and gamma rays (emitted from radioactive sources as cobalt-60 or cesium-137). Treatment effects include killing bacteria, molds, and insect pests, reducing the ripening and spoiling of fruits, and at higher doses inducing sterility. The technology may be compared to pasteurization; it is sometimes called “cold pasteurization”, as the product is not heated.

The irradiation process is not directly related to nuclear energy, but does use radioactive isotopes produced in nuclear reactors. Cobalt-60, for example does not occur naturally and can only be produced through neutron bombardment of cobalt-59. Ionizing radiation at high energy levels is hazardous to life (hence its usefulness in sterilisation); for this reason, irradiation facilities have a heavily shielded irradiation room where the process takes place. Radiation safety procedures are used to ensure that neither the workers in such facilities nor the environment receives any radiation dose above administrative limits. Irradiated food does not and cannot become radioactive, and national and international expert bodies have declared food irradiation as wholesome. However, the wholesomeness of consuming such food is disputed by opponents and consumer organizations. National and international expert bodies have declared food irradiation as "wholesome"; organizations of the United Nations, such as the World Health Organization and Food and Agriculture Organization, endorse food irradiation. International legislation on whether food may be irradiated or not varies worldwide from no regulation to full banning. Irradiation may allow lower-quality or contaminated foods to be rendered marketable.

Approximately 500,000 tons of food items are irradiated per year worldwide in over 40 countries. These are mainly spices and condiments with an increasing segment of fresh fruit irradiated for fruit fly quarantine.

Pulsed Electric Field Electroporation

Pulsed electric field (PEF) electroporation is a method for processing cells by means of brief pulses of a strong electric field. PEF holds potential as a type of low-temperature alternative pasteurization process for sterilizing food products. In PEF processing, a substance is placed between two electrodes, then the pulsed electric field is applied. The electric field enlarges the pores of the cell membranes, which kills the cells and releases their contents. PEF for food processing is a developing technology still being researched. There have been limited industrial applications of PEF processing for the pasteurization of fruit juices. To date, several PEF treated juices are available on the market in Europe. Furthermore, for several years a juice pasteurization application in the US has used PEF. For cell disintegration purposes especially potato processors show great interest in PEF technology as an efficient alternative for their preheaters. Potato applications are already operational in the US and Canada. There are also commercial PEF potato applications in various countries in Europe, as well as in Australia, India and China.

Modified Atmosphere

Modifying atmosphere is a way to preserve food by operating on the atmosphere around it. Salad crops that are notoriously difficult to preserve are now being packaged in sealed bags with an atmosphere modified to reduce the oxygen (O_2) concentration and increase the carbon dioxide (CO_2) concentration. There is concern that, although salad vegetables retain their appearance and texture in such conditions, this method of preservation may not retain nutrients, especially vitamins. There are two methods for preserving grains with carbon dioxide. One method is placing a block of dry ice in the bottom and filling the can with the grain. Another method is purging the container from the bottom by gaseous carbon dioxide from a cylinder or bulk supply vessel.

Carbon dioxide prevents insects and, depending on concentration, mold and oxidation from damaging the grain. Grain stored in this way can remain edible for approximately five years.

Nitrogen gas (N_2) at concentrations of 98% or higher is also used effectively to kill insects in the grain through hypoxia. However, carbon dioxide has an advantage in this respect, as it kills organisms through hypercarbia and hypoxia (depending on concentration), but it requires concentrations of above 35%, or so. This makes carbon dioxide preferable for fumigation in situations where a hermetic seal cannot be maintained.

Controlled Atmospheric Storage (CA): "CA storage is a non-chemical process. Oxygen levels in the sealed rooms are reduced, usually by the infusion of nitrogen gas, from the approximate 21 percent in the air we breathe to 1 percent or 2 percent. Temperatures are kept at a constant 0 to 2 °C (32 to 36 °F). Humidity is maintained at 95 percent and carbon dioxide levels are also controlled. Exact conditions in the rooms are set according to the apple variety. Researchers develop specific regimens for each variety to achieve the best quality. Computers help keep conditions constant." "Eastern Washington, where most of Washington's apples are grown, has enough warehouse storage for 181 million boxes of fruit, according to a report done in 1997 by managers for the Washington State Department of Agriculture Plant Services Division. The storage capacity study shows that 67 percent of that space —enough for 121,008,000 boxes of apples — is CA storage."

Air-tight storage of grains (sometimes called hermetic storage) relies on the respiration of grain, insects, and fungi that can modify the enclosed atmosphere sufficiently to control insect pests. This is a method of great antiquity, as well as having modern equivalents. The success of the method relies on having the correct mix of sealing, grain moisture, and temperature.

A patented process uses fuel cells to exhaust and automatically maintain the exhaustion of oxygen in a shipping container, containing, for example, fresh fish.

Nonthermal Plasma

This process subjects the surface of food to a "flame" of ionized gas molecules, such as helium or nitrogen. This causes micro-organisms to die off on the surface.

High-Pressure Food Preservation

High-pressure food preservation or pascalization refers to the use of a food preservation technique that makes use of high pressure. "Pressed inside a vessel exerting 70,000 pounds per square inch (480 MPa) or more, food can be processed so that it retains its fresh appearance, flavor, texture and nutrients while disabling harmful microorganisms and slowing spoilage." By 2005, the process was being used for products ranging from orange juice to guacamole to deli meats and widely sold.

Biopreservation

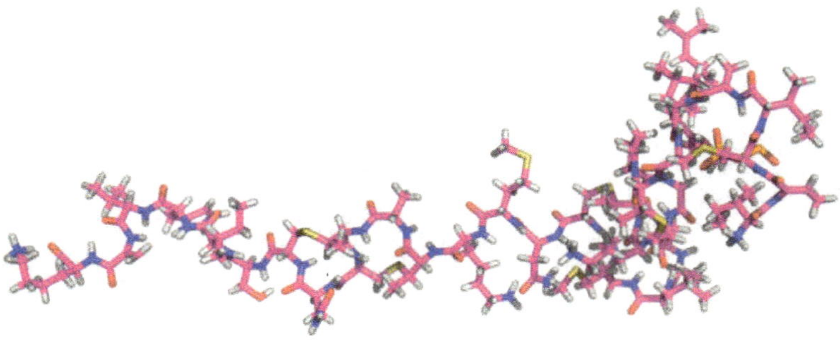

3D stick model of nisin. Some lactic acid bacteria manufacture nisin. It is a particularly effective preservative.

Biopreservation is the use of natural or controlled microbiota or antimicrobials as a way of preserving food and extending its shelf life. Beneficial bacteria or the fermentation products produced by these bacteria are used in biopreservation to control spoilage and render pathogens inactive in food. It is a benign ecological approach which is gaining increasing attention.

Of special interest are lactic acid bacteria (LAB). Lactic acid bacteria have antagonistic properties that make them particularly useful as biopreservatives. When LABs compete for nutrients, their metabolites often include active antimicrobials such as lactic acid, acetic acid, hydrogen peroxide, and peptide bacteriocins. Some LABs produce the antimicrobial nisin, which is a particularly effective preservative.

These days, LAB bacteriocins are used as an integral part of hurdle technology. Using them in combination with other preservative techniques can effectively control spoilage bacteria and other pathogens, and can inhibit the activities of a wide spectrum of organisms, including inherently resistant Gram-negative bacteria.

Hurdle Technology

Hurdle technology is a method of ensuring that pathogens in food products can be eliminated or controlled by combining more than one approach. These approaches can be thought of as "hurdles" the pathogen has to overcome if it is to remain active in the food. The right combination of hurdles can ensure all pathogens are eliminated or rendered harmless in the final product.

Hurdle technology has been defined by Leistner (2000) as an intelligent combination of hurdles that secures the microbial safety and stability as well as the organoleptic and nutritional quality and the economic viability of food products. The organoleptic quality of the food refers to its sensory properties, that is its look, taste, smell, and texture.

Examples of hurdles in a food system are high temperature during processing, low temperature during storage, increasing the acidity, lowering the water activity or redox potential, and the presence of preservatives or biopreservatives. According to the type of pathogens and how risky they are, the intensity of the hurdles can be adjusted individually to meet consumer preferences in an economical way, without sacrificing the safety of the product.

Principal hurdles used for food preservation (after Leistner, 1995)		
Parameter	**Symbol**	**Application**
High temperature	F	Heating
Low temperature	T	Chilling, freezing
Reduced water activity	a_w	Drying, curing, conserving
Increased acidity	pH	Acid addition or formation
Reduced redox potential	E_h	Removal of oxygen or addition of ascorbate
Biopreservatives		Competitive flora such as microbial fermentation
Other preservatives		Sorbates, sulfites, nitrites

REFERENCES

1. "Preserving Food without Freezing or Canning, Chelsea Green Publishing, 1999"
2. Stacy Simon (October 26, 2015). "World Health Organization Says Processed Meat Causes Cancer". Cancer.org.
3. James Gallagher (26 October 2015). "Processed meats do cause cancer - WHO". BBC.
4. "IARC Monographs evaluate consumption of red meat and processed meat" (PDF). International Agency for Research on Cancer. 26 October 2015.
5. Nummer, B. (2002). "Historical Origins of Food Preservation" http://nchfp.uga.edu/publications/nchfp/factsheets/food_pres_hist.html. (Accessed on May 5, 2014)
6. Msagati, T. (2012). "The Chemistry of Food Additives and Preservatives"
7. Nicolas Appert inventeur et humaniste by Jean-Paul Barbier, Paris, 1994 and http://www.appert-aina.com
8. anon., Food Irradation – A technique for preserving and improving the safety of food, WHO, Geneva, 1991
9. World Health Organization. Wholesomeness of irradiated food. Geneva, Technical Report Series No. 659, 1981
10. World Health Organization. High-Dose Irradiation: Wholesomeness of Food Irradiated With Doses Above 10 kGy. Report of a Joint FAO/IAEA/WHO Study Group. Geneva, Switzerland: World Health Organization; 1999. WHO Technical Report Series No. 890
11. Hauther,W. & Worth, M., Zapped! Irradiation and the Death of Food, Food & Water Watch Press, Washington, DC, 2008
12. Consumers International – Home Archived 18 August 2010 at the Wayback Machine.

13. NUCLEUS – Food Irradiation Clearances
14. Food irradiation – Position of ADA J Am Diet Assoc. 2000;100:246-253
15. C.M. Deeley, M. Gao, R. Hunter, D.A.E. Ehlermann, The development of food irradiation in the Asia Pacific, the Americas and Europe; tutorial presented to the International Meeting on Radiation Processing, Kuala Lumpur, 2006. http://www.doubleia.org/index.php?sectionid=43&parentid=13&contentid=494
16. Annis, P.C. and Dowsett, H.A. 1993. Low oxygen disinfestation of grain: exposure periods needed for high mortality. Proc. International Conference on Controlled Atmosphere and Fumigation. Winnipeg, June 1992, Caspit Press, Jerusalem, pp 71-83.
17. Annis, P.C. and Morton, R. 1997. The acute mortality effects of carbon dioxide on various life stages of Sitophilus oryzae. J. Stored Prod.Res. 33. 115-124
18. Controlled Atmospheric Storage (CA) :: Washington State Apple Commission
19. Various authors, Session 1: Natural Air-Tight Storage In: Shejbal, J., ed., Controlled Atmosphere Storage of Grains, Elsevier: Amsterdam, 1-33
20. Annis P.C. and Banks H.J. 1993. Is hermetic storage of grains feasible in modern agricultural systems? In "Pest control and sustainable agriculture" Eds S.A. Corey, D.J. Dall and W.M. Milne. CSIRO, Australia. 479-482
21. Laine Welch (18 May 2013). "Laine Welch: Fuel cell technology boosts long-distance fish shipping". Anchorage Daily News. Archived from the original on 9 June 2013. Retrieved May 19, 2013.
22. NWT magazine, December 2012
23. "High-Pressure Processing Keeps Food Safe". Military.com. Archived from the original on 2008-02-02. Retrieved 2008-12-16. Pressed inside a vessel exerting 70,000 pounds per square inch or more, food can be processed so that it retains its fresh appearance, flavor, texture and nutrients while disabling harmful microorganisms and slowing spoilage.
24. Ananou S, Maqueda M, Martínez-Bueno M and Valdivia E (2007) "Biopreservation, an ecological approach to improve the safety and shelf-life of foods" In: A. Méndez-Vilas (Ed.) Communicating Current Research and Educational Topics and Trends in Applied Microbiology, Formatex. ISBN 978-84-611-9423-0.
25. Yousef AE and Carolyn Carlstrom C (2003) Food microbiology: a laboratory manual Wiley, Page 226. ISBN 978-0-471-39105-0.
26. FAO: Preservation techniques Fisheries and aquaculture department, Rome. Updated 27 May 2005. Retrieved 14 March 2011.
27. Alzamora SM, Tapia MS and López-Malo A (2000) Minimally processed fruits and vegetables: fundamental aspects and applications Springer, Page 266. ISBN 978-0-8342-1672-3.
28. Alasalvar C (2010) Seafood Quality, Safety and Health Applications John Wiley and Sons, Page 203. ISBN 978-1-4051-8070-2.
29. Leistner I (2000) "Basic aspects of food preservation by hurdle technology" International Journal of Food Microbiology, 55:181–186.

30. Leistner L (1995) "Principles and applications of hurdle technology" In Gould GW (Ed.) New Methods of Food Preservation, Springer, pp. 1-21. ISBN 978-0-8342-1341-8.

31. Lee S (2004) "Microbial Safety of Pickled Fruits and Vegetables and Hurdle Technology" Internet Journal of Food Safety, 4: 21–32.

CHAPTER 4

Microbial Food Spoilage

Chapter Contents

- **Introduction**
- **Reasons**
- **Food Rotation System**
- **Preservative**
- **Lactic Acid Fermentation**

Food is considered contaminated when unwanted microorganisms are present. Most of the time the contamination is natural, but sometimes it is artificial. Natural contamination occurs when microorganisms attach themselves to foods while the foods are in their growing stages. For instance, fruits are often contaminated with yeasts because yeasts ferment the carbohydrates in fruits. Artificial contamination occurs when food is handled or processed, such as when fecal bacteria enter food through improper handling procedures.

INTRODUCTION

Spoilage is the process in which food deteriorates to the point in which it is not edible to humans or its quality of edibility becomes reduced. Various external forces are responsible for the spoilage of food. Food that is capable of spoiling is referred to as perishable food.

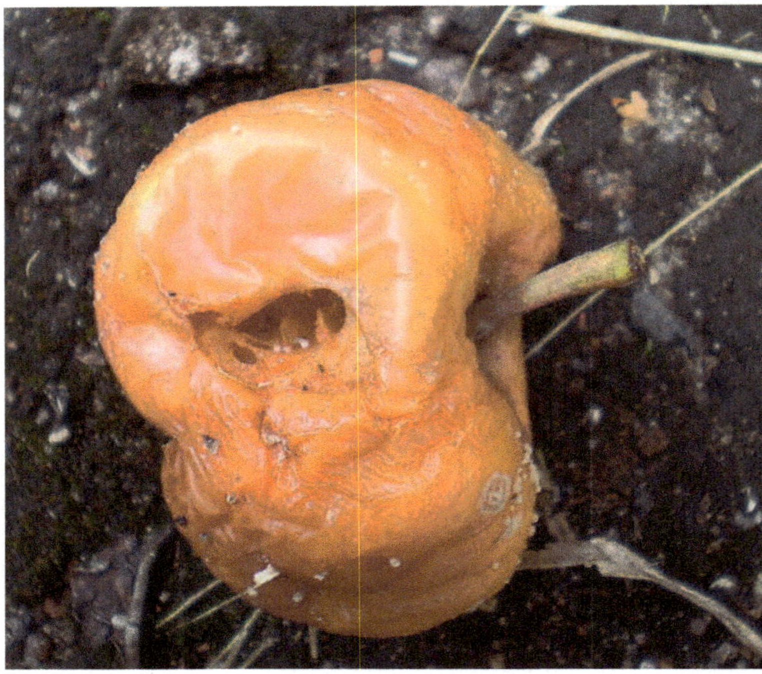

This apple has decomposed to the point that it is not of a quality appealing to humans to eat

REASONS

Harvested foods decompose from the moment they are harvested due to attacks from enzymes, oxidation and microorganisms. These include bacteria, mold, yeast, moisture, temperature and chemical reaction.

Bacteria

Bacteria can be responsible for the spoilage of food. When bacteria breaks down the food, acids and other waste products are created in the process. While the bacteria itself may or may not be harmful, the waste products may be unpleasant to taste or may even be harmful to one's health.

Yeasts

Yeasts can be responsible for the decomposition of food with a high sugar content. The same effect is useful in the production of various types of food and beverages, such as bread, yogurt, cider, and alcoholic beverages.

Signs

Signs of food spoilage may include an appearance different from the food in its fresh form, such as a change in color, a change in texture, an unpleasant odor, or an undesirable taste. The item may become softer than normal. If mold occurs, it is often visible externally on the item.

Consequences

"food poisoning", and more properly as "foodborne illness".

Prevention

A number of methods of prevention can be used that can either totally prevent, delay, or otherwise reduce food spoilage.

Food rotation system uses the first in first out method (FIFO), which ensures that the first item purchased is the first item consumed.

Preservatives can expand the shelf life of food and can lengthen the time long enough for it to be harvested, processed, sold, and kept in the consumer's home for a reasonable length of time.

Refrigeration can increase the shelf life of certain foods and beverages, though with most items, it does not indefinitely expand it. Freezing can preserve food even longer, though even freezing has limitations.

A high-quality vacuum flask (thermos) will keep coffee, soup, and other boiling-hot foods above the danger zone (140F/58C) for over 24 hours.

Canning of food can preserve food for a particularly long period of time, whether canned at home or commercially. Canned food is vacuum packed in order to keep oxygen out of the can that is needed to allow bacteria to break it down. Canning does have limitations, and does not preserve the food indefinitely.

Lactic acid fermentation also preserves food and prevents spoilage.

FOOD ROTATION SYSTEM

A **food rotation system** is a front-loading shelving unit that organizes and rotates food cans on a first-in first-out basis (FIFO). An effective food rotation system is essential for storing food to prepare for catastrophes, preventing foodborne illness and controlling commercial kitchen costs. When used correctly, the first-in first-out food rotation method ensures serving safe food and eliminates spoiled food waste.

Besides the shelving units used for food rotation, other systems exist with the same idea. These systems are especially present in the food and beverage type industries such as restaurants, cafes, bakeries, etc. where food is being produced or being removed from their original package and put into other containers. In order to keep the food safety standard intact with the rotation system, adhesive labels are used to keep track of the date at which it was repackaged and or transferred, as well as the date it must be used by. The labels focus people's attention toward it, so that they are aware to keep maintenance whenever possible. Many factors must be considered when using adhesive labels for a rotation system; such as type of material it is made of, size, shape, training involved and addition information that the label may include. The labels provide a visual aid in assisting employees and managers to rotate containers and maintain a high quality product with minimal waste. Not only does this benefit the consumer, but the owners as well.

Food rotation systems help establishments run more smoothly and efficiently, which is a standard that should be strived for. Other standards, such as the FDA food code are also met when implementing a food rotation system. The system, if done correctly and maintained regularly, one can extract information (for example, length of storage), that may be useful in preventing food borne pathogens from growing and causing sickness.

A benefit, besides following the regulations set out by the FDA, is that it organizes stock and inventory. If the sequences at which items are received are used in the same manner, it will reduce the cost to owners. This cost would otherwise be used to replenish goods and maintain a solid business. Lastly, the food rotation system allows businesses to build their reputation and have confidence in what they are selling to everyday customers.

PRESERVATIVE

A preservative is a substance or a chemical that is added to products such as food, beverages, pharmaceutical drugs, paints, biological samples, cosmetics, wood, and many other products to prevent decomposition by microbial growth or by undesirable chemical changes. In general, preservation is implemented in two modes, chemical and physical. Chemical preservation entails adding chemical compounds to the product. Physical preservation entails processes such as refrigeration or drying. Preservative food additives reduce the risk of foodborne infections, decrease microbial spoilage, and preserve fresh attributes and nutritional quality. Some physical techniques for food preservation include dehydration, UV-C radiation, freeze-drying, and refrigeration. Chemical preservation and physical preservation techniques are sometimes combined.

Antimicrobial Preservatives

Antimicrobial preservatives prevent degradation by bacteria. This method is the most traditional and ancient type of preserving—ancient methods such as pickling and adding honey prevent microorganism growth by modifying the pH level. The most commonly used antimicrobial preservative is lactic acid. Common antimicrobial preservatives are presented in the table. Nitrates and nitrites are also antimicrobial. The detailed mechanism of these chemical compounds range from inhibiting growth of the bacteria to the inhibition of specific enzymes.

E number	chemical compound	comment
E201 – E203	benzoic acid, sodium benzoate	used in acidic foods such as jams, salad dressing, juices, pickles, carbonated drinks, soy sauce
E214 – E219	hydroxybenzoate and derivatives	stable at a broad pH range
E270	lactic acid	-
E249 – E250	nitrite	used in meats to prevent botulism toxin
E251 – E252	nitrate	used in meats
E280 – E283	propionic acid and sodium propionate	baked goods
E220 – E227	sulfur dioxide and sulfites	common for fruits
E200 – E203	sorbic acid and sodium sorbate	common for cheese, wine, baked goods

Antioxidants

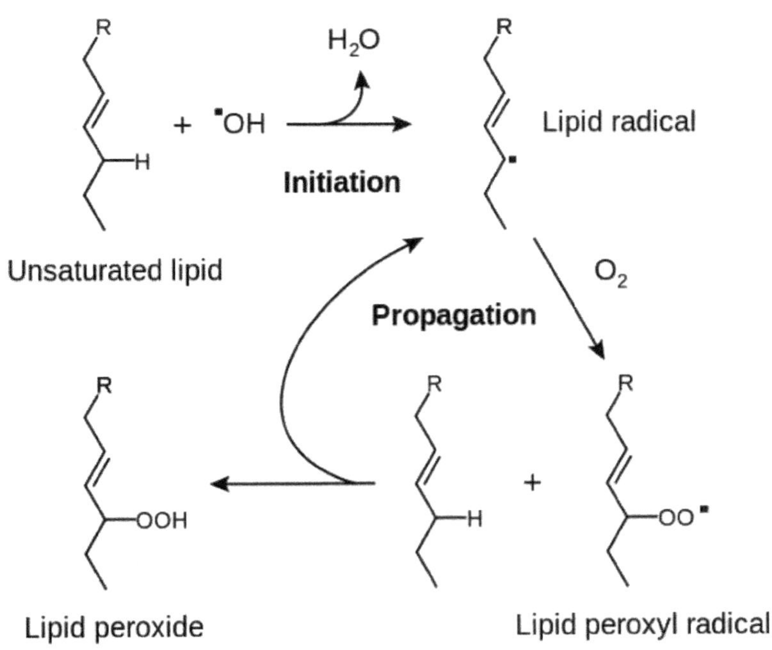

The free radical pathway for the first phase of the oxidative rancidification of fats. This process is slowed by antioxidants.

The oxidation process spoils most food, especially those with a high fat content. Fats quickly turn rancid when exposed to oxygen. Antioxidants prevent or inhibit the oxidation process. The most common antioxidant additives are ascorbic acid (vitamin C) and ascorbates. Thus, antioxidants are commonly added to oils, cheese, and chips. Other antioxidants include the phenol derivatives BHA, BHT, TBHQ and propyl gallate. These agents suppress the formation of hydroperoxides. Other preservatives include ethanol and methylchloroisothiazolinone.

E number	chemical compound	comment
E300-304	ascorbic acid, sodium ascorbate	cheese, chips
E321	butylated hydroxytoluene, butylated hydroxyanisole	also used in food packaging
E310-312	gallic acid and sodium gallate	oxygen scavenger
E220 – E227	sulfur dioxide and sulfites	beverages, wine
E306 – E309	tocopherols	vitamin E activity

A variety of agents are added to sequester (deactivate) metal ions that otherwise catalyze the oxidation of fats. Common sequestering agents are disodium EDTA, citric acid (and citrates), tartaric acid, and lecithin.

Nonsynthetic Compounds for Food Preservation

Citric and ascorbic acids target enzymes that degrade fruits and vegetables, e.g., phenolase which turns surfaces of cut apples and potatoes brown. Ascorbic acid and tocopherol, which are vitamins, are common preservatives. Smoking entails exposing food to a variety of phenols, which are antioxidants. Natural preservatives include rosemary extract, hops, salt, sugar, vinegar, alcohol, diatomaceous earth and castor oil.

Traditional preservatives, such as sodium benzoate have raised health concerns in the past. Benzoate was shown in a study to cause hypersensitivity in some asthma sufferers. This has caused reexamination of natural preservatives which occur in vegetables.

Preservatives have been used since prehistoric times. Smoked meat for example has phenols and other chemicals that retard spoilage. The preservation of foods has evolved greatly over the centuries and has been instrumental in increasing food security. The use of preservatives other than traditional oils, salts, paints, etc. in food began in the late 19th century, but was not widespread until the 20th century.

The use of food preservatives varies greatly depending on the country. Many developing countries that do not have strong governments to regulate food additives face either harmful levels of preservatives in foods or a complete avoidance of foods that are considered unnatural or foreign. These countries have also proven useful in case studies surrounding chemical preservatives, as they have been only recently introduced. In urban slums of highly populated countries, the knowledge about contents of food tends to be extremely low, despite consumption of these imported foods.

Public Awareness of Food Preservation

Public awareness of food preservatives is uneven. Americans have a perception that food-borne illnesses happen more often in other countries. This may be true, but the occurrence of illnesses, hospitalizations, and deaths are still high. It is estimated by the Center for Disease Control (CDC) that each year there are 76 million illnesses, 325,000 hospitalizations, and 5,000 deaths linked to food-borne illness.

The increasing demand for ready-to-eat fresh food products has led to challenges for food distributors regarding the safety and quality of their foods. Artificial preservatives meet some of these challenges by preserving freshness for longer periods of time, but these preservatives can cause negative side-effects as well. Sodium nitrite is a preservative used in lunch meats, hams, sausages, hot dogs, and bacon to prevent botulism. It serves the important function of controlling the bacteria that cause botulism, but sodium nitrite can react with proteins, or during cooking at high heats, to form carcinogenic N-nitrosamines. It has also been linked to cancer in lab animals. The commonly used sodium benzoate has been found to extend the shelf life of bottled tomato paste to 40 weeks without loss of quality. However, it can form the carcinogen benzene when combined with vitamin C. Many food manufacturers have reformed their products to eliminate this combination, but a risk still exists. Consumption of sodium benzoate may also cause hyperactivity. For over 30 years, there has been a debate about whether or not preservatives and other food additives can cause hyperactivity. Studies have found that there may be increases in hyperactivity amongst children who consume artificial colorings and benzoate preservatives and who are already genetically predisposed to hyperactivity, but these studies were not entirely conclusive. Hyperactivity only increased moderately, and it was not determined if the preservatives, colorings, or a combination of the two were responsible for the increase.

LACTIC ACID FERMENTATION

Lactic acid fermentation is a metabolic process by which glucose and other six-carbon sugars (also, disaccharides of six-carbon sugars, e.g. sucrose or lactose) are converted into cellular energy and the metabolite lactate. It is an anaerobic fermentation reaction that occurs in some bacteria and animal cells, such as muscle cells.

If oxygen is present in the cell, many organisms will bypass fermentation and undergo cellular respiration; however, facultative anaerobic organisms will both ferment and undergo respiration in the presence of oxygen. Sometimes even when oxygen is present and aerobic metabolism is happening in the mitochondria, if pyruvate is building up faster than it can be metabolized, the fermentation will happen anyway.

Lactate dehydrogenase catalyzes the interconversion of pyruvate and lactate with concomitant interconversion of NADH and NAD+.

In homolactic fermentation, one molecule of glucose is ultimately converted to two molecules of lactic acid. Heterolactic fermentation, in contrast, yields carbon dioxide and ethanol in addition to lactic acid, in a process called the phosphoketolase pathway.

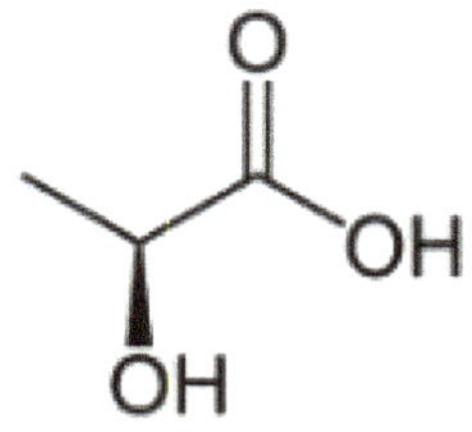

One isomer of lactic acid

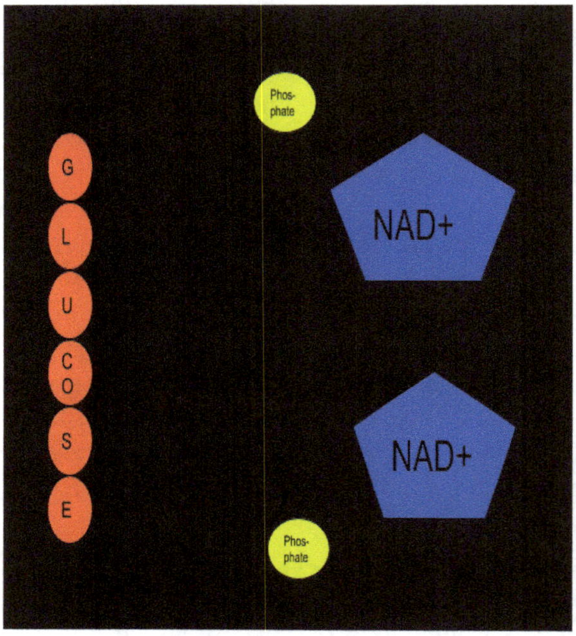

This animation focuses on one molecule of glucose turning into pyruvate then into lactic acid. In the process there is one 6 carbon glucose molecule and 2 NAD+ molecules. 2 phosphates attach to the ends of the glucose molecule, splitting the glucose molecule into 2 pyruvate molecules. The NAD+ molecules add another phosphate onto the open ends of the 2 pyruvate molecules, turning the 2 NAD+ into 2 NADP. Then ADP comes and takes the phosphates, creating 2 ATP molecules.The pyruvate is turned into 2 lactate molecules.The process then repeats, starting with another glucose molecule.

Applications

Lactic acid fermentation is used in many areas of the world to produce foods that cannot be produced through other methods. The most commercially important genus of lactic acid-fermenting bacteria is *Lactobacillus*, though other bacteria and even yeast are sometimes used. Two of the most common applications of lactic acid fermentation are in the production of yogurt and sauerkraut.

Kimchi

Kimchi also uses lactic acid fermentation.

Sauerkraut

Lactic acid fermentation is also used in the production of sauerkraut. The main type of bacteria used in the production of sauerkraut is of the genus *Leuconostoc*.

As in yogurt, when the acidity rises due to lactic acid-fermenting organisms, many other pathogenic microorganisms are killed. The bacteria produce lactic acid, as well as simple alcohols and other hydrocarbons. These may then combine to form esters, contributing to the unique flavor of sauerkraut.

Sour Beer

Lactic acid is a component in the production of sour beers, including Lambics and Berliner Weisses.

Yogurt

The main method of producing yogurt is through the lactic acid fermentation of milk with harmless bacteria. The primary bacteria used are typically *Lactobacillus bulgaricus* and *Streptococcus thermophilus*, and United States law requires all yogurts to contain these two cultures (though others may be added as probiotic cultures). These bacteria produce lactic acid in the milk culture, decreasing its pH and causing it to congeal. The bacteria also produce compounds that give yogurt its distinctive flavor. An additional effect of the lowered pH is the incompatibility of the acidic environment with many other types of harmful bacteria.

For a probiotic yogurt, additional types of bacteria such as *Lactobacillus acidophilus* are also added to the culture.

Physiological

Lactobacillus fermentation and accompanying production of acid provides a protective vaginal microbiome that protects against the proliferation of pathogenic organisms.

REFERENCES

1. Tull, Anita (1997), Food and nutrition (3 ed.), Oxford University Press, p. 154, ISBN 978-0-19-832766-0
2. Tricket, Jill (2001-07-15). The prevention of food poisoning. p. 8. ISBN 978-0-7487-5893-7.
3. Tricket, Jill (2001-07-15). The prevention of food poisoning. p. 9. ISBN 978-0-7487-5893-7.

4. Jeanroy, Amelia; Ward, Karen. Canning & Preserving for Dummies. p. 39.
5. Jeanroy, Amelia; Ward, Karen. Canning & Preserving for Dummies. p. 41.
6. McGinnis, P. (2008). PROTECT YOUR BRAND WITH A FOOD ROTATION PROGRAM, Daydots, pg10-15 Retrieved from https://www.daydots.com/article.asp?HKEY=003&strPRODH=&ArticleCID=82&ArticleID=8
7. U. S. DEPARTMENT OF HEALTH AND HUMAN SERVICES. (2015). Public Health Service: FDA 2015 Food Code. United States: Author. Retrieved from http://www.fda.gov/Food/GuidanceRegulation/RetailFoodProtection/FoodCode/ucm374275.htm
8. Milliorn, M.J. (2006). Adhesive Labels and Indicia For Use in Food Rotation to Enhance Methods of Food Safety in the Food Industry.Daydots Holding Inc. 0207144(A1),pg 1-5 Retrieved from http://www.google.com/patents/about/11_200_726_Adhesive_labels_and_indicia_f.html?id=O8-YAAAAEBAJ
9. Erich Lück and Gert-Wolfhard von Rymon Lipinski "Foods, 3. Food Additives" in Ullmann's Encyclopedia of Industrial Chemistry, 2002, Wiley-VCH, Weinheim. doi: 10.1002/14356007.a11_561
10. Msagati, Titus A. M. (2012). The Chemistry of Food Additives and Preservatives. Retrieved from http://www.eblib.com
11. Dalton, Louisa (November 2002). "Food Preservatives". Chemical and Engineering News. 80 (45): 40. doi:10.1021/cen-v080n045.p040. Retrieved 9 February 2012.
12. "Using Preservatives". Retrieved 9 February 2012.
13. Shaw, Ian C. (2012). Food Safety : The Science of Keeping Food Safe. Retrieved from http://www.eblib.com (306- 334)
14. Field, Simon Quellen (2008). Why There's Antifreeze in Your Toothpaste: The Chemistry of Household Ingredients. Chicago: Chicago Review Press.
15. (Bhat, Rajeev; Alias, Abd Karim; Paliyath, Gopinadham (2011). Progress in Food Preservation. Retrieved from http://www.eblib.com
16. P'EREZ-D'IAZ, I.M; MCFEETERS, R.F (May 2010). "Preservation of Acidified Cucumbers with a Natural Preservative Combination of Fumaric Acid and Allyl Isothiocyanate that Target Lactic Acid Bacteria and Yeasts.". Journal of Food Science. 75 (4): M204–M208. doi:10.1111/j.1750-3841.2010.01587.x.
17. Evans, G., de Challemaison, B., & Cox, D. N. (2010). "Consumers' ratings of the natural and unnatural qualities of foods". Appetite. 54 (3): 557–563. doi:10.1016/j.appet.2010.02.014.
18. Ashagrie, Z. Z., & Abate, D. D. (2012). IMPROVEMENT OF INJERA SHELF LIFE THROUGH THE USE OF CHEMICAL PRESERVATIVES. African Journal Of Food, Agriculture, Nutrition & Development, 12(5), 6409-6423.
19. Kumar, H., Jha, A., Taneja, K. K., Kabra, K., & Sadiq, H. M. (2013). A STUDY ON CONSUMER AWARENESS, SAFETY PERCEPTIONS & PRACTICES ABOUT FOOD PRESERVATIVES AND FLAVOURING AGENTS USED IN PACKED /CANNED FOODS FROM SOUTH INDIA. National Journal Of

Community Medicine, 4(3), 402-406.

20. Kumar, H. N. Harsha; Jha, Anshu Kumar; Taneja, Khushboo K.; Kabra, Krishan; Sadiq, Hafeez M. (2013). A Study On Consumer Awareness, Safety Perceptions & Practices about Food Preservatives and Flavouring Agents used in Packed/ Canned Foods from South India. National Journal of Community Medicine, 4(3), 402.
21. Theron, M. M. & Lues, J. F. (2007). Organic acids and meat preservation: A review. Food Reviews International, 23, 141-158.
22. Antinoro, L. (2008). EN Rates 12 Common Food Additives As Safe Or Sorry Ingredients. (Cover story). Environmental Nutrition, 31(5), 1-4.
23. Barrett, J. R. (2007). "Hyperactive Ingredients?". Environmental Health Perspectives. 115 (12): A578. doi:10.1289/ehp.115-a578.
24. "Fermented Fruits and Vegetables - A Global SO Perspective". United Nations FAO. 1998. Retrieved 2007-06-10.
25. Ohio State University (1998-04-03). "Glycolysis and Fermentation". Retrieved 2010-01-12.
26. Campbell, Neil; Reece, Jane (2005). Biology, 7th Edition. Benjamin Cummings. ISBN 0-8053-7146-X.
27. "Lactic acid fermentation". Retrieved 2010-01-09.
28. "Lactic acid fermentation". Retrieved 2010-01-09.
29. "Lactic acid fermentation in the production of foods from vegetables, cereals and legumes". Antonie van Leeuwenhoek Journal. 1983. Retrieved 2010-06-28.
30. "Sauerkraut Fermentation". University of Wisconsin–Madison. 1999. Retrieved 2010-01-09.
31. Nummer, Brian A. "Brewing With Lactic Acid Bacteria". MoreFlavor Inc. Retrieved 2 October 2013.
32. "Yogurt Production". 2006-12-29. Retrieved 2010-01-09.
33. Nardis, C.; Mastromarino, P.; Mosca, L. (September–October 2013). "Vaginal microbiota and viral sexually transmitted diseases". Annali di Igiene. 25 (5): 443–56. doi:10.7416/ai.2013.1946. PMID 24048183.

CHAPTER 5

Microbial Food Cultures

Chapter Contents

- **Introduction**
- **Function of Microbial Food Cultures in Food**
- **Production of Microbial Food Cultures**

Microbial food cultures are live bacteria, yeasts or moulds used in food production. Microbial food cultures carry out the fermentation process in foodstuffs. ... As of 1995, fermented food represented between one quarter and one third of food consumed in Central Europe.

INTRODUCTION

Microbial food cultures are live bacteria, yeasts or moulds used in food production. Microbial food cultures carry out the fermentation process in foodstuffs. Used by humans since the Neolithic period (around 10 000 years BC) fermentation helps to preserve perishable foods and to improve their nutritional and organoleptic qualities (in this case, taste, sight, smell, touch). As of 1995, fermented food represented between one quarter and one third of food consumed in Central Europe. More than 260 different species of microbial food culture are identified and described for their beneficial use in fermented food products globally, showing the importance of their use.

The scientific rationale of the function of microbes in fermentation started to be built with the discoveries of Louis Pasteur in the second half of the 19th century. Extensive scientific study continues to characterize microbial food cultures traditionally used in food fermentation taxonomically, physiologically, biochemically and genetically. This allows better understanding and improvement of traditional food processing and opens up new fields of applications.

Microorganisms are the earliest form of life on earth, first evolving more than three billion years ago. Our ancestors discovered how to harness the power of microorganisms to make new foods, even if they did not know the science behind what they were doing.

Milestones

1665—Robert Hooke and Antoni Van Leeuwenhoek first observe and describe microorganisms.

1857–1876—Louis Pasteur proves the function of microorganisms in lactic and alcoholic fermentation.

1881—Emil Christian Hansen isolates *Saccharomyces carlsbergensis*, a pure yeast culture, which is today widely used in brewing of lager beers.

1889–1896—Herbert William Conn, Vilhelm Storch and Hermann Weigmann demonstrate that bacteria are responsible for the acidification of milk and of cream.

1897—Eduard von Freudenreich isolates *Lactobacillus brevis*.

1919—Sigurd Orla-Jensen classifies lactic acid bacteria on the basis of the bacteria's physiological response patterns.

Starting from 1970s—production of first industrial concentrated cultures, frozen or freeze-dried cultures, for the direct inoculation of processed milk, improving the regularity of production processes.

FUNCTION OF MICROBIAL FOOD CULTURES IN FOOD

Microbial food cultures preserve food through formation of inhibitory metabolites such as organic acid (lactic acid, acetic acid, formic acid, propionic acid), ethanol, bacteriocins, etc., often in combination with decrease of water activity (by drying or use of salt). Further, microbial food cultures help to improve food safety through inhibition of pathogens or removing of toxic compounds. Microbial food cultures also improve the nutritional value and organoleptic quality of the food.

The microbial food cultures used in food fermentation can be divided into three major groups: bacteria, yeasts and moulds.

Bacteria

Bacterial food cultures can be divided into starter cultures and probiotics.

Starter cultures have mainly a technological function in the food manufacturing. They are used as food ingredients at one or more stages in the food manufacturing process and develop the desired metabolic activity during the fermentation or ripening process. They contribute to the one or multiple unique properties of a foodstuff especially in regard to taste, flavour, colour, texture, safety, preservation, nutritional value, wholesomeness and/ or health benefits.

Probiotics have a functional role, which refers to the ability of certain microbes to confer health benefits to the consumer.

Generally, the bacteria used as starter culture are not the same used as probiotics. There are, however, cases when one bacterium can be used both as starter culture and as probiotic. The scientific community is presently trying to deepen understanding of the roles played by microbes in food processing and human health.

The most important bacteria in food manufacturing are *Lactobacillus* species, belonging to the group of lactic acid bacteria.

Bacterial food cultures are responsible for the aroma, taste and texture of cheeses and fermented milk products such as yogurts, ayran, doogh, skyr or ymer. They contribute to developing the flavour and colour of such fermented products as salami, pepperoni and dried ham. Lactic acid bacteria converts the unstable malic acid that is naturally present in wine into the stable lactic acid. This malolactic fermentation gives the stability that is characteristic of high-quality wines that improve on storage.

Lactic acid bacteria are also used in food supplements as probiotics which help to restore the balance in human intestinal biota.

Yeasts

The most familiar yeast in food production, *Saccharomyces cerevisiae*, has been used in brewing and baking for thousands of years.

S. cerevisiae feeds on the sugars present in the bread dough and produces the gas carbon dioxide. This forms bubbles within the dough, causing it to expand and the bread to rise.

Several different yeasts are used in brewing beer, where they ferment the sugars present in malted barley to produce alcohol. One of the most common is *S. cerevisiae*. The same strain of *S. cerevisiae* which can also be used in breadmaking is used to make ale-type beers. It is known as a top-fermenting yeast because it creates a foam on the top of the brew. Bottom-fermenting yeasts, such as *S. pastorianus*, are more commonly used to make lagers. They ferment more of the sugars in the mixture than top-fermenting yeasts, which gives a cleaner taste.

The alcohol in wine is formed by the fermentation of the sugars in grape juice, with carbon dioxide as a by-product. Yeast is naturally present on grapeskins, and this alone can be sufficient for the fermentation of sugars to alcohol to occur. A pure yeast culture, most often *S. cerevisiae*, is usually added to ensure the fermentation is reliable. Other yeast cultures like *Pichia*, *Torulaspora* and *Kluyveromyces* are naturally present or added to create special flavours in the wine. Sparkling wine, including champagne, is made by adding further yeast to the wine when it is bottled. The carbon dioxide formed in this second fermentation is trapped as bubbles.

Yeasts are also used to produce kefir products, semi-soft ripened cheeses and fermented soy drinks.

Moulds

Three main types of cheese rely on moulds for their characteristic properties: blue cheese, soft ripened cheese (such as camembert and brie) and rind-washed cheese (such as époisses and taleggio).

To make blue cheese, the cheese is treated with a mould, usually *Penicillium roqueforti*, while it is still in the loosely pressed curd form. As the cheese matures, the mould grows, creating blue veins within it which gives the cheese its characteristic flavour. Examples include stilton, roquefort and gorgonzola.

Soft ripened cheese such as brie and camembert are made by allowing *P. camemberti* to grow on the outside of the cheese, which causes them to age from the outside in. The mould forms a soft white crust, and the interior becomes runny with a strong flavour.

Rind-washed cheeses like limburger also ripen inwards, but here, as the name suggests, they are washed with brine and other ingredients such as beer and wine which contain mould. This also makes them attractive to bacteria, which add to the flavour.

Traditionally, inoculations of sausages with moulds were done with the indigenous biota of the slaughters. Different moulds (such as *P. chrysogenum* and *P. nalgiovense*) can be used to ripen surfaces of sausages. The mould cultures develop the aroma and improve the texture of the sausages. They also contribute to shortening of the ripening period and preserving the natural quality. This expands the shelf life of the meat product.

In the past, soy sauce has been made by mixing soybeans and other grains with a mould (*Aspergillus oryzae* or *A. sojae*) and yeast. This mixture was then left to ferment in the sun.Today soy sauce is made under controlled conditions. The key flavour ingredients formed in this process are salts of the amino acid glutamic acid, notably monosodium glutamate.

PRODUCTION OF MICROBIAL FOOD CULTURES

The industrial production of microbial food cultures is carried out after careful selection process and under strictly controlled conditions. First, the microbiology laboratory, where the original strains are kept, prepares the inoculation material, which is a small quantity of microbes of a single (pure) strain. Then, the inoculation material is multiplied and grown either in fermenters (liquid) or on a surface (solid) under defined and monitored conditions. Grown cells of pure culture are harvested, eventually blended with other cultures and, finally, formulated (preserved) for subsequent transportation and storage. They are sold in liquid, frozen or freeze-dried formats.

Another and traditional way of starting a food fermentation is often referred to as spontaneous fermentation. Cultures come from raw milk, i.e. milk that has not undergone any sanitation treatment or from the reuse of a fraction of the previous production (back-slopping). The composition of such cultures is complex and extremely variable. The use of such techniques is steadily decreasing in developed countries. Some countries even prohibit the back-slopping technique because of the “potential to magnify pathogen loads to very dangerous levels”.

Safety and Regulatory Aspects

Microbial food cultures are considered as traditional food ingredients and are permitted in the production of foodstuffs all over the world under general food laws.

Commercially available microbial food cultures are sold as preparations, which are formulations, consisting of concentrates of one or more microbial species and/or strains including unavoidable media components carried over from the fermentation and components, which are necessary for their survival, storage, standardisation and to facilitate their application in the food production process.

Safety of microbial food cultures, depending on their characteristics and use, can be based on genus, species or strain levels.

Microorganisms with Documented History of Safe Use in Food

The first (non-exhaustive) inventory of microorganisms with a documented history of use in food was for the first time compiled in 2001 by the International Dairy Federation (IDF) and the European Food and Feed Cultures Association (EFFCA).

In 2012, this inventory was updated. It now covers a wide range of food applications (including dairy, fish, meat, beverages and vinegar) and features a reviewed taxonomy of microorganisms.

US

In the United States of America, microbial food cultures are regulated under the Food, Drug and Cosmetic Act. Section 409 of the 1958 Food Additives Amendment of the Food, Drug and Cosmetic Act, exempts from the definition of food additives substances generally recognized by experts as safe (GRAS) under conditions of their intended use. These substances do not require premarket approval by the US Food and Drug Administration.

Because there are various ways to obtain GRAS status for microbial food cultures, there is no exhaustive list of microbial food cultures having GRAS status in the US.

European Union

Within the European Union, microbial food cultures are regarded as food ingredients and are regulated by Regulation 178/2002, commonly referred to as the General Food Law.

Since 2007, the European Food Safety Authority (EFSA) has been maintaining a list of microorganisms having qualified presumption of safety (QPS). The QPS list covers only a limited number of microorganisms, which have been referred to EFSA for safety assessment. It has been conceived as an internal evaluation tool for microorganisms used in the food production chain (e.g. feed cultures, cell factories producing enzymes or additives, plant protection) that need an evaluation by EFSA scientific panels before being marketed in the EU. Microbial food cultures with a long history of safe use are, however, considered to be traditional food ingredients and are legally permitted for use in human food without EFSA evaluation.

Denmark

From 1974 to 2010 Denmark required premarket approval of microbial food cultures. The positive list of microbial food cultures is available on the website of the Danish Veterinary and Food Administration.

In 2010, the regulation changed. Approval is no longer needed but a notification should be made to the Veterinary and Food Administration.

REFERENCES

1. Prajapati, J.B., Nair, B.M. (2003). Farnworth, E.R., ed. The history of fermented foods in Fermented Functional Foods. CRC Press, Boca Raton, New York, London, Washington DC. pp. 1–25.
2. Holzapfel, W.H., U. Schillinger, and R. Geisen (January 1995). "Biological Preservation of Foods with Reference to Protective Cultures, Bacteriocins and Food-Grade Enzymes". International Journal of Food Microbiology. 24 (3): 343–362. doi:10.1016/0168-1605(94)00036-6.
3. Bourdichon, F., Casaregola, S., Farrokh, C., Frisvad, J.C., Gerds, M.L., Hammes, W.P., Harnett, J., Huys, G., Laulund, S., Ouwehand, A., Powell, I.B., Prajapati, J.B., Seto, Y., Ter Schure, E., Van Boven, A., Vankerckhoven, V., Zgoda, A., Tuijtelaars, S., Bech Hansen, E. (2012). "Food fermentations: Microorganisms with technological beneficial use". International Journal of Food Microbiology. 154: 87–97. doi:10.1016/j.ijfoodmicro.2011.12.030.
4. Wyman, J. (1862). "Spontaneous generation". British Medical Journal. 2 (90): 311–312. doi:10.1136/bmj.2.90.311. PMC 2288299 . PMID 20744126.
5. Farley, J., Geison, G.L., J; Geison, GL (1974). "Science, politics and spontaneous generation in nineteenth-century France: the Pasteur-Pouchet debate". Bulletin of the History of Medicine. 48 (2): 161–198. PMID 4617616.
6. Schopf J (2006). "Fossil evidence of Archaean life" (PDF). Philos Trans R Soc Lond B Biol Sci. 361 (1470): 869–85. doi:10.1098/rstb.2006.1834. PMC 1578735 . PMID 16754604.
7. Altermann W, Kazmierczak J (2003). "Archean microfossils: a reappraisal of early life on Earth". Res Microbiol. 154 (9): 611–7. doi:10.1016/j.resmic.2003.08.006. PMID 14596897.
8. Cavalier-Smith T (2006). "Cell evolution and Earth history: stasis and revolution" (PDF). Philos Trans R Soc Lond B Biol Sci. 361 (1470): 969–1006. doi:10.1098/rstb.2006.1842. PMC 1578732 . PMID 16754610.
9. McGovern, P. E.; Zhang, J.; Tang, J.; Zhang, Z.; Hall, G. R.; Moreau, R. A.; Nunez, A.; Butrym, E. D.; Richards, M. P.; Wang, C. -S.; Cheng, G.; Zhao, Z.; Wang, C. (2004). "Fermented beverages of pre- and proto-historic China".

Proceedings of the National Academy of Sciences. 101 (51): 17593–17598. doi:10.1073/pnas.0407921102. PMC 539767 . PMID 15590771.

10. "8,000-year-old wine unearthed in Georgia". The Independent. 2003-12-28. Retrieved 2007-01-28.
11. "Now on display ... world's oldest known wine jar". Retrieved 2007-01-28.
12. "Fermented fruits and vegetables. A global perspective". FAO Agricultural Services Bulletins - 134. Archived from the original on January 19, 2007. Retrieved 2007-01-28.
13. Cavalieri, D; McGovern P.E.; Hartl D.L.; Mortimer R.; Polsinelli M. (2003). "Evidence for S. cerevisiae fermentation in ancient wine." (PDF). Journal of Molecular Evolution. 57 Suppl 1: S226–32. doi:10.1007/s00239-003-0031-2. PMID 15008419. 15008419. Archived from the original (PDF) on December 9, 2006. Retrieved 2007-01-28.
14. Gest, H., H (2004). "The discovery of microorganisms by Robert Hooke and Antoni van Leeuwenhoek, Fellows of The Royal Society". Notes and Records of the Royal Society of London. 58 (2): 187–201. doi:10.1098/rsnr.2004.0055. PMID 15209075.
15. John Long Wilson. "Stanford University School of Medicine and the Predecessor Schools: An Historical Perspective". Retrieved 8 August 2012.
16. "Emile Christian Hansen". Encyclopædia Britannica.
17. Jespersen, L., Josephsen, J. (2004). Hui, Y.H.; et al., eds. Starter Cultures and Fermented Products in Handbook of Food and Beverage Fermentation Technology. CRC Press. ISBN 978-0-8247-4780-0.
18. "La biodiversité des microorganismes des produits laitiers". Les microorganismes bénéfiques de l'industrie de transformation du lait. INRA. Retrieved 8 August 2012.
19. "Sigurd Orla-Jensen". Biokemisk Forening.
20. Ross, R.P., Morgan, S., Hill, C. (2002). "Preservation and fermentation: past, present and future". International Journal of Food Microbiology. 79: 3–16. doi:10.1016/s0168-1605(02)00174-5.
21. Gaggia, F., Di Gioia, D., Baffoni, L., Biavati, B. (2011). "The role of protective and probiotics cultures in food and feed and their impact on food safety". Trends in Food Science and Technology. 22: S58–S66. doi:10.1016/j.tifs.2011.03.003.
22. Adams, M., Mitchell, R. (2002). "Fermentation and pathogen control: a risk assessment approach". International Journal of Food Microbiology. 79: 75–83. doi:10.1016/s0168-1605(02)00181-2.
23. Adams, M.R., Nicolaides, L. (2008). "Review of the sensitivity of different foodborne pathogens to fermentation". Food Control. 8: 227–239. doi:10.1016/s0956-7135(97)00016-9.
24. Hammes, W.P., Tichaczek, P.S. (1994). "The potential of lactic acid bacteria for the production of safe and wholesome food". Zeitschrift für Lebensmittel-Untersuchung und -Forschung. 198: 193–201. doi:10.1007/bf01192595.

25. van Boekel, M., Fogliano, V., Pellegrini, N., Stanton, C., Scholz, G., Lalljie, S., Somoza, V., Knorr, D., Jasti, P.R., Eisenbrand, G. (2010). "A review on the beneficial aspects of food processing". Molecular Nutrition & Food Research. 54: 1215–1247. doi:10.1002/mnfr.200900608.
26. Poutanen, K., Flander, L., Katina, K. (2009). "Sourdough and cereal fermentation in an nutritional perspective". Food Microbiology. 7: 693–699. doi:10.1016/j.fm.2009.07.011.
27. Marilley, L., Casey, M.G. (2004). "Flavors of cheese products: metabolic pathways, analytical tools and identification of producing strains". International Journal of Food Microbiology. 90: 139–159. doi:10.1016/s0168-1605(03)00304-0.
28. Smit, G., Smit, B.A., Engels, W.J. (2005). "Flavor formation by lactic acid bacteria and biochemical flavor profiling of cheese products". FEMS Microbiology Reviews. 29: 591–610. doi:10.1016/j.femsre.2005.04.002.
29. Lacroix, N., St Gelais, D., Champagne, C.P., Fortin, J., Vuillemard, J.C. (2010). "Characterization of aromatic properties of old-style cheese starters". Journal of Dairy Science. 93: 3427–3441. doi:10.3168/jds.2009-2795.
30. Sicard, D., Legras, J.L. (2011). "Bread, beer and wine: yeast domestication in the Saccharomyces sensu strict complex". Comptes Rendus Biologies. 334 (3): 229–236. doi:10.1016/j.crvi.2010.12.016.
31. "Raw-fermented sausages". Food and Agriculture Organization of the United Nations (FAO). Retrieved 8 August 2012.
32. Wu, Z.-Y., Zhang, W.-X., Zhang, Q.-S., Hu, C., Wang, R., Liu, Z.-H. (2009). "Developing New Sacchariferous Starters for Liquor Production Based on Functional Strains Isolated from the Pits of Several Famous Luzhou-flavor Liquor Brewers". Journal of the institute of brewing. 115 (2): 111–115. doi:10.1002/j.2050-0416.2009.tb00354.x.
33. Mogra, R., Choudhry, M. (2008). "Effect of starter culture on the development of curd". J. Dairying, Foods & H.S. 27 (2): 130–133.
34. "Health and Nutritional Properties of Probiotics in Food including Powder Milk with Live Lactic Acid Bacteria" (PDF). Report of a Joint FAO/WHO Expert Consultation on Evaluation of Health and Nutritional Properties of Probiotics in Food Including Powder Milk with Live Lactic Acid Bacteria. World Health Organisation of the United nations (WHO). Retrieved 8 August 2012.
35. Rijkers, G.T., de Vos, W.M., Brummer, R.-J., Morelli, L., Corthier, G., Marteau, P. (2011). "Health benefits and health claims of probiotics: bridging science and marketing". British Journal of Nutrition. 106: 1291–6. doi:10.1017/s000711451100287x. PMID 21861940.
36. Heller, K.J. "Probiotic bacteria in fermented foods: product characteristics and starter organisms". American Society for Clinical Nutrition. Retrieved 8 August 2012.
37. Vinderola, C.G., Reinheimer, J.A. (2003). "actic acid starter and probiotic bacteria: a comparative "in vitro" study of probiotic characteristics and biological barrier

resistance". Food Research International. 36 (9-10): 895–904. doi:10.1016/s0963-9969(03)00098-x.

38. Szabo, L. (updated 5/8/2012). "New research on probiotics shows promise". USA Today. Retrieved 8 August 2012. Check date values in: |date= (help)
39. "Human Microbiome Project". Retrieved 8 Mar 2012.
40. "Fermented frutis and vegetables. A global perspective". Chapter 5 - Bacterial fermentations. Food and Agriculture Organization of the United Nations (FAO). Retrieved 8 August 2012.
41. Ribéreau-Gayon, P., Dubourdieu, D., Donèche, B., Lonvaud, A. (2006). Handbook of Enology, Volume 1: The microbiology of wine and vinifications. J.Wiley & Sond Ltd., Chichester, U.K.
42. Lonvaud-Funel, A. (1999). "Lactic acid bacteria in the quality improvement and depreciation of wine". Antonie van Leeuwenhoek. 76: 317–331. doi:10.1007/978-94-017-2027-4_16.
43. Gueimonde, M., de Los Reyes- Gavilán, C.G., Borja Sánchez, B. (2011). Von Wright, A., ed. Lactic Acid Bacteria, Microbiological and Functional Aspects, Fourth Edition. CRC Press. ISBN 978-1-4398-3677-4.
44. Yabaya, A., Jatau, E.D. (2009). "Investigating Wild Yeast Baking Potentials". Middle-East Journal of Scientific Research. 4 (4): 320–322.
45. "Biochemistry of yeast fermentation" (PDF). University of British Columbia. Retrieved 8 August 2012.
46. Libkinda, D., Hittingerb, C.T., Valériod, E., Gonçalvesd, C., Doverb, J., Johnstonb, M., Gonçalvesd, P., Sampaiod, J.P. "Microbe domestication and the identification of the wild genetic stock of lager-brewing yeast". Proceedings of the National Academy of Sciences of the United States of America. Retrieved 8 August 2012.
47. Mills, D.A., Phister, T., Neeley, E., Johannsen, E. (2008). Cocolin, L., Ercolini, D., ed. Wine Fermentation in Molecular Techniques in the Microbial Ecology of Fermented Foods. Springer.
48. McCarthy, E., Ewing-Mulligan, M. "The Methods of Producing Sparkling Wine". John Wiley & Sons, Inc. Retrieved 8 August 2012.
49. "Kefir, The champagne of Dairy Products". Armand-Frappier Museum.
50. Boekhout, T., Robert, V. (2003). Yeasts in food. Woodhead. ISBN 9781855737068.
51. Nelson, J.H. (1970). "Production of Blue cheese flavor via submerged fermentation by Penicillium roqueforti". Journal of Agricultural and Food Chemistry. 18 (4): 567–569. doi:10.1021/jf60170a024.
52. Leclercq-Perlat, M.N.; et al. (2004). "Controlled production of Camembert-type cheeses.". Journal of Dairy Research. 71 (3).
53. "Washed Rind Cheese". Dairy Australia. Retrieved 9 August 2012.
54. Ludemann, V., Pose, G., Moavro, A., Maliaviabarrena, M.G., Fandiño, F., Ripoll, G., Basílico, J.C., Pardo, A.G. (September 2009). "Toxicological assessment of Penicillium nalgiovense strains for use as starter cultures in the manufacture of

dry fermented sausages". Journal of food protection. 72 (8): 1666–70.

55. Marianski, S., Mariański, A. (2009). The Art of Making Fermented Sausages. Bookmagic LLC.
56. Lund, B., Baird-Parker, A.C., Gould, G.W. (2000). Microbiological Safety and Quality of Food. Aspen Publishers Inc.
57. Machida, M., Yamada, O., Gomi, K. (2008). "Genomics of Aspergillus oryzae: Learning from the History of Koji Mold and Exploration of Its Future". DNA Research. 15: 173–183. doi:10.1093/dnares/dsn020.
58. "MSG". New South Wales (Australia) Food Authority.
59. Gaggia, F., Di Gioia, D., Baffoni, L., Biavati, B. (2011). "The role of protective and probiotic cultures in food and feed and their impact in food safety". Trends in Food Science & Technology. 22 (1): S58–S66. doi:10.1016/j.tifs.2011.03.003.
60. "Microbiology of starter cultures". Dairy Science Food Technology. Retrieved 9 August 2012.
61. Varnam, A., Sutherland,J.M. (1995). Meat and Meat Products: Technology, Chemistry and Microbiology. Chapman & Hall, UK.
62. Ross, T., Shadbolt, C.T. "Predicting Escherichia coli inactivation in uncooked comminuted fermented meat products, Final Report" (PDF). Meat & Livestock Australia.
63. Health Canada, 2003. Amendment (Schedule No. 948) to Division 28 of the Food and Drug Regulations, Sections B.28.001–003. Food and Drugs Regulations
64. Mogensen, G., Salminen, S., O'Brien, J., Ouwehand, A., Holzapfel, W., Shortt, C., Fonden, R., Miller, G.D., Donohue, D., Playne, M., Crittenden, R., Salvadori, B., Zink, R. (2002). "Inventory of microorganisms with a documented history of use in food". Bulletin of IDF. 377: 10–19.
65. "Federal Food, Drug, and Cosmetic Act (FD&C Act)". US Food and Drug Administration. Retrieved 10 August 2012.
66. "How U.S. FDA's GRAS Notification Program Works". US Food and Drug Administration. Retrieved 10 August 2012.
67. Stevens, H., O'Brien Nabors, L. (2009). "Microbial Food Cultures:a regulatory update" (PDF). Food Technology: 36–41.
68. "Regulation (EC) no 178/2002 of the European Parliament and of the Council of 28 January 2002 laying down the general principles and requirements of food law, establishing the European Food Safety Authority and laying down procedures in matters of food safety". OJ EC. L31/1. 2002.
69. Herody, C., Soyeux, Y., Bech Hansen, E., Gillies, K. (2010). "The legal status of microbial food cultures in the European Union: an overview". European Food and Feed Law Review. 5: 258–269.
70. "Qualified presumption of safety (QPS)". European Food Safety Authority. Retrieved 10 August 2012.

71. Anon, 2005. EFSA Scientific Colloquium—Microorganisms in Food and Feed:Qualified Presumption of Safety — 13–14 December 2004, Brussels, Belgium. ISSN 1830-4737, http://www.efsa.europa.eu/en/supporting/pub/109e.htm.

72. Leuschner, R.-G.K., Robinson, T., Hugas, M., Cocconcelli, P.S., Richard-Forget, F., Klein, G., Licht, T.R., Nguyen-The, C., Querol, A., Richardson, M., Suarez, J.E., Vlak, J.M., von Wright, A. (2010). "Qualified presumption of safety (QPS): a generic risk assessment approach for biological agents notified to the European Food Safety Authority (EFSA)". Trends in Food Science and Technology. 21: 425–435. doi:10.1016/j.tifs.2010.07.003.

73. "Liste over anmeldte mikrobielle kulturer" (PDF). Ministeriet for Fødevarer, Landbrug og Fiskeri. Retrieved 10 August 2012.

74. "Anmeldelsesordning for kulturer af bakterier samt gær- og skimmelsvampe". Ministeriet for Fødevarer, Landbrug og Fiskeri.

Fermentation in Food Processing

Chapter Contents

- **Introduction**
- **Uses**
- **Fermented Foods by Region**

Fermentation is the conversion of carbohydrates into alcohol and carbon dioxide. This process happens using bacteria or yeasts, or a combination of the two under anaerobic conditions. Occasionally, the term fermentation may also include the chemical conversion of sugars into ethanol. This process is used to make beer, wine, and cider. Food fermentation is also involved in the process of leavening bread and the process of producing lactic acid in foods such as dry sausages, sauerkraut, yogurt, pickles, and kimchi.

INTRODUCTION

Fermentation in food processing is the process of converting carbohydrates to alcohol or organic acids using microorganisms—yeasts or bacteria—under anaerobic conditions. Fermentation usually implies that the action of microorganisms is desired. The science of fermentation is known as zymology or zymurgy.

The term fermentation sometimes refers specifically to the chemical conversion of sugars into ethanol, producing alcoholic drinks such as wine, beer, and cider. However, similar processes take place in the leavening of bread (CO_2 produced by yeast activity), and in the preservation of sour foods with the production of lactic acid, such as in sauerkraut and yogurt.

Apart from alcohol, widely consumed fermented foods include vinegar, olives, yogurt, bread, and cheese. In various parts of the world, more localised foods prepared by fermentation may also be based on beans, dough, grain, vegetables, fruit, honey, dairy products, fish, meat, or tea.

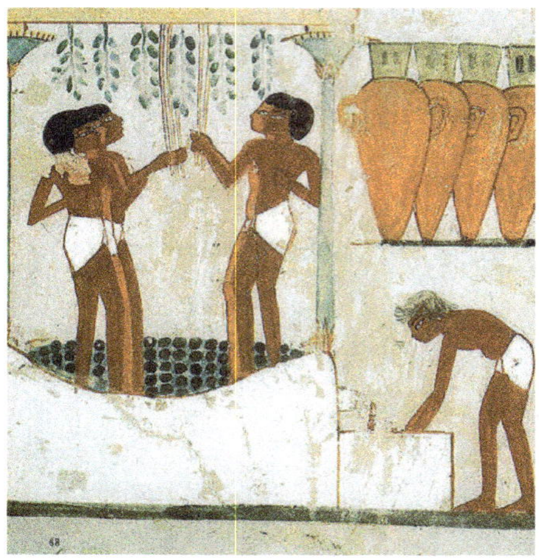

Grapes being trodden to extract the juice and made into wine in storage jars. Tomb of Nakht, 18th dynasty, Thebes, Ancient Egypt

Natural fermentation precedes human history. Since ancient times, humans have exploited the fermentation process. The earliest evidence of an alcoholic drink, made from fruit, rice, and honey, dates from 7000 to 6600 BC, in the Neolithic Chinese village of Jiahu, and winemaking dates from 6000 BC, in Georgia, in the Caucasus area. Seven-thousand-year-old jars containing the remains of wine, now on display at the University of Pennsylvania, were excavated in the Zagros Mountains in Iran. There is strong evidence that people were fermenting alcoholic drinks in Babylon c. 3000 BC, ancient Egypt c. 3150 BC, pre-Hispanic Mexico c. 2000 BC, and Sudan c. 1500 BC.

The French chemist Louis Pasteur founded zymology, when in 1856 he connected yeast to fermentation. When studying the fermentation of sugar to alcohol by yeast, Pasteur concluded that the fermentation was catalyzed by a vital force, called "ferments", within the yeast cells. The "ferments" were thought to function only within living organisms. "Alcoholic fermentation is an act correlated with the life and organization of the yeast cells, not with the death or putrefaction of the cells", he wrote.

Nevertheless, it was known that yeast extracts can ferment sugar even in the absence of living yeast cells. While studying this process in 1897, Eduard Buchner of Humboldt University of Berlin, Germany, found that sugar was fermented even when there were no living yeast cells in the mixture, by a yeast secreted enzyme complex that he termed *zymase*. In 1907 he received the Nobel Prize in Chemistry for his research and discovery of "cell-free fermentation".

One year earlier, in 1906, ethanol fermentation studies led to the early discovery of NAD^+.

USES

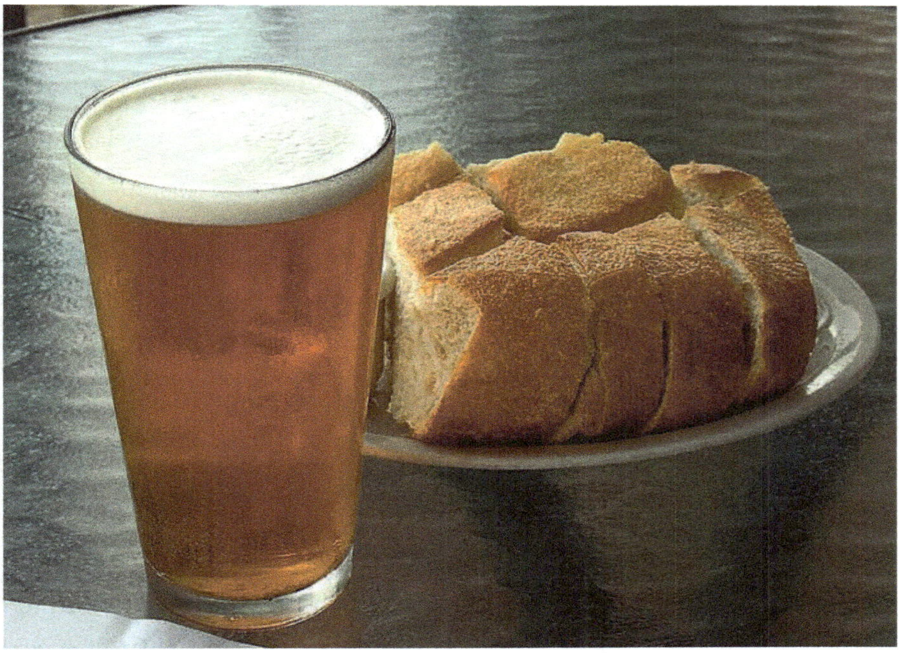

Beer and bread, two major uses of fermentation in food

Food fermentation is the conversion of sugars and other carbohydrates into alcohol or preservative organic acids and carbon dioxide. All three products have found human uses. The production of alcohol is made use of when fruit juices are converted to wine, when grains are made into beer, and when foods rich in starch, such as potatoes, are fermented and then distilled to make spirits such as gin and vodka. The production of carbon dioxide is used to leaven bread. The production of organic acids is exploited to preserve and flavor vegetables and dairy products.

Food fermentation serves five main purposes: to enrich the diet through development of a diversity of flavors, aromas, and textures in food substrates; to preserve substantial amounts of food through lactic acid, alcohol, acetic acid, and alkaline fermentations; to enrich food substrates with protein, essential amino acids, and vitamins; to eliminate antinutrients; and to reduce cooking time and the associated use of fuel.

FERMENTED FOODS BY REGION

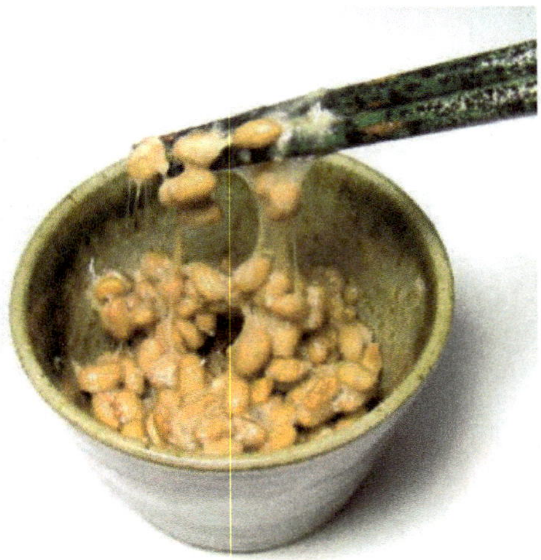

Nattō, a Japanese fermented soybean food

- **Worldwide:** alcohol(beer, wine), vinegar, olives, yogurt, bread, cheese
- **Asia**
- **East and Southeast Asia:** amazake, atchara, bai-ming, belacan, burong mangga, com ruou, dalok, doenjang, douchi, jeruk, lambanog, kimchi, kombucha, leppet-so, narezushi, miang, miso, nata de coco, nata de pina, natto, naw-mai-dong, oncom, pak-siam-dong, paw-tsaynob, prahok, ruou nep, sake, seokbakji, soju, soy sauce, stinky tofu, szechwan cabbage, tai-tan tsoi, chiraki, tape, tempeh, totkal kimchi, yen tsai, zha cai
- **Central Asia:** kumis (mare milk), kefir, shubat (camel milk)
- **South Asia:** achar, appam, dosa, dhokla, dahi (yogurt), idli, kaanji, mixed pickle, ngari, hawaichaar, jaand (rice beer), sinki, tongba, paneer
- **Africa:** fermented millet porridge, garri, hibiscus seed, hot pepper sauce, injera, lamoun makbouss, laxoox, mageu, mauoloh, msir, mslalla, oilseed, ogi, ogili, ogiri, iru
- **Americas:** sourdough bread, cultured milk, chicha, elderberry wine, kombucha, pickling (pickled vegetables), sauerkraut, lupin seed, oilseed, chocolate, vanilla, tabasco, tibicos, pulque, mikyuk (fermented bowhead whale)
- **Middle East:** kushuk, lamoun makbouss, mekhalel, torshi, boza
- **Europe:** rakfisk, sauerkraut, pickled cucumber, surströmming, mead, elderberry wine, salami, sucuk, prosciutto, cultured milk products such as quark, kefir, filmjölk, crème fraîche, smetana, skyr, rakı, tupí.
- **Oceania:** poi, kaanga pirau (rotten corn), sago

List of Fermented Foods

This is a **list of fermented foods**, which are foods produced or preserved by the action of microorganisms. In this context, fermentation typically refers to the fermentation of sugar to alcohol using yeast, but other fermentation processes involve the use of bacteria such as lactobacillus, including the making of foods such as yogurt and sauerkraut. The science of fermentation is known as zymology.

Many pickled or soured foods are fermented as part of the pickling or souring process, but many are simply processed with brine, vinegar, or another acid such as lemon juice.

Fermented Foods

Name	Image	Origin	Description
Amasi	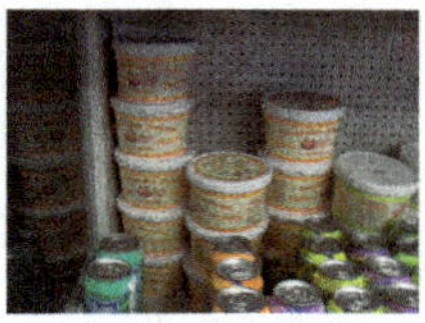		A word for fermented milk that tastes like cottage cheese or plain yogurt. It is very popular in South Africa.
Amazake	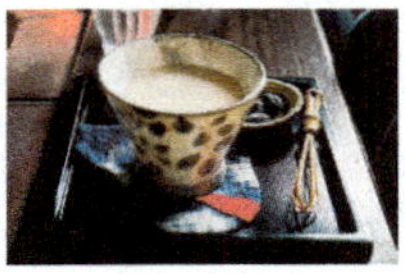	Japan	A traditional sweet, low- or non-alcohol (depending on recipes) Japanese drink made from fermented rice.
Appam	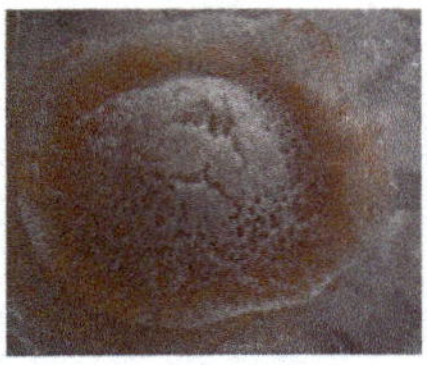	India	A type of South Indian pancake made with fermented rice batter and coconut milk. It is a popular food in South Indian states of Kerala and Tamil Nadu. It is also very popular in Sri Lanka where it is commonly referred to by its anglicized name as Hoppers.
Atchara	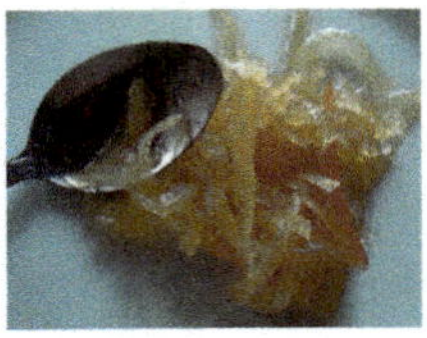		A pickle made from grated unripe papaya that is popular in the Philippines. It is often served as a side dish for fried or grilled foods such as pork barbecue. The name may come from several names for South Asian pickle and is related to *acar* from neighbouring Indonesia and Malaysia.
Ayran	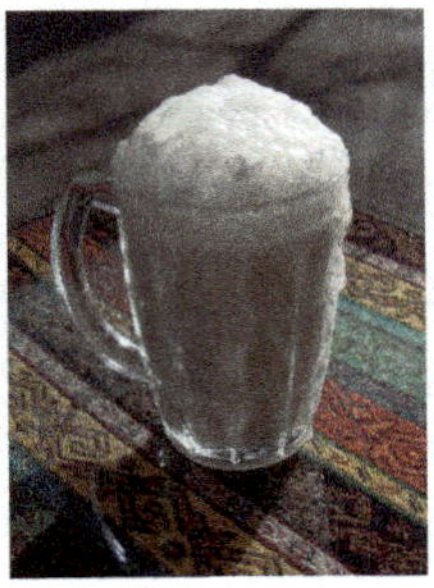		A cold yogurt beverage mixed with salt. In addition to Turkey, where it is considered a national drink, ayran is found in Iran (here called *doogh*), Afghanistan, Armenia (here called *tan*), Azerbaijan, the Balkans, Kazakhstan, Kyrgyzstan, Lebanon, Syria and across the Caucasus. Its primary ingredients are water and yogurt.

Name	Image	Origin	Description
Bagoong	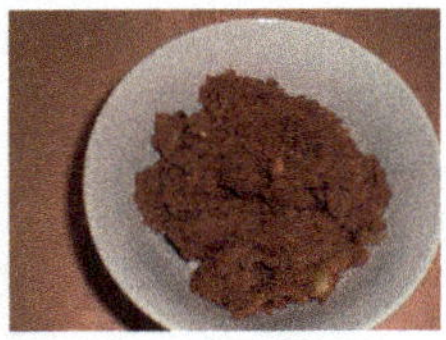	Philippines	A Philippine condiment made of partially or completely fermented fish or shrimp and salt. The fermentation process also results in fish sauce (known as *patis*).
Bagoong monamon	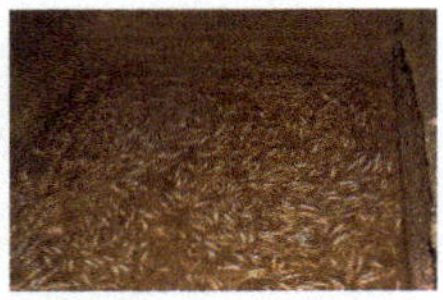		Prepared by fermenting salted anchovies
Bagoong terong	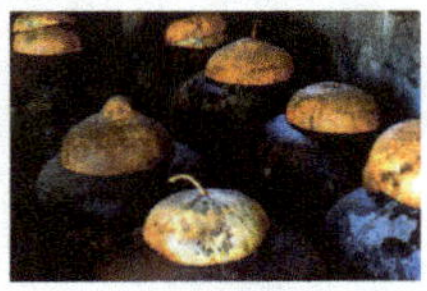		Made by salting and fermenting the bonnet mouth fish
Bánh cuốn	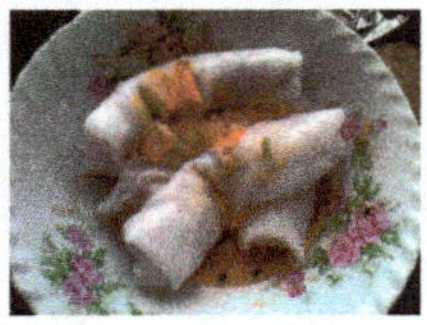	Northern Vietnam.	Made from a thin, wide sheet of steamed fermented rice batter filled with seasoned ground pork, minced wood ear mushroom, and minced shallots.
Blaand			A fermented milk product made from whey. It is similar in alcohol content to wine.
Boza	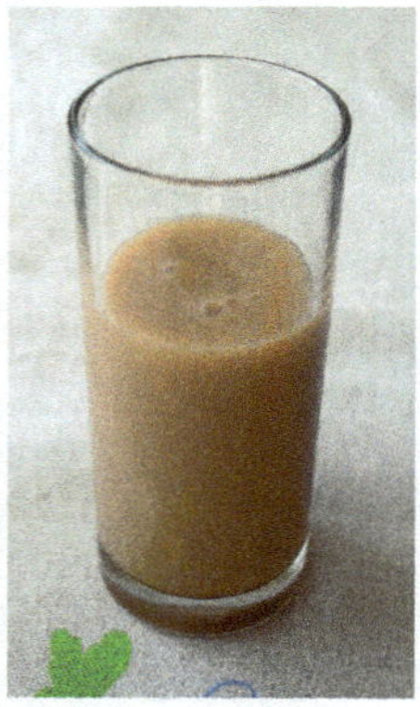		A traditional fermented drink with alcohol found in many countries
Bread	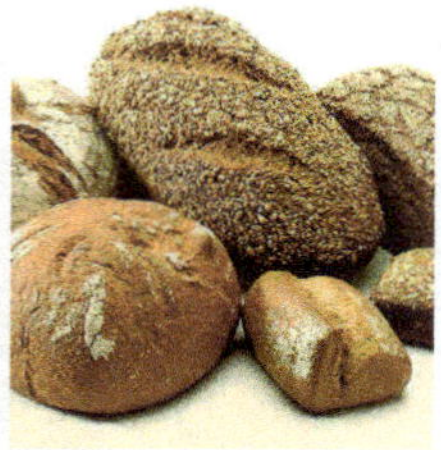		Some breads, such as sourdough, use dough that is fermented

Name	Image	Origin	Description
Brem	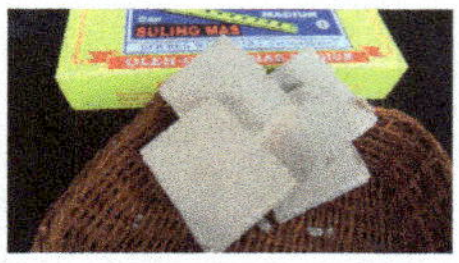	Indonesia	A traditional fermented food of Indonesia that uses rice.
Burong mangga		Philippines	Made by mixing sugar, salt, and water to mangoes that have previously been salted
Calpis		Japan	An uncarbonated soft drink, manufactured by Calpis Co., Ltd. that is produced using lactic acid fermentation
Chass		Gujarat, India	The word used for buttermilk in Rajasthani and Gujarati. Chass is the traditional Gujarati beverage from Gujarat, India.
Cheese	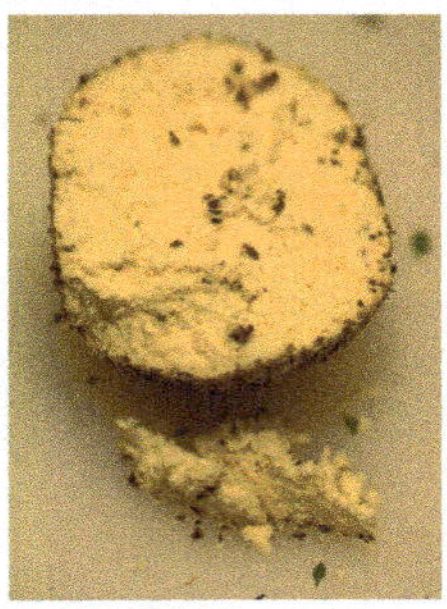		Some cheeses, such as Shanklish (pictured), are fermented as part of their production
Cheonggukjang	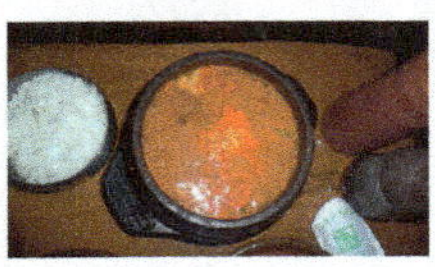	Korea	A fermented soybean paste used in Korean cuisine that contains both whole and ground soybeans
Chicha	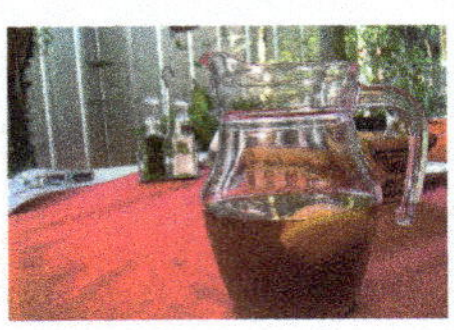		In South America and Central America, chicha is a fermented or non-fermented beverage usually derived from maize. Chicha includes corn beer known as chicha de jora and non-alcoholic beverages such as chicha morada.
Chinese pickles			Various vegetables or fruits, which have been fermented by pickling with salt and brine or marinated in mixtures based on soy sauce or savory bean pastes
Cocoa	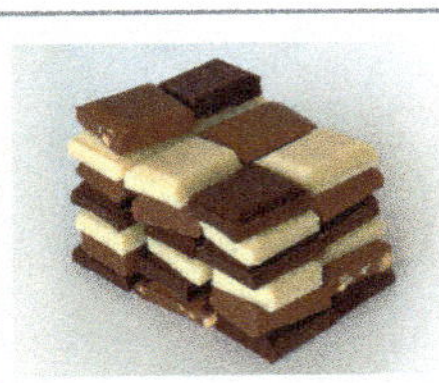		Cocoa bean fermentation for chocolate, and other cocoa products

Name	Image	Origin	Description
Cod liver oil (Traditional preparation method)			Cod liver oil was traditionally manufactured by filling a wooden barrel with fresh cod livers and seawater and allowing the mixture to ferment for up to a year before removing the oil.
Crème fraîche	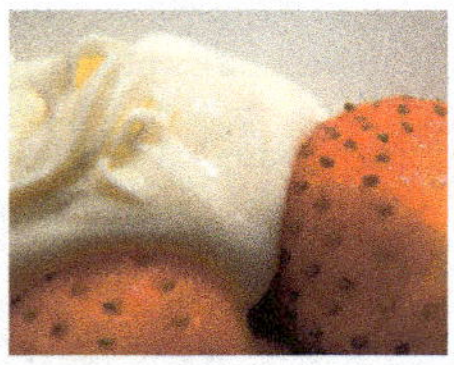		A soured cream containing 30–45% butterfat and having a pH of around 4.5. It is soured with bacterial culture, but is less sour than U.S.-style sour cream, and has a lower viscosity and a higher fat content.
Curtido	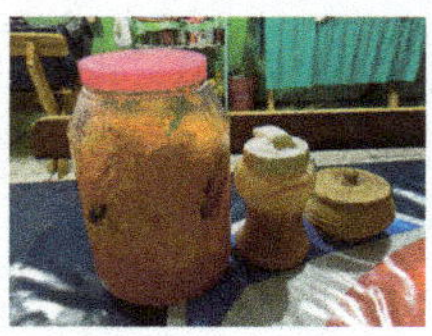		A type of lightly fermented cabbage relish. It is typical in Salvadoran cuisine and that of other Central American countries, and is usually made with cabbage, onions, carrots, and sometimes lime juice
Dhokla	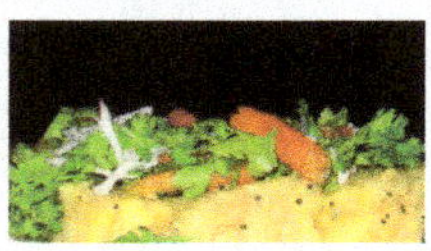	Gujarat, India	A vegetarian food item made with a fermented batter derived from rice and chickpea splits.
Doenjang	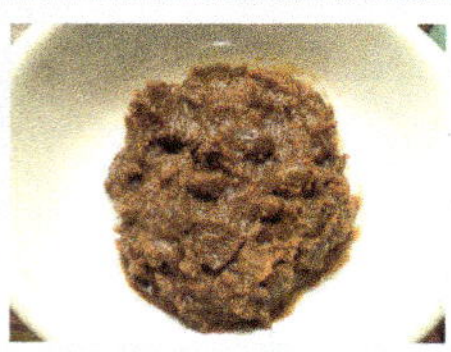	Korea	A thick bean paste that includes fermentation in its preparation
Doogh	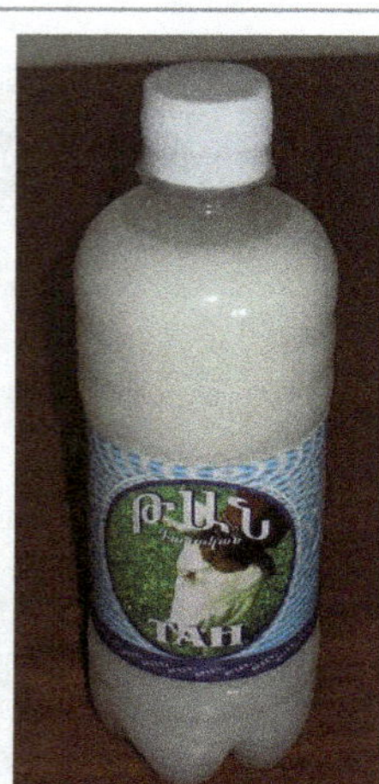	Ancient Persia	A savory yogurt-based beverage
Dosa	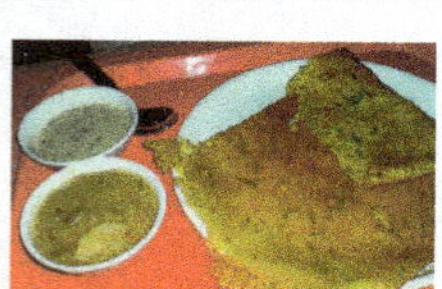	India	A fermented crepe or pancake made from rice batter and black lentils. It is a staple food in many parts of India. Pictured is *Rava dosa*, a type of Dosa dish.Plain dosa and Masala dosa are better fermented dishes.The batter is fermented for 8 to 10 hrs.

Name	Image	Origin	Description
Doubanjiang	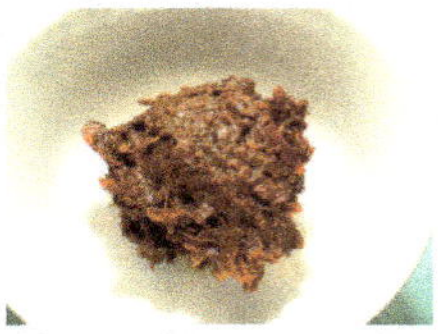		A spicy, salty paste made from fermented broad beans, soybeans, salt, rice, and various spices
Douchi	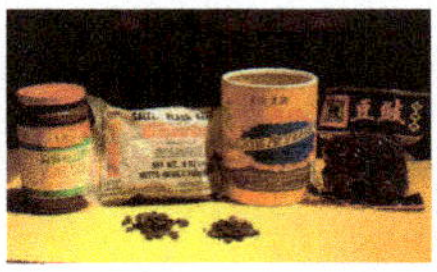		A type of fermented and salted black soybean
Fermented bean curd	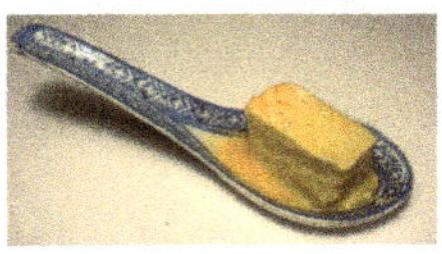		Fermented tofu (pictured) is a type of Fermented bean curd
Fermented bean paste	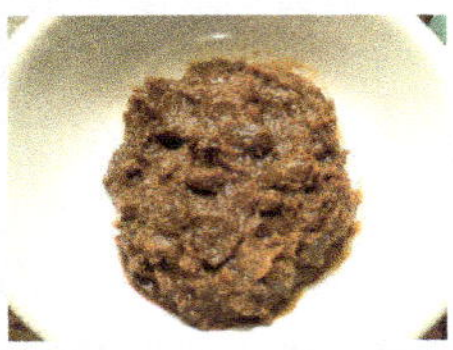		A category of fermented foods typically made from ground soybeans, which are indigenous to the cuisines of East and Southeast Asia. In some cases, such as in the production of *miso*, other varieties of beans such as broad beans, may also be used.
Fermented fish	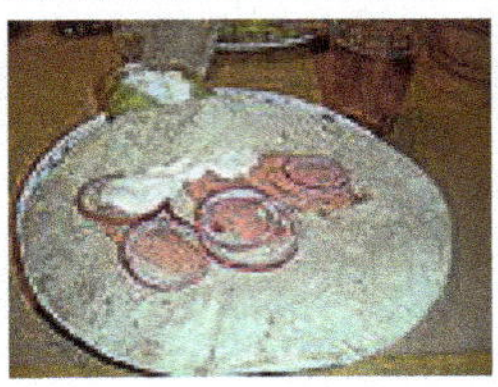		A traditional preparation of fish. Before refrigeration, canning and other modern preservation techniques became available, fermenting was an important preservation method.
Fermented milk products			Also known as cultured dairy foods, cultured dairy products, or cultured milk products, fermented milk products are dairy foods that have been fermented with lactic acid bacteria such as Lactobacillus, Lactococcus, and Leuconostoc. Pictured is matzoon, a fermented milk product of Armenian origin.
Filmjölk	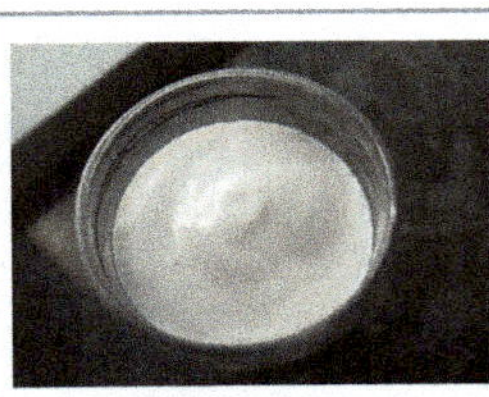	Nordic countries	A mesophilic fermented milk product that is made by fermenting cow's milk with a variety of bacteria from the species *Lactococcus lactis* and *Leuconostoc mesenteroides*.
Fish sauce	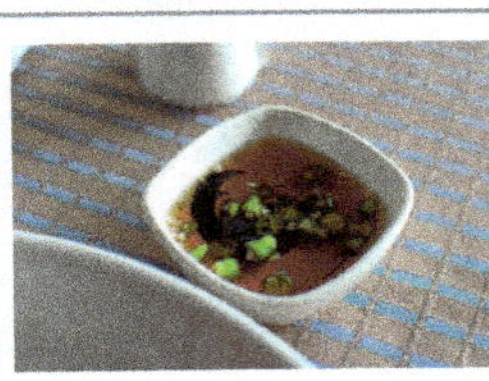		

Name	Image	Origin	Description
Ganjang	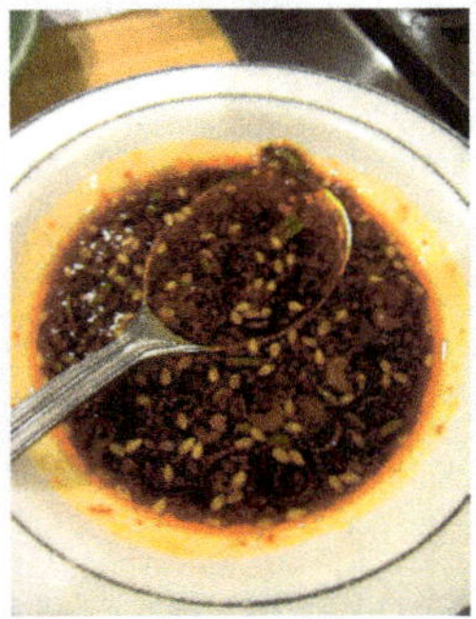	Korea	a kind of Korean soy sauce made from fermented soybeans Ganjang is a uniquely Korean condiment
Garri	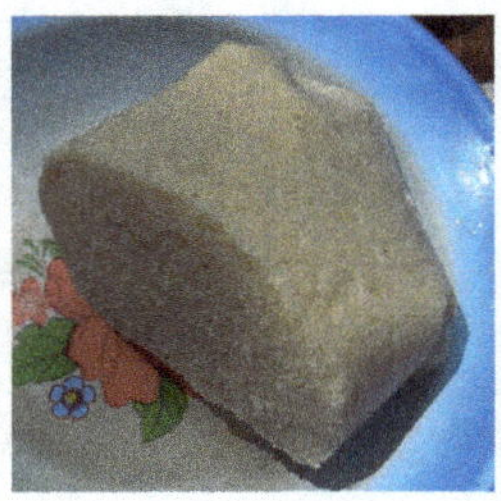		
Garum			Garum was a fish sauce made from the fermentation of fish entrails, used as a condiment in the cuisines of ancient Greece, Rome, and Byzantium. It is believed to have resembled the fermented anchovy sauce colatura di alici still produced today in Campania, Italy.
Gejang	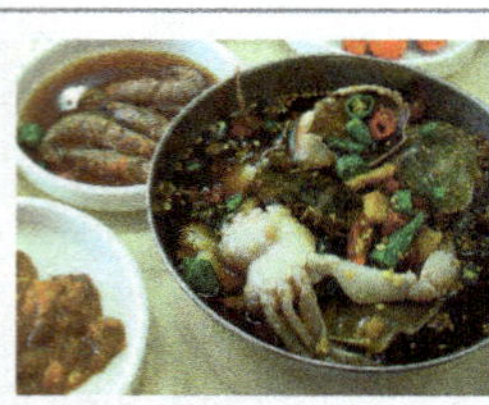	Korea	
Gochujang	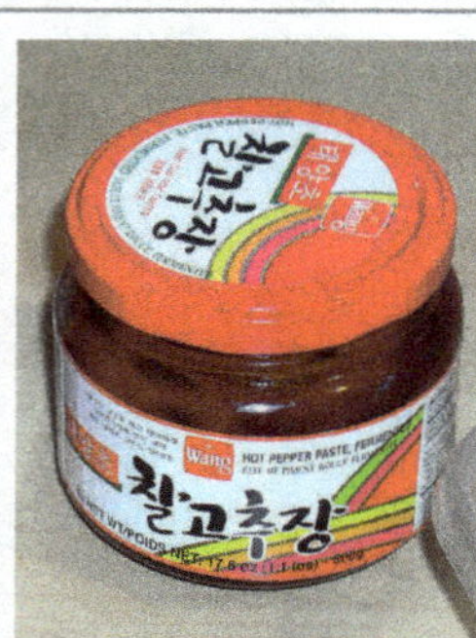	Korea	

Name	Image	Origin	Description
Gundruk	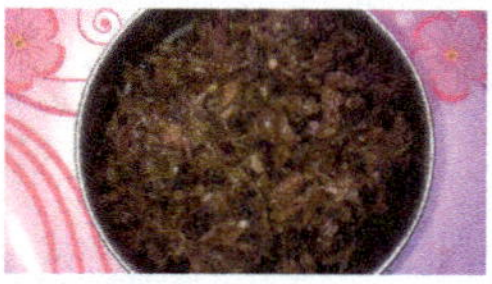	- Nepal	Gundruk is made by fermenting leaves of vegetables of Brassica family.
Hákarl	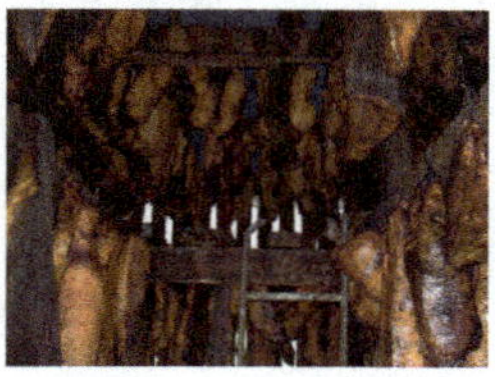	Iceland	Made by fermenting shark meat, then hanging it to dry. Pictured is Hákarl hanging to dry in Iceland
Hongeohoe	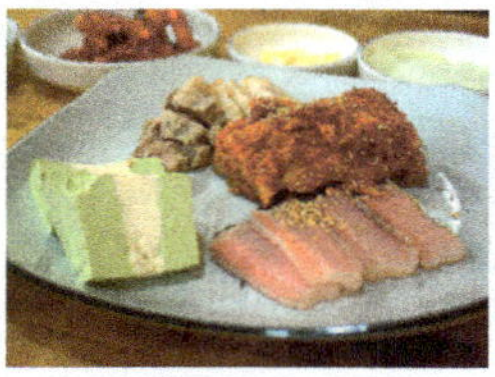	Korea	
Idli	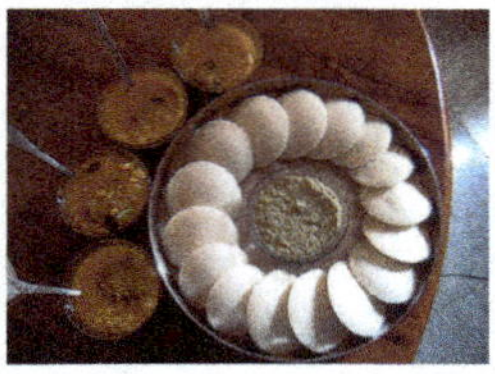	India	
Igunaq	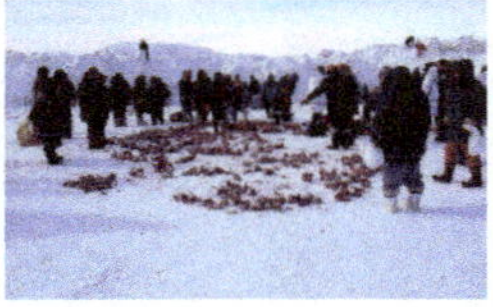		
Injera	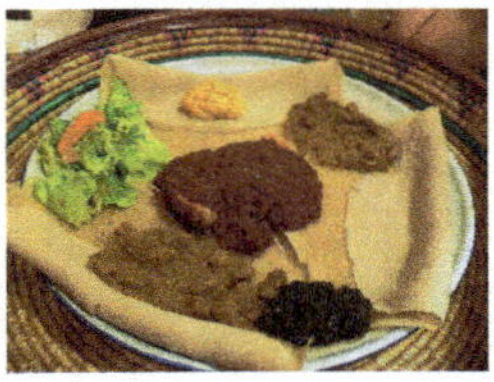		A sourdough-risen flatbread with a unique, slightly spongy texture. Traditionally made out of teff flour, it is a national dish in Ethiopia and Eritrea.
Iru (food)	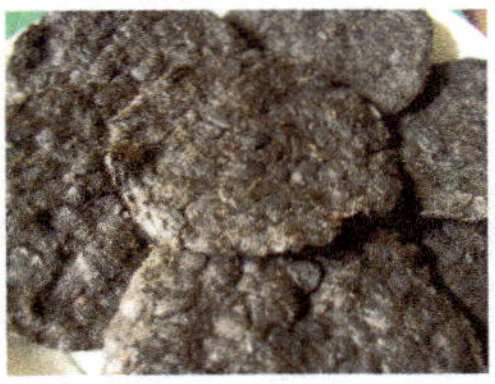		

Name	Image	Origin	Description
Jeotgal	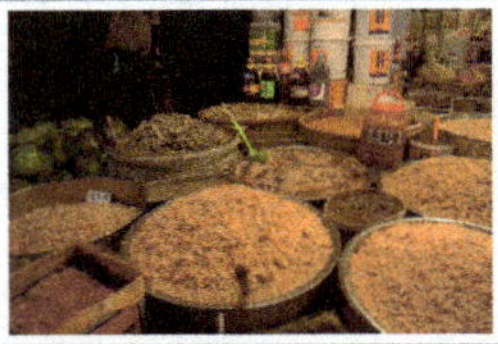	Korea	
Jogijeot	Made with fish in Korea.	Korea	
Kapusta kiszona duszona	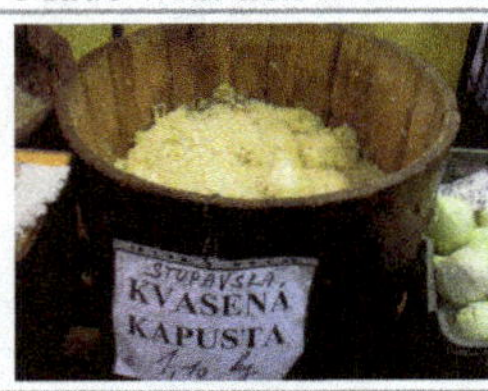	Poland	
Katsuobushi	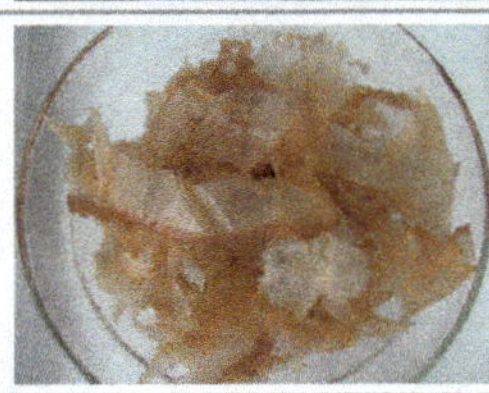	Japan	
Kaymak			
Kefir	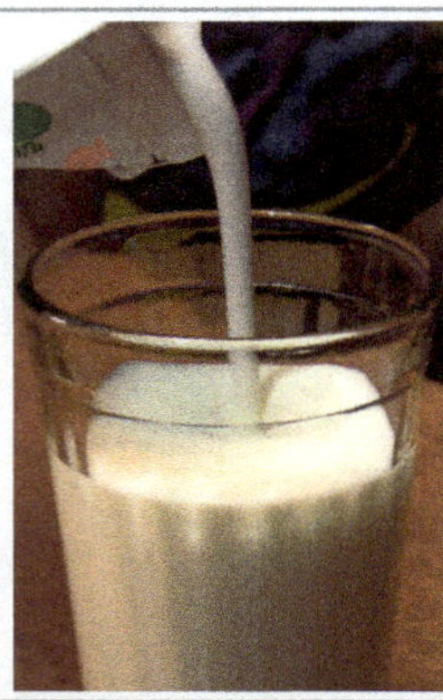		A fermented milk product
Kenkey	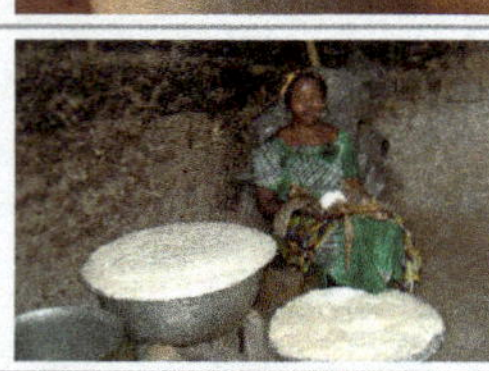		
Ketchup	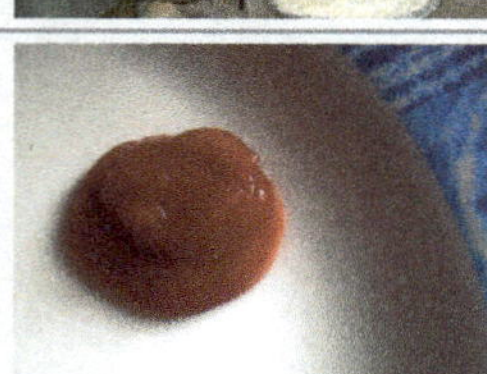		In Indonesian cuisine, which is similar to Malay, the term *kecap* refers to fermented savory sauces.
Khanom chin	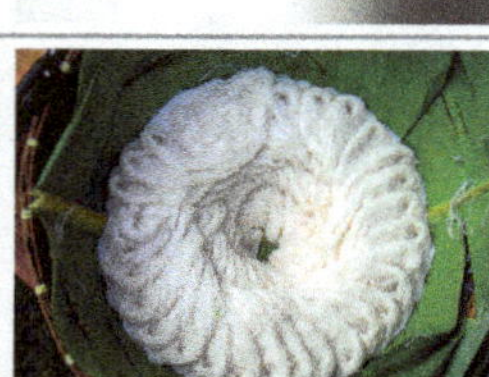		

Name	Image	Origin	Description
Kimchi	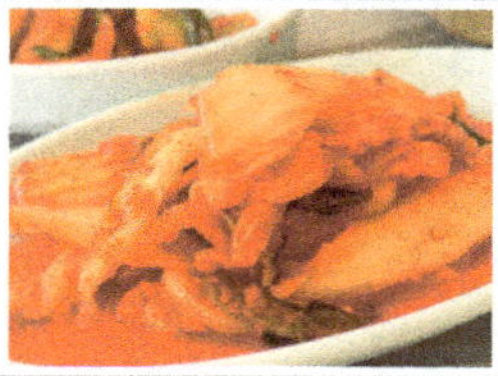	Korea	
Kisela repa			Fermented shreds of turnip, used in bean soup or as a side usually in winter meals in continental Croatian cuisine.
Kiviak			Kiviak or kiviaq is a traditional wintertime Inuit food from Greenland that is made of auks preserved in the hollowed-out body of a seal.
Kombucha	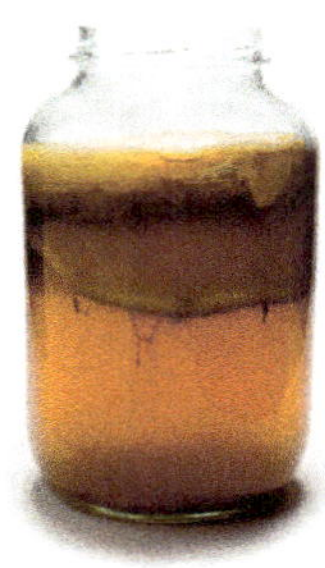		
Kumis	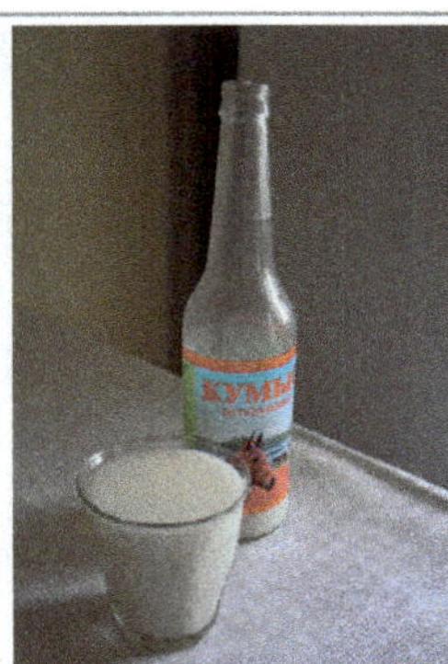		
Kusaya		Japan	A traditional salted and fermented fish dish originating in the Izu Islands, and often eaten with sake, shōchū, or a local drink called Shima Jiman.
Kuzhi paniyaram	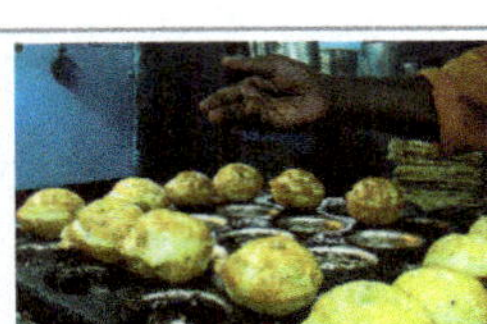		

Name	Image	Origin	Description
Kvass	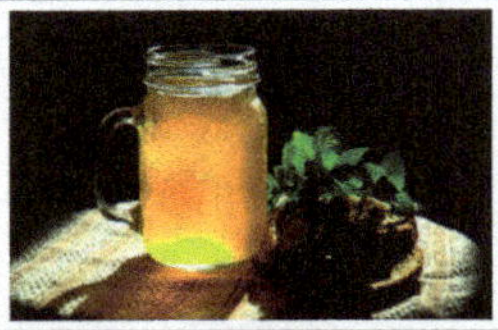		
Lassi	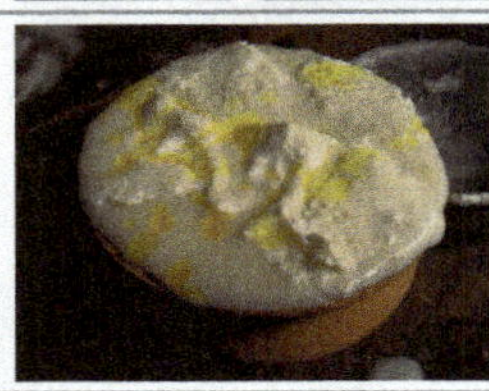		
Leben (milk product)			
Lufu (food)			
Mageu	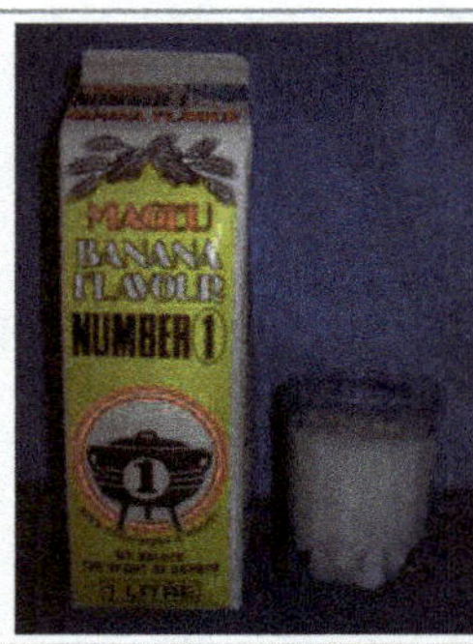		
Meigan cai	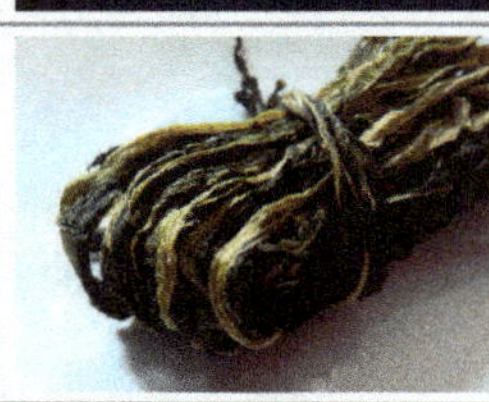		
Miso	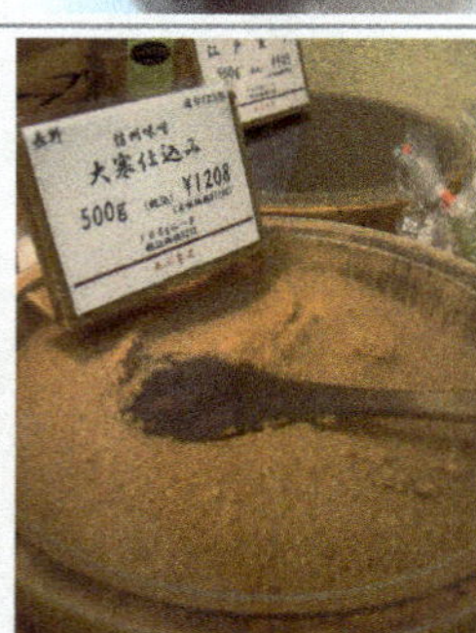		
Mixian (noodle)	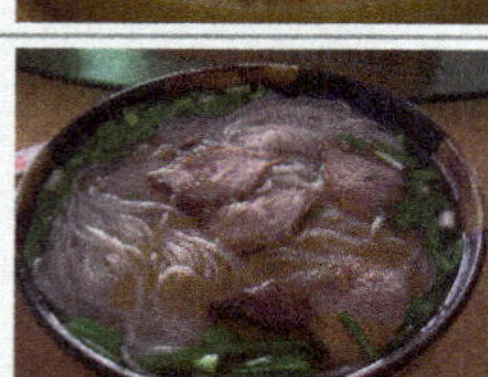		

Name	Image	Origin	Description
Mohnyin tjin	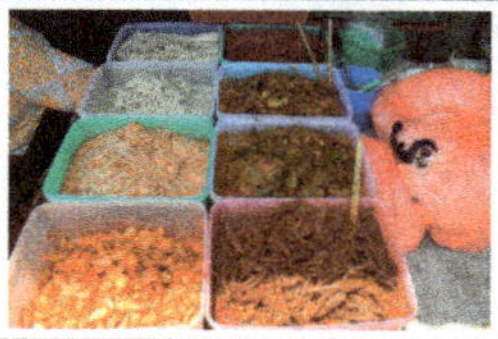		
Murri (condiment)			
Mursik			
Myeolchijeot	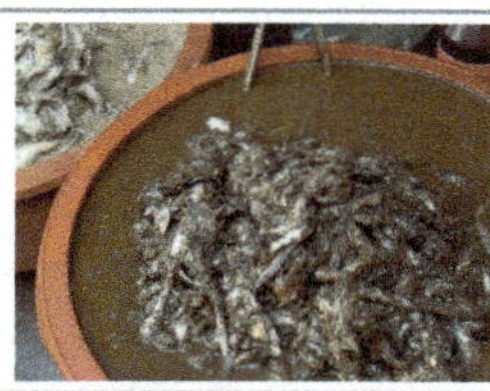	Korea	
Myeongran		Korea	
Nata de coco	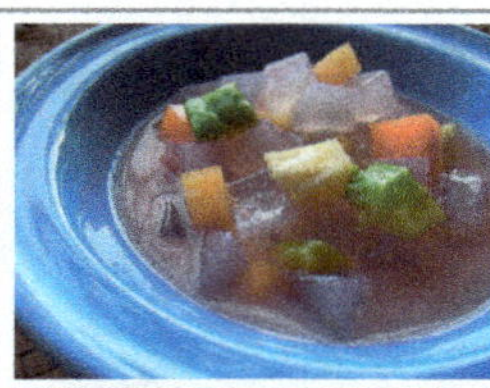		
Nattō	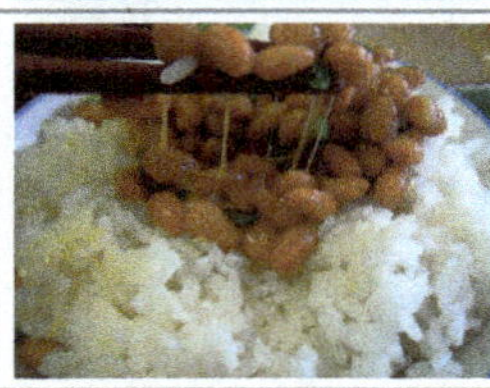	Japan	
Nem chua	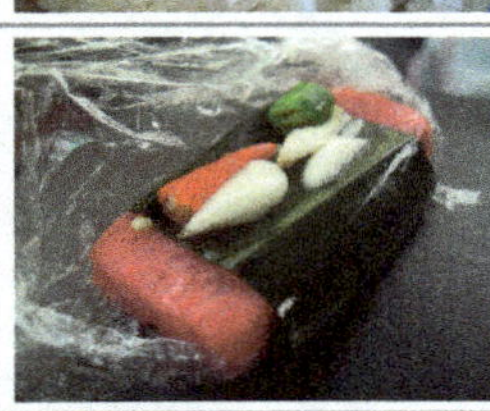	Vietnam	Nem chua is a Vietnamese fermented pork dish, usually rolled or cut in bite sizes. The meat is sweet, sour, salty and spicy. It is often served with bird's eye chili, garlic and Vietnamese coriander.
Ngapi	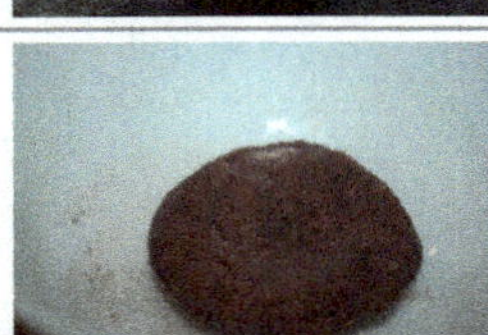		
Ogi (cereal ferment)			
Ogiri			

Name	Image	Origin	Description
Oncom	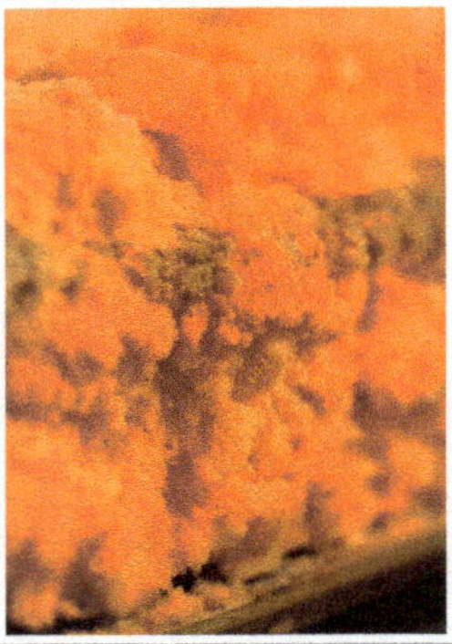		
Palappam			
Pesaha Appam	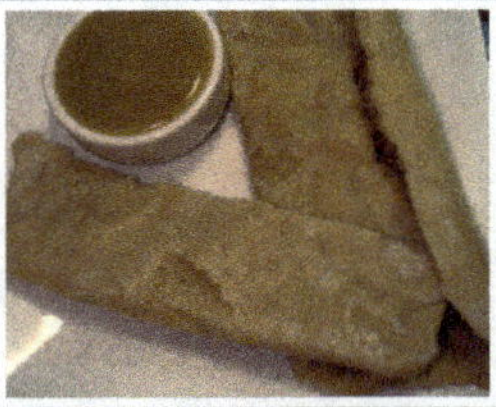		
Peuyeum	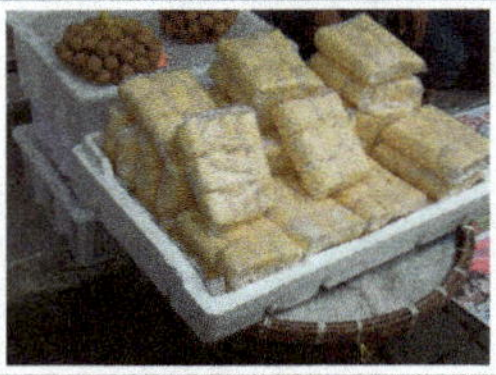		
Pickles	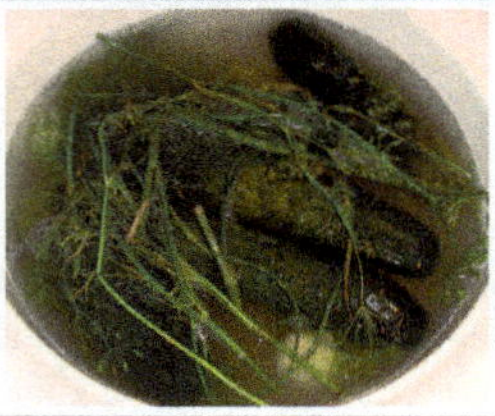		
Podpiwek		Poland, Lithuania	Soft drink usually made from grain coffee, hops, yeast, water and sugar, which undergo fermentation.
Poi (food)	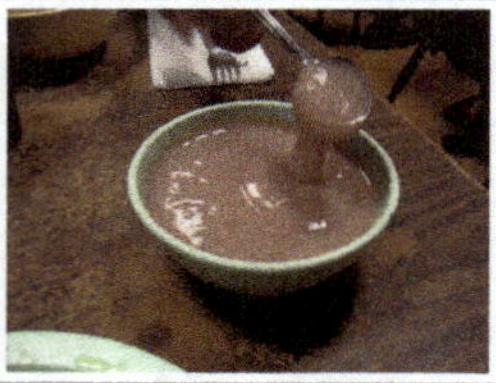		

Name	Image	Origin	Description
Pulque	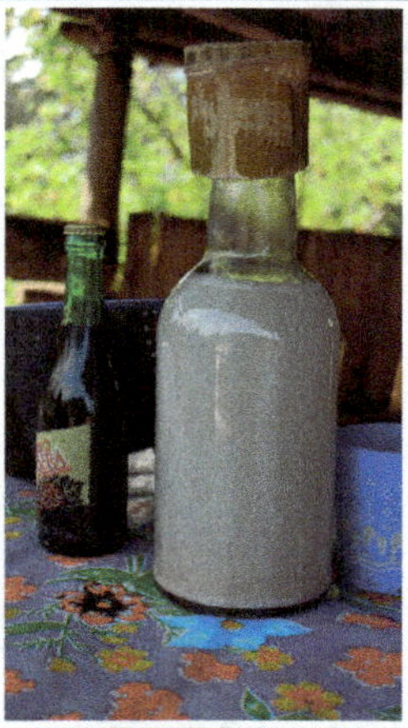		
Puto	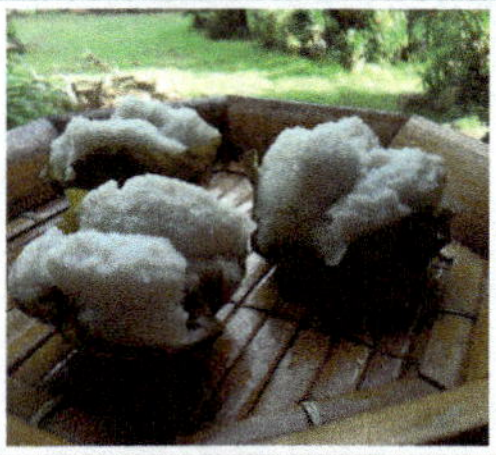		Pictured is puto in banana leaf
Rakfisk	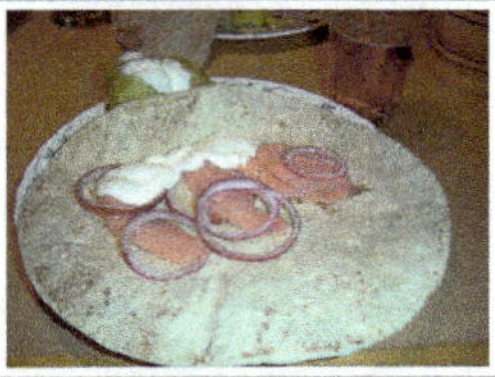		
Rượu nếp	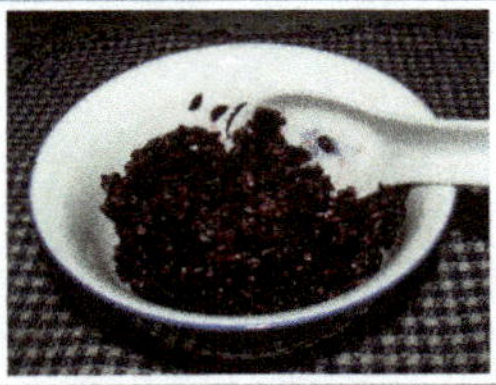		
Ryazhenka	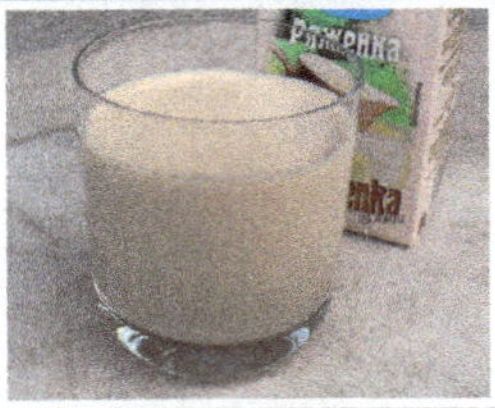		
Saeujeot	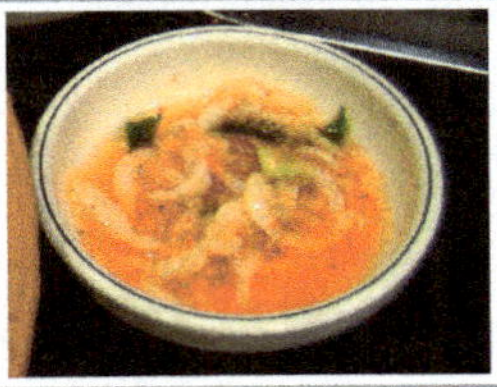	Korea	
Salami		Italy	

Name	Image	Origin	Description
Sauerkraut	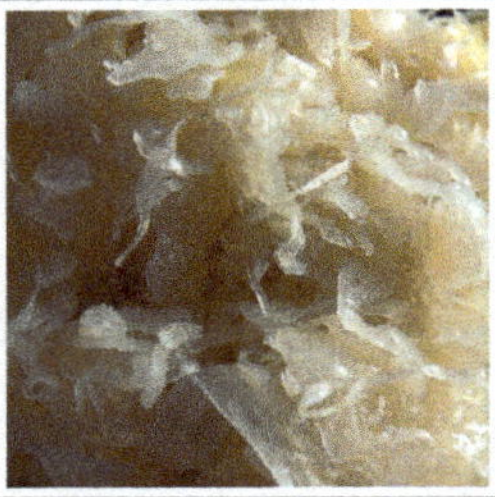		Finely cut cabbage that has been fermented by various lactic acid bacteria, including *Leuconostoc*, *Lactobacillus*, and *Pediococcus*. It has a long shelf life and a distinctive sour flavor, both of which result from the lactic acid that forms when the bacteria ferment the sugars in the cabbage.
SCOBY			
Şalgam	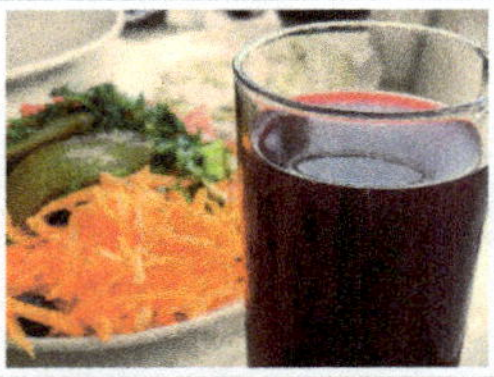	Turkey	Şalgam is a popular beverage from southern Turkey's cities of Adana and Mersin. It is made with the juice of red carrot pickles, salted, spiced, and flavoured with aromatic turnip (çelem) fermented in barrels with the addition of ground bulgur.
Shark meat	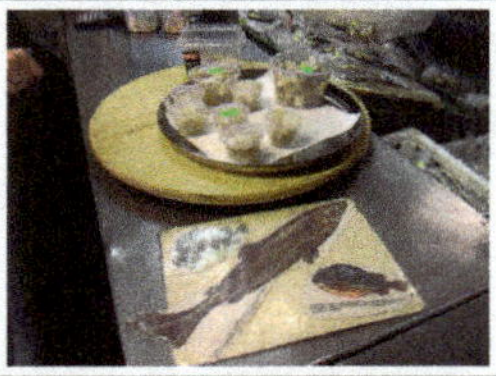		Shark meat is sometimes fermented.
Shiokara	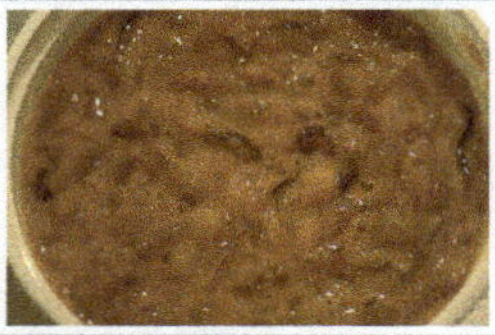		
Shrimp paste	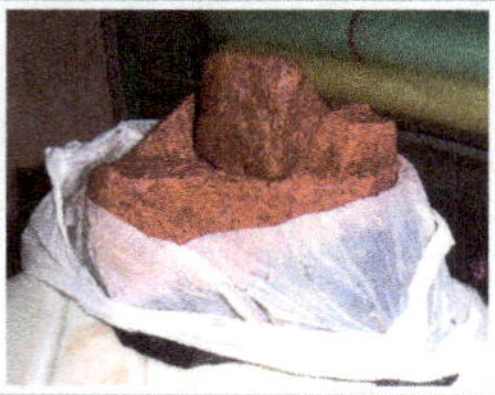		
Sinki (food)			
Skyr	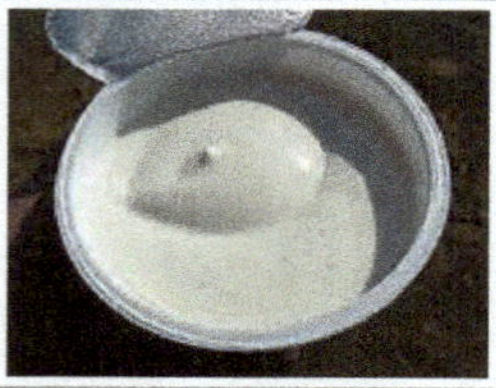		
Smântână	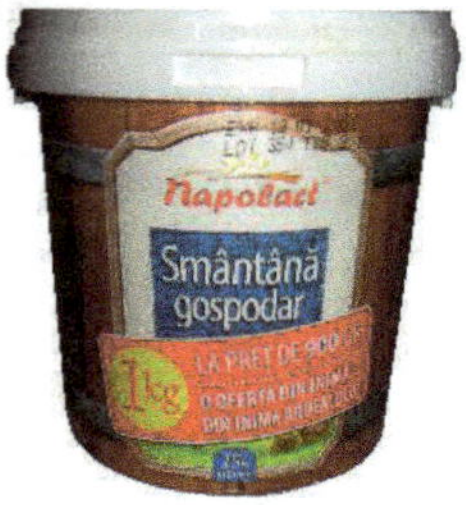		

Name	Image	Origin	Description
Smetana (dairy product)	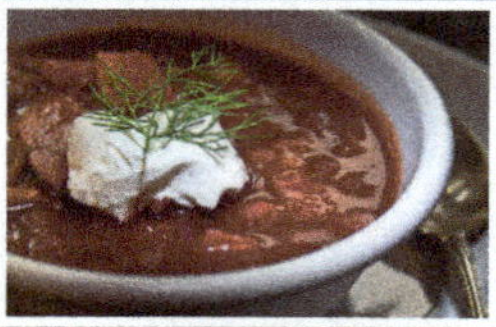		
Som moo	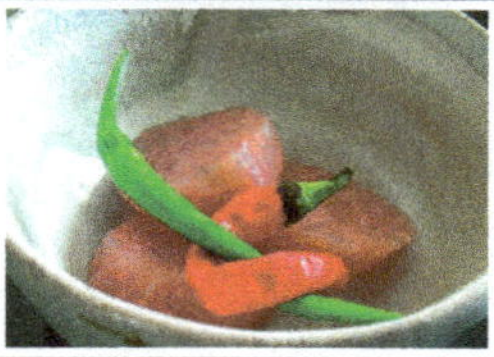		
Sour cabbage			Vegetable preserve similar to sauerkraut, with the difference that it is prepared through the lacto-fermentation of whole heads of cabbage (Brassica Oleracea var.capitata), not separate leaves or grated mass.
Sour cream	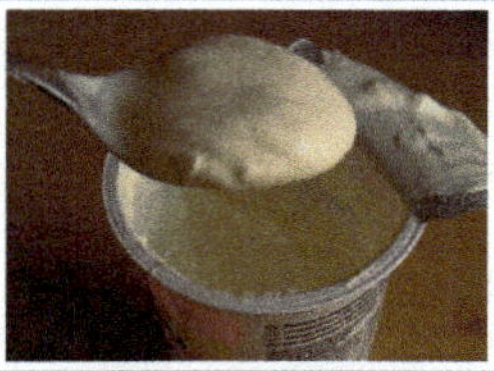		Obtained by fermenting a regular cream with certain kinds of lactic acid bacteria. The bacterial culture, which is introduced either deliberately or naturally, sours and thickens the cream. Pictured is Smetana.
Soured milk	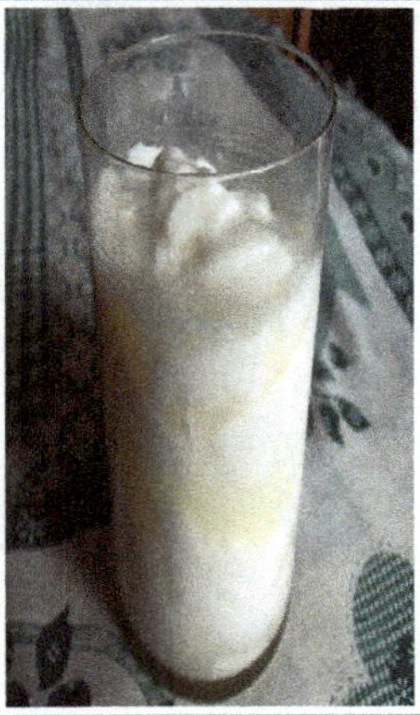		
Sowans			
Soy sauce	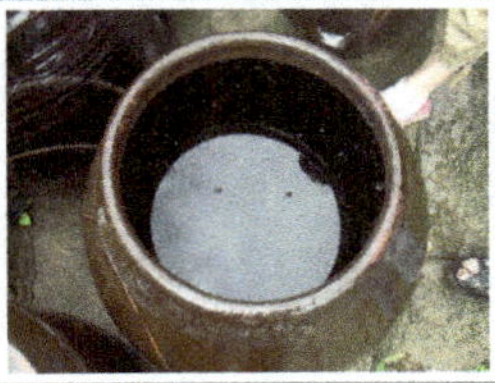	Korea, Japan, China	Pictured is traditional Korean soy sauce

Name	Image	Origin	Description
Ssamjang	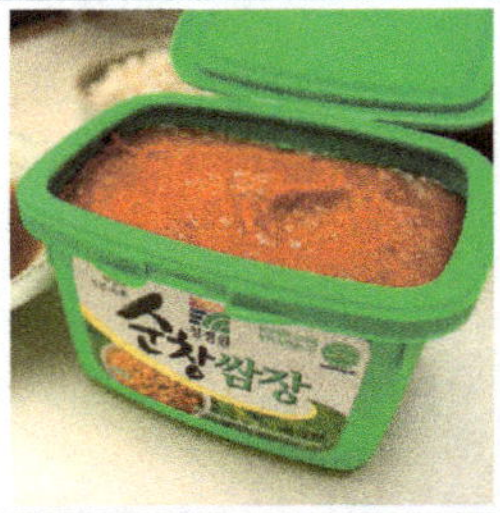	Korea	
Stinky tofu	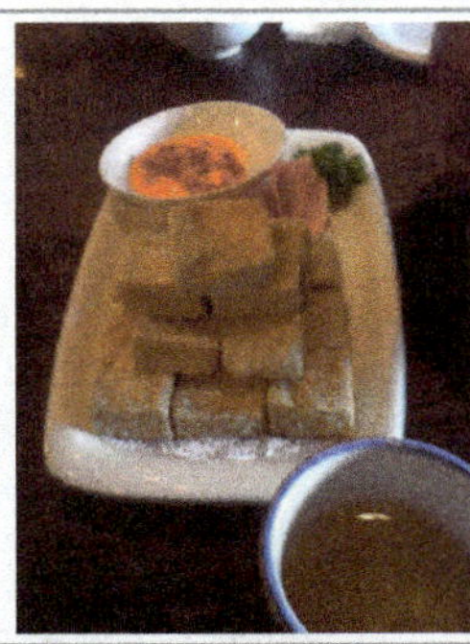		
Strained yogurt	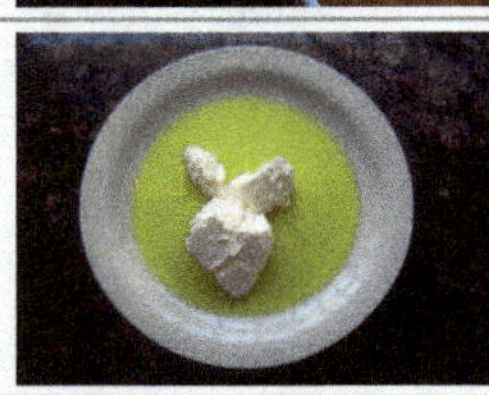		
Suan cai	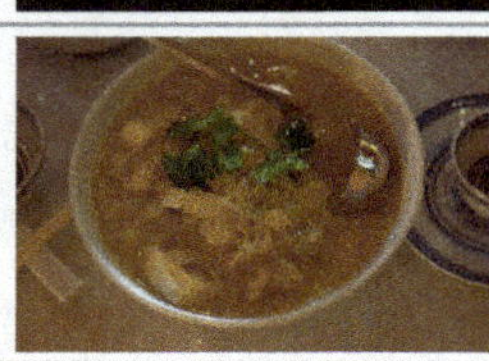		
Sumbala			
Súrmjólk			
Surströmming	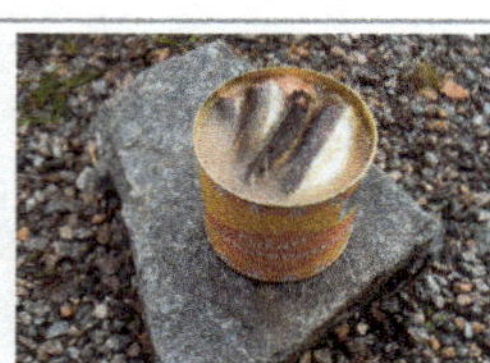		
Tabasco sauce	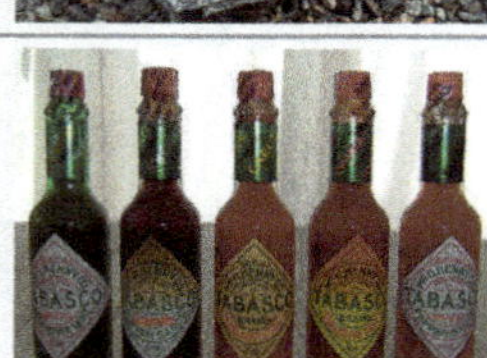		

Name	Image	Origin	Description
Tapai	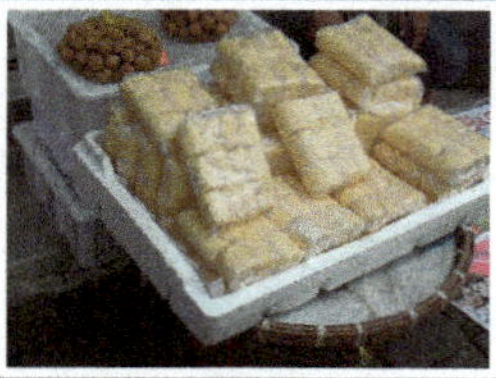		
Tarhana	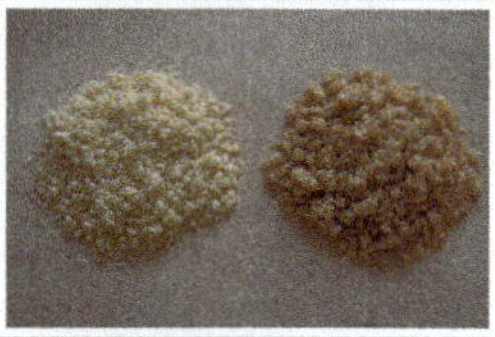		
Tempeh	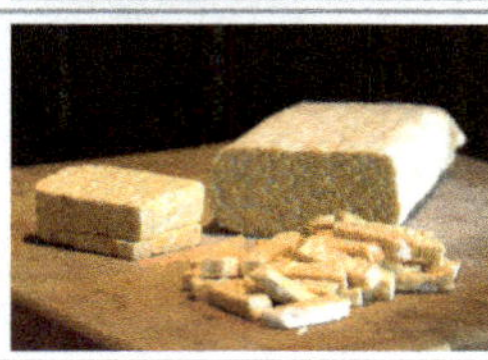	Indonesia	A traditional soy product originally from Indonesia that is made by a natural culturing and controlled fermentation process that binds soybeans into a cake form
Tesgüino			
Tianjin preserved vegetable	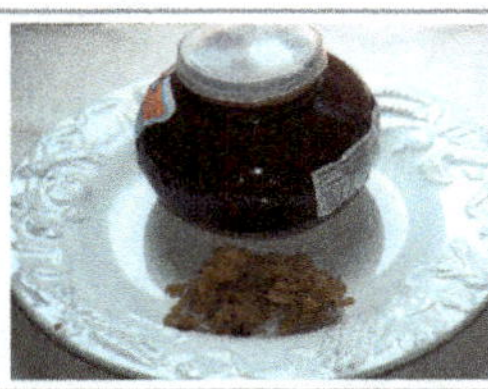		
Tianmianjiang	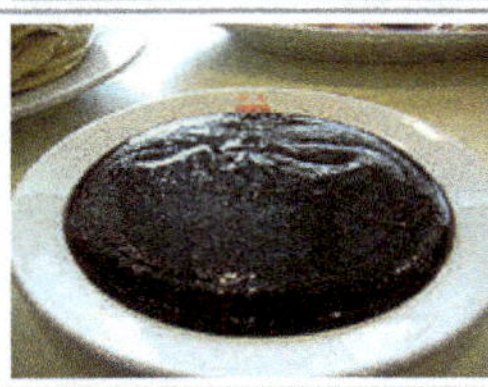		
Tibicos	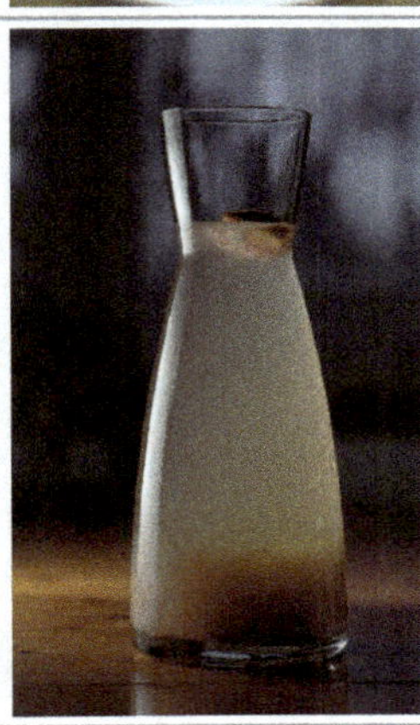		

Name	Image	Origin	Description
Tsukemono	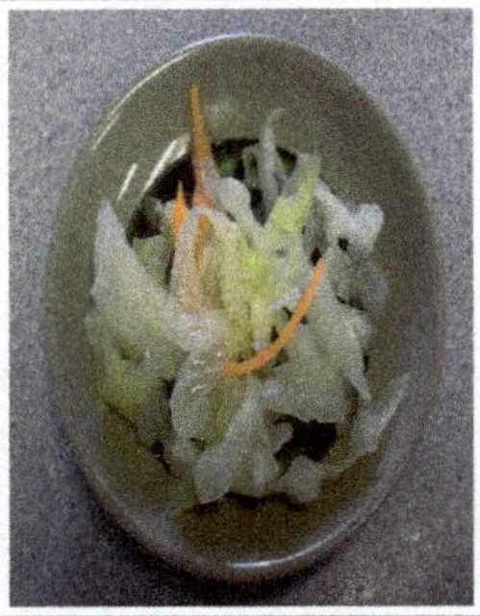		
Tương			
Viili			
White sugar sponge cake	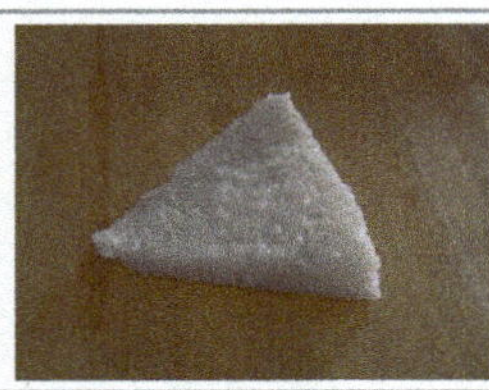		
Worcestershire sauce	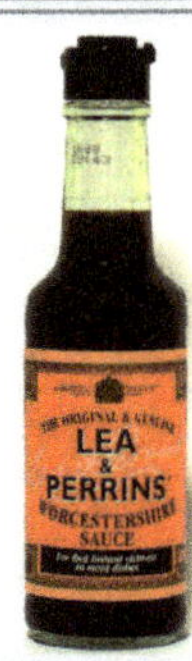		
Yakult	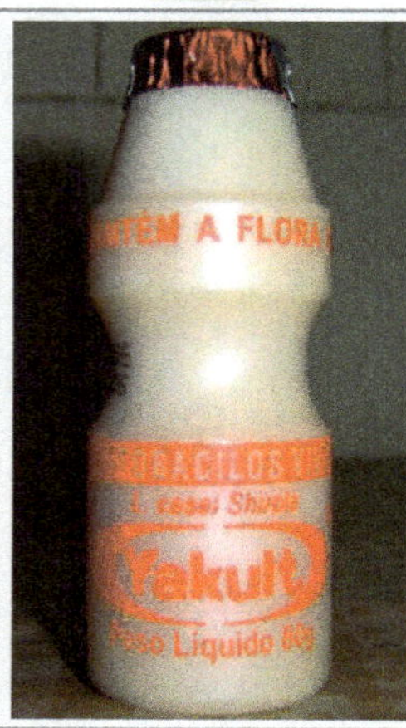		
Yellow soybean paste			

Name	Image	Origin	Description
Yogurt	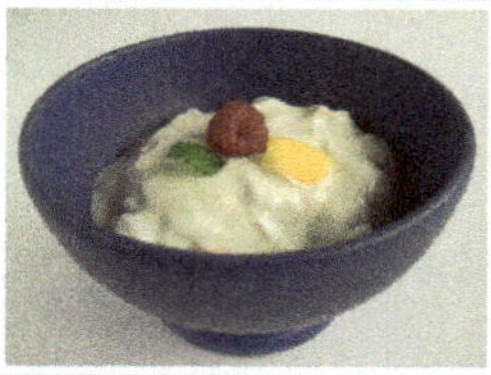		A fermented milk product produced by the bacterial fermentation of milk
Zha cai	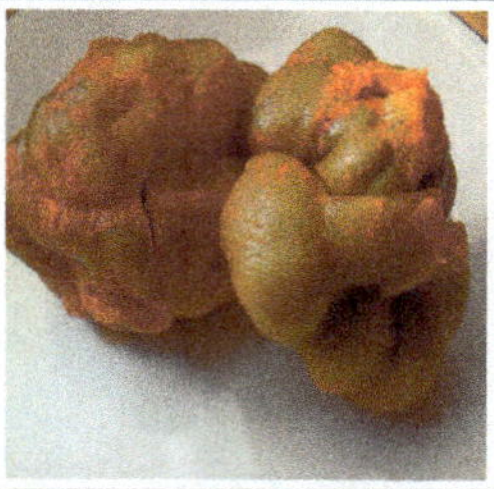		
Chakuli pitha	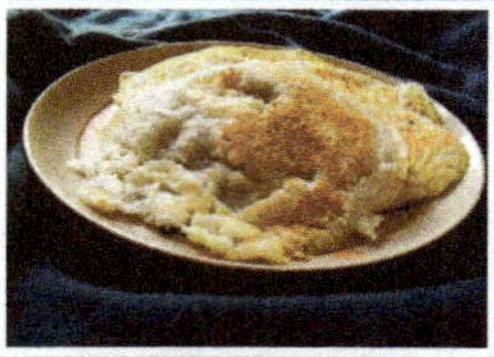	India	A rice-based fried pancake traditionally made in the Indian state of Odisha. It is made from fermented rice and black gram
Enduri Pitha	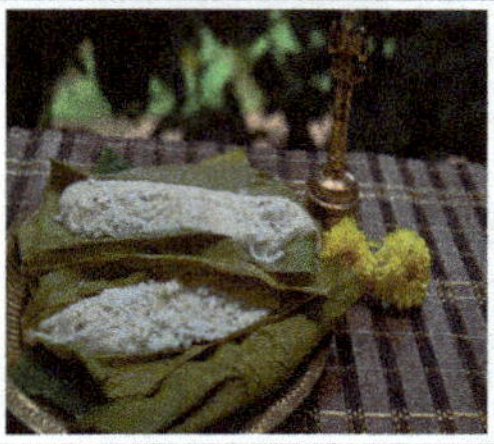	India	A traditional *pitha* made in the northern and central region Indian state of Odisha. A fermented batter made of rice and black gram is steamed with/without stuffing made of coconut, jaggery and black pepper.
Žinčica		Žinčica (in Slovakia), Žinčice (in the Czech Republic), Żentyca (in Poland)	A drink made of sheep milk whey as a by-product in the process of making *bryndza* cheese..

Fermented Foods by Type

Bean-Based

Cheonggukjang, doenjang, miso, natto, soy sauce, stinky tofu, tempeh, oncom, soybean paste, Beijing mung bean milk, kinama, iru

Dough-Based

Proofing (baking technique)

Grain-Based

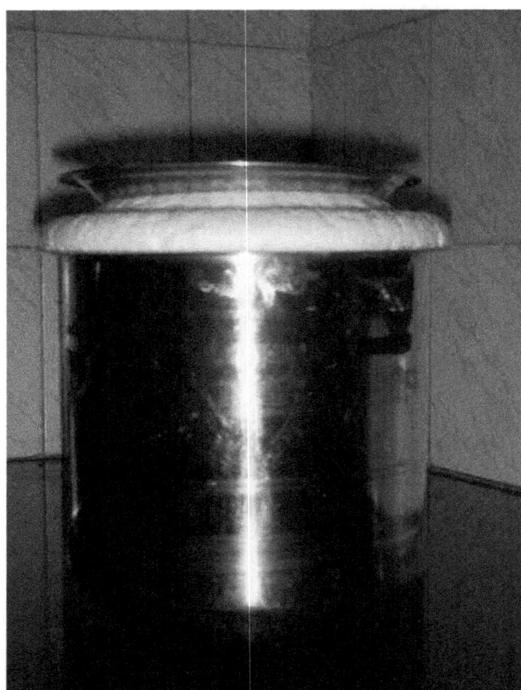

Batter made from rice and lentil (*Vigna mungo*) prepared and fermented for baking idlis and dosas

Amazake, beer, bread, choujiu, gamju, injera, kvass, makgeolli, murri, ogi, rejuvelac, sake, sikhye, sourdough, sowans, rice wine, malt whisky, grain whisky, idli, dosa, vodka, boza

Vegetable-Based

Kimchi, mixed pickle, sauerkraut, Indian pickle, gundruk, tursu

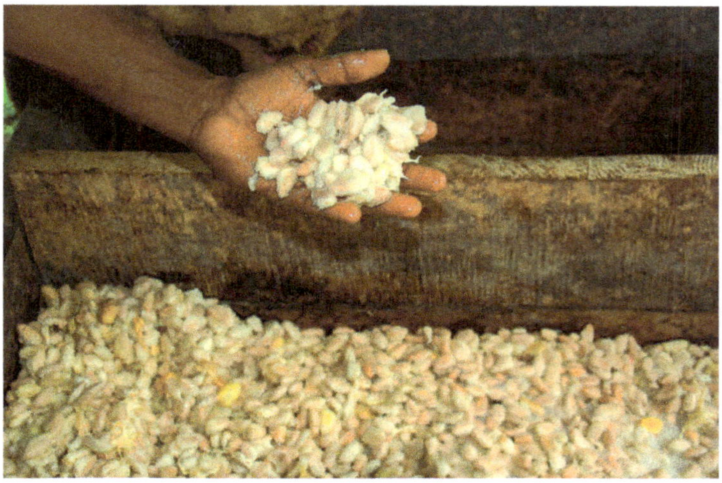

Fermenting cocoa beans

Fruit-Based

Wine, vinegar, cider, perry, brandy, atchara, nata de coco, burong mangga, asinan, pickling, vişinată, chocolate, rakı

Honey-Based

Mead, metheglin

Dairy-Based

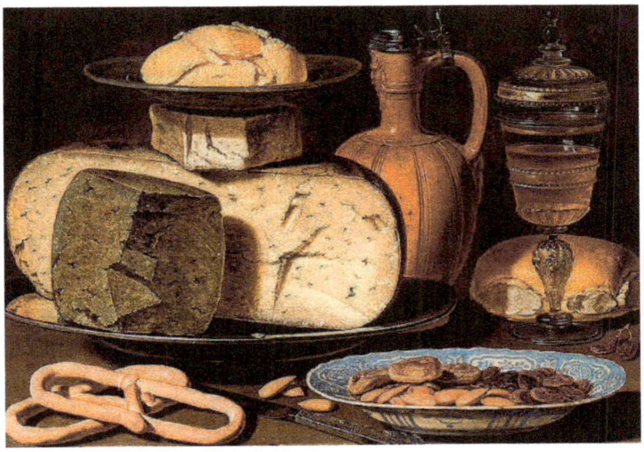

Cheeses in art: *Still Life with Cheeses, Almonds and Pretzels*, Clara Peeters, c. 1615

Some kinds of cheese also, kefir, kumis (mare milk), shubat (camel milk), cultured milk products such as quark, filmjölk, crème fraîche, smetana, skyr, and yogurt

Fish-Based

Bagoong, faseekh, fish sauce, Garum, Hákarl, jeotgal, rakfisk, shrimp paste, surströmming, shidal

Meat-Based

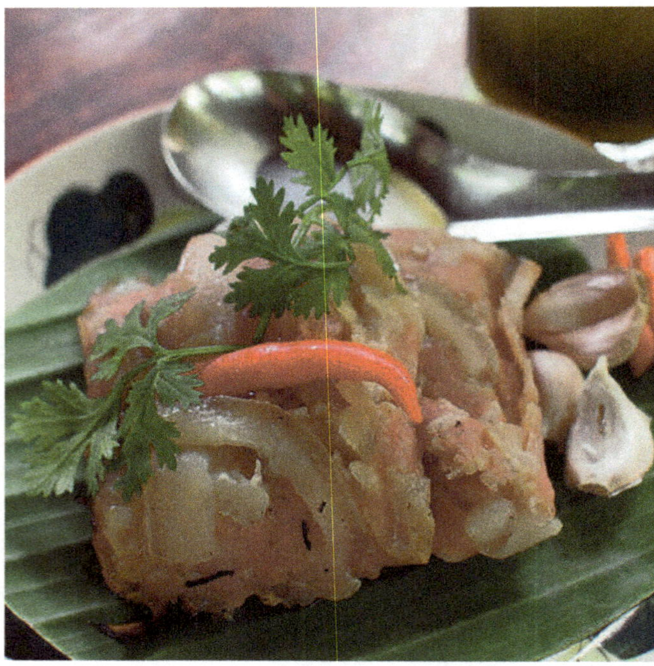

Chin som mok is a northern Thai speciality made with grilled, banana leaf-wrapped pork (both skin and meat) that has been fermented with glutinous rice

Chorizo, salami, sucuk, pepperoni, nem chua, som moo, saucisson

Tea-Based

Pu-erh tea, Kombucha

Risks

Alaska has witnessed a steady increase of cases of botulism since 1985. It has more cases of botulism than any other state in the United States of America. This is caused by the traditional Eskimo practice of allowing animal products such as whole fish, fish heads, walrus, sea lion, and whale flippers, beaver tails, seal oil, and birds, to ferment for an extended period of time before being consumed. The risk is exacerbated when a plastic container is used for this purpose instead of the old-fashioned, traditional method, a grass-lined hole, as the *Clostridium botulinum* bacteria thrive in the anaerobic conditions created by the air-tight enclosure in plastic.

The World Health Organization has classified pickled foods as possibly carcinogenic, based on epidemiological studies. Other research found that fermented food contains a carcinogenic by-product, ethyl carbamate (urethane). "A 2009 review of the existing studies conducted across Asia concluded that regularly eating pickled vegetables roughly doubles a person's risk for esophageal squamous cell carcinoma."

REFERENCES

1. McGovern, P. E.; Zhang, J.; Tang, J.; Zhang, Z.; Hall, G. R.; Moreau, R. A.; Nunez, A.; Butrym, E. D.; Richards, M. P.; Wang, C. -S.; Cheng, G.; Zhao, Z.; Wang, C. (2004). "Fermented beverages of pre- and proto-historic China". Proceedings of the National Academy of Sciences. 101 (51): 17593–17598. doi:10.1073/pnas.0407921102. PMC 539767 . PMID 15590771.
2. "8,000-year-old wine unearthed in Georgia". The Independent. 2003-12-28. Retrieved 2007-01-28.
3. "Now on display ... world's oldest known wine jar". Retrieved 2007-01-28.
4. "Fermented fruits and vegetables. A global perspective". FAO Agricultural Services Bulletins - 134. Archived from the original on January 19, 2007. Retrieved 2007-01-28.
5. Cavalieri, D.; McGovern P.E.; Hartl D.L.; Mortimer R.; Polsinelli M. (2003). "Evidence for S. cerevisiae fermentation in ancient wine." (PDF). Journal of Molecular Evolution. 57 Suppl 1: S226–32. doi:10.1007/s00239-003-0031-2. PMID 15008419. 15008419. Archived from the original (PDF) on December 9, 2006. Retrieved 2007-01-28.
6. Dirar, H. (1993). The Indigenous Fermented Foods of the Sudan: A Study in African Food and Nutrition. CAB International.
7. "Fermentation" (PDF). Archived from the original (PDF) on 2012-05-30.
8. Dubos, J. (1951). "Louis Pasteur: Free Lance of Science, Gollancz. Quoted in Manchester K. L. (1995) Louis Pasteur (1822–1895)--chance and the prepared mind". Trends in Biotechnology. 13 (12): 511–515. doi:10.1016/S0167-7799(00)89014-9. PMID 8595136.
9. Nobel Laureate Biography of Eduard Buchner at http://nobelprize.org
10. "The Nobel Prize in Chemistry 1929". Retrieved 2007-01-28.
11. Harden, A.; Young, W.J. (October 1906). "The Alcoholic Ferment of Yeast-Juice". Proceedings of the Royal Society of London (Series B, Containing Papers of a Biological Character ed.). 78 (526): 369–375.
12. Hui YH, Meunier-Goddik L, Josephsen J, Nip WK, Stanfield PS (2004). Handbook

of Food and Beverage Fermentation Technology. CRC Press. pp. 27 and passim. ISBN 978-0-8247-5122-7.

13. Steinkraus, K.H., ed. (1995). Handbook of Indigenous Fermented Foods. Marcel Dekker.
14. "Why does Alaska have more botulism". Centers for Disease Control and Prevention (U.S. federal agency). Archived from the original on 7 August 2006. Retrieved 18 July 2011.
15. "Agents Classified by the IARC Monographs, Volumes 1–105" (PDF). International Agency for Research on Cancer (United Nations World Health Organization agency). Retrieved 10 October 2012.
16. "New Link Between Wine, Fermented Food And Cancer". ScienceDaily. Retrieved 10 October 2012.
17. "The WHO Says Cellphones—and Pickles—May Cause Cancer". Slate. Retrieved 10 October 2012.s

CHAPTER 7

Foodborne Illness Food Pathogens

Chapter Contents

- **Introduction**
- **Causes**
- **Epidemiology**
- **Society and Culture**

A foodborne illness is any illness that results from consuming food contaminated with pathogenic microorganisms, or toxic compounds released by microorganisms. The disease-causing microorganisms are most often bacteria, but can also include fungi, viruses and protozoa. Your food usually travels a long distance from its origin before it gets to your plate. It can be handled by many different people and exposed to many different conditions. This results in many potential points where food can become contaminated.

Some microbes responsible for foodborne illnesses are members of the normal microflora of the food organism. So, for example, the bacteria that are naturally found in the cow intestinal tract can end up contaminating the slabs of beef during butchering. This kind of contamination can occur during slaughter or during any point in the food's processing.

Vegetables and fruits are not immune to contamination with foodborne pathogens, despite the fact that they are picked, not slaughtered. Irrigation water or fertilizers sprayed on crops can be contaminated with animal or human waste containing foodborne pathogens.

INTRODUCTION

Foodborne illness (also foodborne disease and colloquially referred to as food poisoning) is any illness resulting from the food spoilage of contaminated food, pathogenic bacteria, viruses, or parasites that contaminate food, as well as chemical or natural toxins such as poisonous mushrooms and various species of beans that have not been boiled for at least 10 minutes.

Symptoms vary depending on the cause, and are described below in this article. A few broad generalizations can be made, e.g.: The incubation period ranges from hours to days, depending on the cause and on how much was consumed. The incubation period tends to cause sufferers to not associate the symptoms with the item consumed, and so to cause sufferers to attribute the symptoms to gastroenteritis for example. Symptoms often include vomiting, fever, and aches, and may include diarrhea. Bouts of vomiting can be repeated with an extended delay in between, because even if infected food was eliminated from the stomach in the first bout, microbes (if applicable) can pass through the stomach into the intestine via cells lining the intestinal walls and begin to multiply. Some types of microbes stay in the intestine, some produce a toxin that is absorbed into the bloodstream, and some can directly invade deeper body tissues.

CAUSES

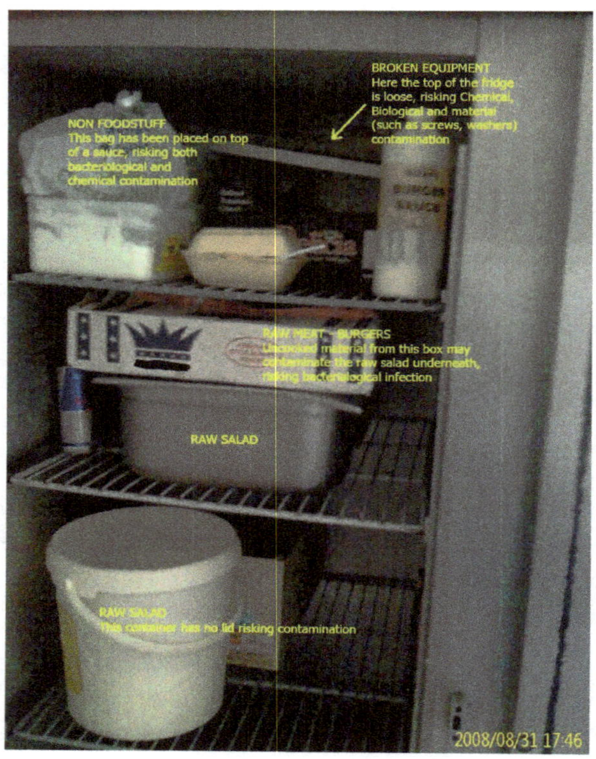

Poorly stored food in a refrigerator

Foodborne illness usually arises from improper handling, preparation, or food storage. Good hygiene practices before, during, and after food preparation can reduce the chances of contracting an illness. There is a consensus in the public health community that regular hand-washing is one of the most effective defenses against the spread of foodborne illness. The action of monitoring food to ensure that it will not cause foodborne illness is known as food safety. Foodborne disease can also be caused by a large variety of toxins that affect the environment.

Foodborne illness can also be caused by pesticides or medicines in food and naturally toxic substances such as poisonous mushrooms or reef fish.

Bacteria

Bacteria are a common cause of foodborne illness. In the United Kingdom during 2000, the individual bacteria involved were the following: *Campylobacter jejuni* 77.3%, *Salmonella* 20.9%, *Escherichia coli* O157:H7 1.4%, and all others less than 0.56%. In the past, bacterial infections were thought to be more prevalent because few places had the capability to test for norovirus and no active surveillance was being done for this particular agent. Toxins from bacterial infections are delayed because the bacteria need time to multiply. As a result, symptoms associated with intoxication are usually not seen until 12–72 hours or more after eating contaminated food. However, in some cases, such as Staphylococcal food poisoning, the onset of illness can be as soon as 30 minutes after ingesting contaminated food.

Most common bacterial foodborne pathogens are:

- *Campylobacter jejuni* which can lead to secondary Guillain–Barré syndrome and periodontitis
- *Clostridium perfringens*, the "cafeteria germ"
- *Salmonella* spp. – its *S. typhimurium* infection is caused by consumption of eggs or poultry that are not adequately cooked or by other interactive human-animal pathogens

Salmonella

- *Escherichia coli O157:H7* enterohemorrhagic (EHEC) which can cause hemolytic-uremic syndrome

Other common bacterial foodborne pathogens are:

- *Bacillus cereus*
- *Escherichia coli*, other virulence properties, such as enteroinvasive (EIEC), enteropathogenic (EPEC), enterotoxigenic (ETEC), enteroaggregative (EAEC or EAgEC)
- *Listeria monocytogenes*
- *Shigella* spp.
- *Staphylococcus aureus*

- *Staphylococcal enteritis*
- *Streptococcus*
- *Vibrio cholerae*, including O1 and non-O1
- *Vibrio parahaemolyticus*
- *Vibrio vulnificus*
- *Yersinia enterocolitica* and *Yersinia pseudotuberculosis*

Less common bacterial agents:

- *Brucella* spp.
- *Corynebacterium ulcerans*
- *Coxiella burnetii* or Q fever
- *Plesiomonas shigelloides*

Enterotoxins

In addition to disease caused by direct bacterial infection, some foodborne illnesses are caused by enterotoxins (exotoxins targeting the intestines). Enterotoxins can produce illness even when the microbes that produced them have been killed. Symptom appearance varies with the toxin but may be rapid in onset, as in the case of enterotoxins of *Staphylococcus aureus* in which symptoms appear in one to six hours. This causes intense vomiting including or not including diarrhea (resulting in staphylococcal enteritis), and staphylococcal enterotoxins (most commonly staphylococcal enterotoxin A but also including staphylococcal enterotoxin B) are the most commonly reported enterotoxins although cases of poisoning are likely underestimated. It occurs mainly in cooked and processed foods due to competition with other biota in raw foods, and humans are the main cause of contamination as a substantial percentage of humans are persistent carriers of *S. aureus*. The CDC has estimated about 240,000 cases per year in the United States.

- Clostridium botulinum
- Clostridium perfringens
- Bacillus cereus

The rare but potentially deadly disease botulism occurs when the anaerobic bacterium *Clostridium botulinum* grows in improperly canned low-acid foods and produces botulin, a powerful paralytic toxin.

Pseudoalteromonas tetraodonis, certain species of Pseudomonas and Vibrio, and some other bacteria, produce the lethal tetrodotoxin, which is present in the tissues of some living animal species rather than being a product of decomposition.

Emerging Foodborne Pathogens

Many foodborne illnesses remain poorly understood.

- *Aeromonas hydrophila*, *Aeromonas caviae*, *Aeromonas sobria*

Preventing Bacterial Food Poisoning

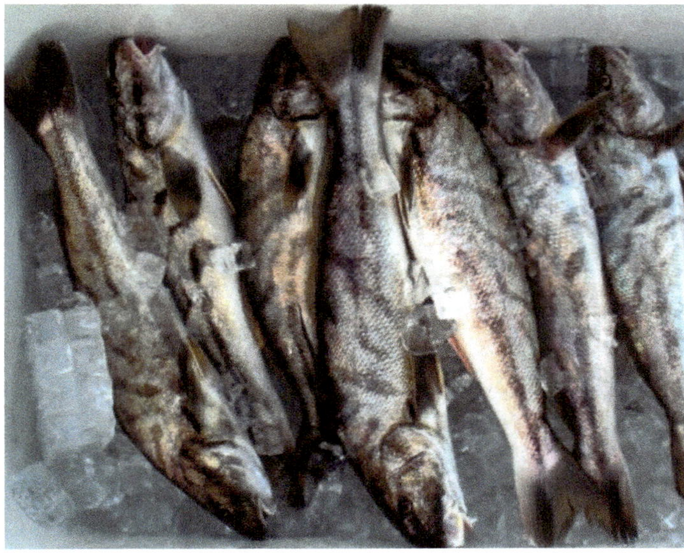

Proper storage and refrigeration of food help in the prevention of food poisoning

Prevention is mainly the role of the state, through the definition of strict rules of hygiene and a public services of veterinary surveying of animal products in the food chain, from farming to the transformation industry and delivery (shops and restaurants). This regulation includes:

- traceability: in a final product, it must be possible to know the origin of the ingredients (originating farm, identification of the harvesting or of the animal) and where and when it was processed; the origin of the illness can thus be tracked and solved (and possibly penalized), and the final products can be removed from the sale if a problem is detected;
- enforcement of hygiene procedures such as HACCP and the "cold chain";
- power of control and of law enforcement of veterinarians.

In August 2006, the United States Food and Drug Administration approved Phage therapy which involves spraying meat with viruses that infect bacteria, and thus preventing infection. This has raised concerns, because without mandatory labelling consumers would not be aware that meat and poultry products have been treated with the spray.

At home, prevention mainly consists of good food safety practices. Many forms of bacterial poisoning can be prevented by cooking it sufficiently, and either eating it quickly or refrigerating it effectively. Many toxins, however, are not destroyed by heat treatment.

Techniques that help prevent food borne illness in the kitchen are hand washing, rinsing produce, preventing cross-contamination, proper storage, and maintaining cooking temperatures. In general, freezing or refrigerating prevents virtually all bacteria from growing, and heating food sufficiently kills parasites, viruses, and most bacteria. Bacteria grow most rapidly at the range of temperatures between 40 °F and 140 °F, called the "danger zone". Storing food below or above the "danger zone" can effectively limit the production of toxins. For storing leftovers, the food must be put in shallow containers for quick cooling and must be refrigerated within two hours. When food is reheated, it must reach an internal temperature of 165 °F (74 °C) or until hot or steaming to kill bacteria.

Mycotoxins and Alimentary Mycotoxicoses

The term alimentary mycotoxicoses refers to the effect of poisoning by Mycotoxins (The term 'mycotoxin' is usually reserved for the toxic chemical products produced by fungi that readily colonize crops) through food consumption. Mycotoxins sometimes have important effects on human and animal health. For example, an outbreak which occurred in the UK in 1960 caused the death of 100,000 turkeys which had consumed aflatoxin-contaminated peanut meal. In the USSR in World War II, 5,000 people died due to Alimentary Toxic Aleukia (ALA). The common foodborne Mycotoxins include:

- Aflatoxins – originated from Aspergillus parasiticus and Aspergillus flavus. They are frequently found in tree nuts, peanuts, maize, sorghum and other oilseeds, including corn and cottonseeds. The pronounced forms of Aflatoxins are those of B1, B2, G1, and G2, amongst which Aflatoxin B1 predominantly targets the liver, which will result in necrosis, cirrhosis, and carcinoma. In the US, the acceptable level of total aflatoxins in foods is less than 20 μg/kg, except for Aflatoxin M1 in milk, which should be less than 0.5 μg/kg. The official document can be found at FDA›s website.
- Altertoxins – are those of Alternariol (AOH), Alternariol methyl ether (AME), Altenuene (ALT), Altertoxin-1 (ATX-1), Tenuazonic acid (TeA) and Radicinin (RAD), originated from Alternaria spp. Some of the toxins can be present in sorghum, ragi, wheat and tomatoes. Some research has shown that the toxins can be easily cross-contaminated between grain commodities, suggesting that manufacturing and storage of grain commodities is a critical practice.
- Citrinin
- Citreoviridin
- Cyclopiazonic acid
- Cytochalasins
- Ergot alkaloids / Ergopeptine alkaloids – Ergotamine
- Fumonisins – Crop corn can be easily contaminated by the fungi Fusarium moniliforme, and its Fumonisin B1 will cause Leukoencephalomalacia (LEM) in horses, Pulmonary edema syndrome (PES) in pigs, liver cancer in rats and Esophageal cancer in humans. For human and animal health, both the FDA and the EC have regulated the content levels of toxins in food and animal feed.
- Fusaric acid
- Fusarochromanone
- Kojic acid
- Lolitrem alkaloids

- Moniliformin
- 3-Nitropropionic acid
- Nivalenol
- Ochratoxins – In Australia, The Limit of Reporting (LOR) level for Ochratoxin A (OTA) analyses in 20th Australian Total Diet Survey was 1 μg/kg, whereas the EC restricts the content of OTA to 5 μg/kg in cereal commodities, 3 μg/kg in processed products and 10 μg/kg in dried vine fruits.
- Oosporeine
- Patulin – Currently, this toxin has been advisably regulated on fruit products. The EC and the FDA have limited it to under 50 μg/kg for fruit juice and fruit nectar, while limits of 25 μg/kg for solid-contained fruit products and 10 μg/kg for baby foods were specified by the EC.
- Phomopsins
- Sporidesmin A
- Sterigmatocystin
- Tremorgenic mycotoxins – Five of them have been reported to be associated with molds found in fermented meats. These are Fumitremorgen B, Paxilline, Penitrem A, Verrucosidin, and Verruculogen.
- Trichothecenes – sourced from Cephalosporium, Fusarium, Myrothecium, Stachybotrys and Trichoderma. The toxins are usually found in molded maize, wheat, corn, peanuts and rice, or animal feed of hay and straw. Four trichothecenes, T-2 toxin, HT-2 toxin, diacetoxyscirpenol (DAS) and deoxynivalenol (DON) have been most commonly encountered by humans and animals. The consequences of oral intake of, or dermal exposure to, the toxins will result in Alimentary toxic aleukia, neutropenia, aplastic anemia, thrombocytopenia and/or skin irritation. In 1993, the FDA issued a document for the content limits of DON in food and animal feed at an advisory level. In 2003, US published a patent that is very promising for farmers to produce a trichothecene-resistant crop.
- Zearalenone
- Zearalenols

Viruses

Viral infections make up perhaps one third of cases of food poisoning in developed countries. In the US, more than 50% of cases are viral and noroviruses are the most common foodborne illness, causing 57% of outbreaks in 2004. Foodborne viral infection are usually of intermediate (1–3 days) incubation period, causing illnesses which are self-limited in otherwise healthy individuals; they are similar to the bacterial forms described above.

- Enterovirus
- Hepatitis A is distinguished from other viral causes by its prolonged (2–6 week)

incubation period and its ability to spread beyond the stomach and intestines into the liver. It often results in jaundice, or yellowing of the skin, but rarely leads to chronic liver dysfunction. The virus has been found to cause infection due to the consumption of fresh-cut produce which has fecal contamination.

- Hepatitis E
- Norovirus
- Rotavirus

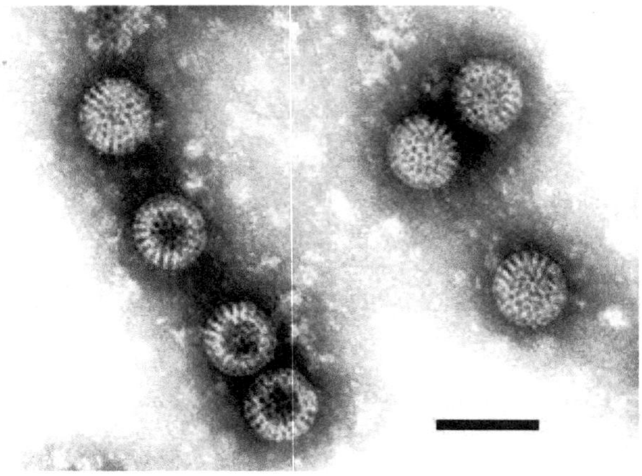

Rotavirus

Parasites

Most foodborne parasites are zoonoses.

- Platyhelminthes:
- *Diphyllobothrium* sp.
- *Nanophyetus* sp.
- *Taenia saginata*
- *Taenia solium*
- *Fasciola hepatica*
- Nematode:
- *Anisakis* sp.
- *Ascaris lumbricoides*
- *Eustrongylides* sp.
- *Trichinella spiralis*
- *Trichuris trichiura*
- *Protozoa:*
- *Acanthamoeba* and other free-living amoebae

- *Cryptosporidium parvum*
- *Cyclospora cayetanensis*
- *Entamoeba histolytica*
- *Giardia lamblia*

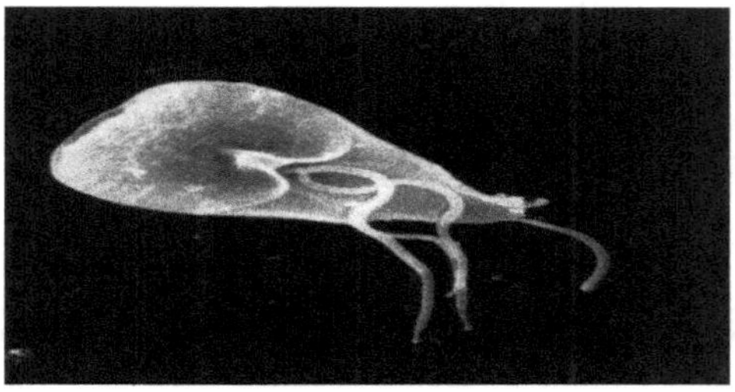

Giardia lamblia

- *Sarcocystis hominis*
- *Sarcocystis suihominis*
- *Toxoplasma gondii*

Natural Toxins

Several foods can naturally contain toxins, many of which are not produced by bacteria. Plants in particular may be toxic; animals which are naturally poisonous to eat are rare. In evolutionary terms, animals can escape being eaten by fleeing; plants can use only passive defenses such as poisons and distasteful substances, for example capsaicin in chili peppers and pungent sulfur compounds in garlic and onions. Most animal poisons are not synthesised by the animal, but acquired by eating poisonous plants to which the animal is immune, or by bacterial action.

- Alkaloids
- Ciguatera poisoning
- Grayanotoxin (honey intoxication)
- Mushroom toxins
- Phytohaemagglutinin (red kidney bean poisoning; destroyed by boiling)
- Pyrrolizidine alkaloids
- Shellfish toxin, including paralytic shellfish poisoning, diarrhetic shellfish poisoning, neurotoxic shellfish poisoning, amnesic shellfish poisoning and ciguatera fish poisoning
- Scombrotoxin
- Tetrodotoxin (fugu fish poisoning)

Some plants contain substances which are toxic in large doses, but have therapeutic properties in appropriate dosages.

- Foxglove contains cardiac glycosides.
- Poisonous hemlock (conium) has medicinal uses.

Other Pathogenic Agents

- Prions, resulting in Creutzfeldt–Jakob disease

"Ptomaine Poisoning"

In 1883, the Italian professor Salmi, of Bologna, introduced the generic name *ptomaine* (from Greek *ptōma*, "fall, fallen body, corpse") for alkaloids found in decaying animal and vegetable matter, especially (as reflected in their names) putrescine and cadaverine. The 1892 *Merck's Bulletin* stated, "We name such products of bacterial origin ptomaines; and the special alkaloid produced by the comma bacillus is variously named Cadaverine, Putrescine, etc.» While *The Lancet* stated, "The chemical ferments produced in the system, the...ptomaines which may exercise so disastrous an influence.» It is now known that the «disastrous...influence» is due to the direct action of bacteria and only slightly to the alkaloids. Thus, the use of the phrase «ptomaine poisoning» is now obsolete.

Tainted potato salad sickening hundreds at a Communist political convention in Massillon, Ohio, and aboard a Washington DC cruise boat in separate incidents during a single week in 1932 drew national attention to the dangers of so-called «ptomaine poisoning» in the pages of the American news weekly, *Time.* Another newspaper article from 1944 told of more than 150 persons being hospitalized in Chicago with ptomaine poisoning apparently from rice pudding served by a chain of restaurants.

Mechanism

Incubation Period

The delay between consumption of a contaminated food and appearance of the first symptoms of illness is called the incubation period. This ranges from hours to days (and rarely months or even years, such as in the case of listeriosis or bovine spongiform encephalopathy), depending on the agent, and on how much was consumed. If symptoms occur within one to six hours after eating the food, it suggests that it is caused by a bacterial toxin or a chemical rather than live bacteria.

The long incubation period of many foodborne illnesses tends to cause sufferers to attribute their symptoms to gastroenteritis.

During the incubation period, microbes pass through the stomach into the intestine, attach to the cells lining the intestinal walls, and begin to multiply there. Some types of microbes stay in the intestine, some produce a toxin that is absorbed into the bloodstream, and some can directly invade the deeper body tissues. The symptoms produced depend on the type of microbe.

Infectious Dose

The infectious dose is the amount of agent that must be consumed to give rise to symptoms of foodborne illness, and varies according to the agent and the consumer's age and overall health. Pathogens vary in minimum infectious dose; for example, *Shigella sonnei* has a low estimated minimum dose of < 500 colony-forming units (CFU) while *Staphylococcus aureus* has a relatively high estimate.

In the case of *Salmonella* a relatively large inoculum of 1 million to 1 billion organisms is necessary to produce symptoms in healthy human volunteers, as *Salmonellae* are very sensitive to acid. An unusually high stomach pH level (low acidity) greatly reduces the number of bacteria required to cause symptoms by a factor of between 10 and 100.

EPIDEMIOLOGY

Asymptomatic subclinical infection may help spread these diseases, particularly *Staphylococcus aureus*, *Campylobacter, Salmonella, Shigella, V. cholerae,* and *Yersini*. For example, as of 1984 it was estimated that in the United States, 200,000 people were asymptomatic carriers of Salmonella.

United States

In the United States, using FoodNet data from 2000–2007, the CDCP estimated there were 47.8 million foodborne illnesses per year (16,000 cases for 100,000 inhabitants) with 9.4 million of these caused by 31 known identified pathogens.

- 127,839 were hospitalized (43 per 100,000 inhabitants per year).
- 3,037 people died (1.0 per 100,000 inhabitants per year).

Causes of foodborne illness in U. S.

	Cause	**Annual cases**	**Rate (per 100,000 inhabitants)**
1	*Norovirus*	5,461,731 cases	X
2	*Salmonella*	1,027,561 cases	X
3	*Clostridium perfringens*	965,958 cases	X
4	Campylobacter	845,024 cases	X

Causes of death by foodborne illness in U. S.

	Cause	**Annual deaths**	**Rate (per 100,000 inhabitants)**
1	*Salmonella*	378 cases	0.126
2	*Toxoplasma gondii*	327 cases	0.109
3	*Listeria*	255 cases	0.085
4	*Norovirus*	149 cases	0.050

France

This data pertains to reported medical cases of 23 specific pathogens, as opposed to total population estimates of all food-borne illness for the United States.

In France, for 750,000 cases (1210 per 100,000 inhabitants):

- 70,000 people consulted in the emergency department of an hospital (113 per 100,000 inhabitants.);
- 113,000 people were hospitalized (182 per 100,000 inhabitants);
- 460 people died (0.75 per 100,000 inhabitants).

Causes of foodborne illness in France

	Cause	Annual hospitalizations	Rate (per 100,000 inhabitants)
1	*Salmonella*	~8,000 cases	13
2	*Campylobacter*	~3,000 cases	4.8
3	Parasites incl. Toxoplasma	~500 cases ~400 cases	0.8 0.65
4	*Listeria*	~300 cases	0.5
5	Hepatitis A	~60 cases	0.1

Causes of death by foodborne illness in France

	Cause	Annual	Rate (per 100,000 inhabitants)
1	*Salmonella*	~300 cases	0.5
2	*Listeria*	~80 cases	0.13
3	Parasites	~37 cases	0.06 (95% due to toxoplasma)
4	*Campylobacter*	~15 cases	0.02
5	Hepatitis A	~2 cases	0.003

Australia

A study by the Australian National University, published in November 2014, found in 2010 that there were an estimated 4.1 million cases of foodborne gastroenteritis acquired in Australia on average each year, along with 5,140 cases of non-gastrointestinal illness. The study was funded by the Australian Department of Health, Food Standards Australia New Zealand and the NSW Food Authority.

The main causes were Norovirus, pathogenic Escherichia coli, Campylobacter spp. and non-typhoidal Salmonella spp., although the causes of approximately 80% of illnesses were unknown. Approximately 25% (90% CrI: 13%–42%) of the 15.9 million episodes of gastroenteritis that occur in Australia were estimated to be transmitted by contaminated food. This equates to an average of approximately one episode of foodborne gastroenteritis every five years per person. Data on the number of hospitalisations and deaths represent the occurrence of serious foodborne illness. Including gastroenteritis, non-gastroenteritis and sequelae, there were an estimated annual 31,920 (90% CrI: 29,500–35,500) hospitalisations due to foodborne illness and 86 (90% CrI: 70–105) deaths due to foodborne illness circa 2010. This study concludes that these rates are similar to recent estimates in the US and Canada.

A main aim of this study was to compare if foodborne illness incidence had increased over time. In this study, similar methods of assessment were applied to data from circa 2000, which showed that the rate of foodborne gastroenteritis had not changed significantly over time. Two key estimates were the total number of gastroenteritis episodes each year, and the proportion considered foodborne. In circa 2010, it was estimated that 25% of all episodes of gastroenteritis were foodborne. By applying this proportion of episodes due to food to the incidence of gastroenteritis circa 2000, there were an estimated 4.3 million (90% CrI: 2.2–7.3 million) episodes of foodborne gastroenteritis circa 2000, although credible intervals overlap with 2010. Taking into account changes in population size, applying these equivalent methods suggests a 17% decrease in the rate of foodborne gastroenteritis between 2000 and 2010, with considerable overlap of the 90% credible intervals.

This study replaces a previous estimate of 5.4 million cases of food-borne illness in Australia every year, causing:

- 18,000 hospitalizations
- 120 deaths (0.5 deaths per 100,000 inhabitants)
- 2.1 million lost days off work
- 1.2 million doctor consultations
- 300,000 prescriptions for antibiotics.

Most foodborne disease outbreaks in Australia have been linked to raw or minimally cooked eggs or poultry. The Australian Food Safety Information Council estimates that one third of cases of food poisoning occur in the home

Comparison between Countries

Country	Annual deaths per 100,000 inhabitants	Annual hospitalization per 100,000 inhabitants
USA	1.0	43
France	0.75	182
Australia	0.5	82

Outbreaks

The vast majority of reported cases of foodborne illness occur as individual or sporadic cases. The origin of most sporadic cases is undetermined. In the United States, where people eat outside the home frequently, 58% of cases originate from commercial food facilities (2004 FoodNet data). An outbreak is defined as occurring when two or more people experience similar illness after consuming food from a common source.

Often, a combination of events contributes to an outbreak, for example, food might be left at room temperature for many hours, allowing bacteria to multiply which is compounded by inadequate cooking which results in a failure to kill the dangerously elevated bacterial levels.

Outbreaks are usually identified when those affected know each other. However, more and more, outbreaks are identified by public health staff from unexpected increases in laboratory results for certain strains of bacteria. Outbreak detection and investigation in the United States is primarily handled by local health jurisdictions and is inconsistent from district to district. It is estimated that 1–2% of outbreaks are detected.

SOCIETY AND CULTURE

United Kingdom

In postwar Aberdeen (1964) a large-scale (>400 cases) outbreak of typhoid occurred, caused by contaminated corned beef which had been imported from Argentina. The corned beef was placed in cans and because the cooling plant had failed, cold river water from the Plate estuary was used to cool the cans. One of the cans had a defect and the meat inside was contaminated. This meat was then sliced using a meat slicer in a shop in Aberdeen, and a lack of cleaning the machinery led to spreading the contamination to other meats cut in the slicer. These meats were then eaten by the people of Aberdeen who then became ill.

Serious outbreaks of foodborne illness since the 1970s prompted key changes in UK food safety law. These included the death of 19 patients in the Stanley Royd Hospital outbreak and the bovine spongiform encephalopathy (BSE, mad cow disease) outbreak identified in the 1980s. The death of 17 people in the 1996 Wishaw outbreak of *E. coli* O157 was a precursor to the establishment of the Food Standards Agency which, according to Tony Blair in the 1998 white paper *A Force for Change* Cm 3830, "would be powerful, open and dedicated to the interests of consumers".

In May 2015, for the second year running, England's Food Standards Agency devoted its annual Food Safety Week to – "The Chicken Challenge". The focus was on the handling of raw chicken in the home and in catering facilities in a drive to reduce the worryingly high levels of food poisoning from the *campylobacter* bacterium. Anne Hardy argues that widespread public education of food hygiene can be useful, particularly through media (T.V cookery programmes) and advertisement. She points to the examples set by Scandinavian societies.

United States

In 2001, the Center for Science in the Public Interest petitioned the United States Department of Agriculture to require meat packers to remove spinal cords before processing cattle carcasses for human consumption, a measure designed to lessen the risk of infection by variant Creutzfeldt–Jakob disease. The petition was supported by the American Public Health Association, the Consumer Federation of America, the Government Accountability Project, the National Consumers League, and Safe Tables Our Priority. This was opposed by the National Cattlemen's Beef Association, the National Renderers Association, the National Meat Association, the Pork Producers Council, sheep raisers, milk producers, the Turkey Federation, and eight other organizations from the animal-derived food industry.

None of the US Department of Health and Human Services targets regarding incidence of foodborne infections were reached in 2007.

Organizations

The World Health Organization Department of Food Safety and Zoonoses (FOS) provides scientific advice for organizations and the public on issues concerning the safety of food. Its mission is to lower the burden of foodborne disease, thereby strengthening the health security and sustainable development of Member States. Foodborne and waterborne diarrhoeal diseases kill an estimated 2.2 million people annually, most of whom are children. WHO works closely with the Food and Agriculture Organization of the United Nations (FAO) to address food safety issues along the entire food production chain—from production to consumption—using new methods of risk analysis. These methods provide efficient, science-based tools to improve food safety, thereby benefiting both public health and economic development.

International Food Safety Authorities Network (INFOSAN)

The International Food Safety Authorities Network (INFOSAN) is a joint program of the WHO and FAO. INFOSAN has been connecting national authorities from around the globe since 2004, with the goal of preventing the international spread of contaminated food and foodborne disease and strengthening food safety systems globally. This is done by:

- Promoting the rapid exchange of information during food safety events;
- Sharing information on important food safety issues of global interest;
- Promoting partnership and collaboration between countries; and
- Helping countries strengthen their capacity to manage food safety risks.

Membership to INFOSAN is voluntary, but is restricted to representatives from national and regional government authorities and requires an official letter of designation. INFOSAN seeks to reflect the multidisciplinary nature of food safety and promote intersectoral collaboration by requesting the designation of Focal Points in each of the respective national authorities with a stake in food safety, and a single Emergency Contact Point in the national authority with the responsibility for coordinating national food safety emergencies; countries choosing to be members of INFOSAN are committed to sharing information between their respective food safety authorities and other INFOSAN members. The operational definition of a food safety authority includes those authorities involved in: food policy; risk assessment; food control and management; food inspection services; foodborne disease surveillance and response; laboratory services for monitoring and surveillance of foods and foodborne diseases; and food safety information, education and communication across the farm-to-table continuum.

Regulatory Steps

Food may be contaminated during all stages of food production and retailing. In order to prevent viral contamination, regulatory authorities in Europe have enacted several measures:

- European Commission Regulation (EC) No 2073/2005 of November 15, 2005
- European Committee for Standardization (CEN): Standard method for the detection of norovirus and hepatitis A virus in food products (shellfish, fruits and vegetables, surfaces and bottled water)
- CODEX Committee on Food Hygiene (CCFH): Guideline for the application of general principles of food hygiene for the control of viruses in food

REFERENCES

1. "food poisoning" at Dorland's Medical Dictionary
2. "Foodborne Illness - Frequently Asked Questions". US Centers for Disease Control and Prevention. Archived from the original on March 3, 2011. Retrieved 3 July 2016.
3. For foodborne illness caused by chemicals, see Food contaminants.
4. "Reducing the risk from E. coli 0157 – controlling cross-contamination". Food Standards Agency, United Kingdom. February 2011. Archived from the original on April 16, 2014. Retrieved 14 August 2016.
5. "Staphylococcal Food Poisoning". U.S. Centers for Disease Control and Prevention. Retrieved 3 July 2016.
6. Humphrey T, O'Brien S, Madsen M (2007). "Campylobacters as zoonotic pathogens: a food production perspective". International Journal of Food Microbiology. 117 (3): 237–57. doi:10.1016/j.ijfoodmicro.2007.01.006. PMID 17368847.
7. "Foodborne Illness: What Consumers Need to Know". USDA.gov. Retrieved 14 August 2016.
8. Tribe, Ingrid G; Cowell, David; Cameron, Peter; Cameron, Scott (2002). "An outbreak of Salmonella Typhimurium phage type 135 infection linked to the consumption of raw shell eggs in an aged care facility". Communicable Diseases Intelligence. 26 (1): 38–9. PMID 11950200. Archived from the original on February 17, 2014.
9. "Salmonella Infection (salmonellosis) and Animals". Centers for Disease Control and Prevention. Retrieved August 12, 2007.
10. Doyle, M. P.; Erickson, M. C. (2006). "Reducing the carriage of foodborne pathogens in livestock and poultry". Poultry science. 85 (6): 960–73. doi:10.1093/ps/85.6.960. PMID 16776463.
11. Food poisoning: Causes. Mayo Clinic.
12. Argudín M, Mendoza MC, Rodicio MR (2010). "Food poisoning and Staphylococcus aureus enterotoxins". Toxins (Basel). 2 (7): 1751–73. doi:10.3390/

toxins2071751. PMC 3153270 . PMID 22069659.

13. Staphylococcus aureus: A Problem When Food Is Left Out Too Long. Ohio State University Extension HYG-5564-11].
14. "FDA Says Viruses Safe for Treating Meat". Archived from the original on August 25, 2006. Retrieved September 2, 2014.
15. DeRusha, Jason. "Good Question: Does Washing Fruit Do Anything?". Retrieved 2016-09-18.
16. How Temperatures Affect Food. U.D. Department of Agriculture
17. Mount, Michael. "Fungi and Mycotoxins" (PDF). vetmed.ucdavis.edu. Retrieved August 11, 2007.
18. "Aflatoxins". Center for Food Safety & Applied Nutrition. Retrieved August 12, 2007.
19. "GASGA Technical Leaflet – 3 Mycotoxins in Grain". Food and Agriculture Organization of the United Nations. Retrieved August 12, 2007.
20. "Chapter 2 Foodborne Hazards in Basic Food Safety for Health Workers" (PDF). World Health Organization. Retrieved August 12, 2007.
21. "Sec. 683.100 Action Levels for Aflatoxins in Animal Feeds (CPG 7126.33)". Food and Drug Administration. Retrieved August 13, 2007.
22. Henry, Michael H. "Mycotoxins in Feeds: CVM's Perspective". FDA.gov. Retrieved January 1, 2012.
23. Webley DJ, Jackson KL, Mullins JD, Hocking AD, Pitt JI (1997). "Alternaria toxins in weather-damaged wheat and sorghum in the 1995–1996 Australian harvest". Australian Journal of Agricultural Research. 48 (8): 1249–56. doi:10.1071/A97005.
24. Li F, Yoshizawa T (2000). "Alternaria mycotoxins in weathered wheat from China". J. Agric. Food Chem. 48 (7): 2920–4. doi:10.1021/jf0000171. PMID 10898645.
25. Motta SD, Valente Soares LM (2001). "Survey of Brazilian tomato products for alternariol, alternariol monomethyl ether, tenuazonic acid and cyclopiazonic acid". Food Addit Contam. 18 (7): 630–4. doi:10.1080/02652030117707. PMID 11469319.
26. Li FQ, Toyazaki N, Yoshizawa T (2001). "Production of alternaria mycotoxins by Alternaria alternata isolated from weather-damaged wheat". J. Food Prot. 64 (4): 567–71. PMID 11307900.
27. Marasas WF (1995). "Fumonisins: their implications for human and animal health". Nat. Toxins. 3 (4): 193–8; discussion 221. doi:10.1002/nt.2620030405. PMID 7582616.
28. Soriano, J.M. (2004). "Occurrence of fumonisins in foods". Food Research International. 37 (10): 985–1000. doi:10.1016/j.foodres.2004.06.009.
29. "CVM and Fumonisins". Food and Drug Administration. Archived from the

original on August 12, 2007. Retrieved August 13, 2007.

30. "More contaminated maize meal products withdrawn from sale". Food Standards Agency. Retrieved August 12, 2007.
31. "20th Australian Total Diet Survey – Part B". Food Standards Australia New Zealand. Retrieved August 13, 2007.
32. "Worldwide regulations for mycotoxins in food and feed in 2003". FAO FOOD AND NUTRITION PAPER 81. Retrieved August 13, 2007.
33. "Patulin in Apple Juice, Apple Juice Concentrates and Apple Juice Products". Food and Drug Administration. Retrieved August 16, 2007.
34. Sabater-Vilar M, Nijmeijer S, Fink-Gremmels J (2003). "Genotoxicity assessment of five tremorgenic mycotoxins (fumitremorgen B, paxilline, penitrem A, verruculogen, and verrucosidin) produced by molds isolated from fermented meats". J. Food Prot. 66 (11): 2123–9. PMID 14627292.
35. Adejumo TO, Hettwer U, Karlovsky P (May 2007). "Occurrence of Fusarium species and trichothecenes in Nigerian maize". Int. J. Food Microbiol. 116 (3): 350–7. doi:10.1016/j.ijfoodmicro.2007.02.009. PMID 17412440.
36. Mazur LJ, Kim J (2006). "Spectrum of noninfectious health effects from molds". Pediatrics. 118 (6): e1909–26. doi:10.1542/peds.2006-2829. PMID 17142508.
37. Froquet R, Sibiril Y, Parent-Massin D (2001). "Trichothecene toxicity on human megakaryocyte progenitors (CFU-MK)". Hum Exp Toxicol. 20 (2): 84–9. doi:10.1191/096032701677428611. PMID 11327514.
38. Joffe AZ, Yagen B (1977). "Comparative study of the yield of T-2 toxic produced by Fusarium poae, F. sporotrichioides and F. sporotrichioides var. tricinctum strains from different sources". Mycopathologia. 60 (2): 93–7. doi:10.1007/bf00490378. PMID 846559.
39. Hay, R. J. (2007). "Fusarium infections of the skin". Current Opinion in Infectious Diseases. 20 (2): 115. doi:10.1097/QCO.0b013e328014392d.
40. "Guidance for Industry and FDA – Letter to State Agricultural Directors, State Feed Control Officials, and Food, Feed, and Grain Trade Organizations". Food and Drug Administration. Archived from the original on June 9, 2007. Retrieved August 13, 2007.
41. Hohn, Thomas M. "Trichothecene-resistant transgenic plants". U.S. Patent 6,646,184. Priority date March 31, 1999.
42. Dubois E, Hennechart C, Deboosère N, et al. (April 2006). "Intra-laboratory validation of a concentration method adapted for the enumeration of infectious F-specific RNA coliphage, enterovirus, and hepatitis A virus from inoculated leaves of salad vegetables". Int. J. Food Microbiol. 108 (2): 164–71. doi:10.1016/j.ijfoodmicro.2005.11.007. PMID 16387377.
43. Schmidt, Heather Martin. "Improving the microbilological quality and safety of fresh-cut tomatoes by low dose dlectron beam irradiation – Master thesis" (PDF). Retrieved August 11, 2007.
44. Oxford English Dictionary (First ed.). London: Oxford University Press. 1933.

p. 1557.

45. Merck's Bulletin, Volume 5, William Henry Porter, 1892.
46. Lancet, 3 Oct 1891, page 752
47. "Report Next Week," Evening Independent (Massillon, OH), July 22, 1932, pg. 6
48. "Medicine: Potato Salad," Time, August 1, 1932.
49. "Poisoning Hits 150 in Chicago". Kenosha Evening News. May 27, 1944.
50. "Food-Related Diseases". US Centers for Disease Control and Prevention.
51. Greig, Judy D. "Infective Doses and Pathogen Carriage". Public Health Agency of Canada.
52. Owens, Michael D (January 2014) Salmonella Infection in Emergency Medicine. emedicine.com
53. Scallan E, Griffin PM, Angulo FJ, Tauxe RV, Hoekstra RM (2011). "Foodborne illness acquired in the United States—unspecified agents". Emerging Infectious Diseases. 17 (1): 16–22. doi:10.3201/eid1701.P21101. PMC 3204615 . PMID 21192849.
54. Scallan E, Hoekstra RM, Angulo FJ, Tauxe RV, Widdowson MA, Roy SL, et al. (2011). "Foodborne illness acquired in the United States—major pathogens". Emerging Infectious Diseases. 17 (1): 7–15. doi:10.3201/eid1701.P11101. PMC 3375761 . PMID 21192848.
55. "Obama Proposes Single Overseer for Food Safety". New York Times. February 20, 2015. Retrieved 2015-02-22. According to the C.D.C., an estimated 87 million Americans are sickened each year by contaminated food, 371,000 are hospitalized with food-related illness and 5,700 die from food-related disease
56. Sabrina Tavernise (July 26, 2013). "F.D.A. Says Importers Must Audit Food Safety". New York Times. Retrieved July 27, 2013. One in every six Americans becomes ill from eating contaminated food each year, Dr. Margaret A. Hamburg, F.D.A. commissioner, estimated. About 130,000 are hospitalized and 3,000 die.
57. Stephanie Strom (January 4, 2013). "F.D.A. Offers Sweeping Rules to Fight Food Contamination". New York Times. Retrieved January 5, 2013. One in six Americans becomes ill from eating contaminated food each year, the government estimates; of those, roughly 130,000 are hospitalized and 3,000 die.
58. "Report of the French sanitary agencies" (PDF) (in French). INVS/Afssa.
59. "Summary of Report of the French sanitary agencies"(PDF) (in French). INVS/ Afssa.
60. Kirk, Martyn; et al. "Foodborne illness in Australia: Annual incidence circa 2010 pp7-9". Australia Department of Health. Australian National University. Retrieved 13 September 2015.
61. "Food borne illness in Australia" (PDF). OzFoodNet.
62. Astridge, K; McPherson, M; Kirk, M; et al. (2011). "Foodborne disease outbreaks in Australia 2001-2009". Food Australia. 63 (12): 44–50.
63. "Food Hygiene". BUPA. Retrieved 13 September 2015.

64. Smith, David F.; Diack, H. Lesley and Pennington, T. Hugh (2005) Food Poisoning, Policy and Politics : Corned Beef and Typhoid in Britain in the 1960s. Boydell Press. ISBN 1-84383-138-4

65. Brian Deer (February 24, 1985). "Food poison deaths probe may reveal NHS flaws". The Sunday Times.

66. Cowden JM, Ahmed S, Donaghy M, Riley A (2001). "Epidemiological investigation of the Central Scotland outbreak of Escherichia coli O157 infection, November to December 1996" (PDF). Epidemiol. Infect. 126: 335–341. doi:10.1017/S0950268801005520. PMC 2869700 . PMID 11467789.

67. "The Food Standards Agency: A Force for Change". gov.uk. Food Standards Agency, United Kingdom. January 14, 1998. Retrieved 14 August 2016.

68. Hardy, Anne (13 January 2016). "Food Poisoning: An On-going Saga". History and Policy. History and Policy. Retrieved 4 July 2016.

69. "Meat Produced by Advanced Meat/Bone Separation Machinery and Meat Recovery (AMR) Systems". Federal Register. U.S. National Archive and Records Administration. Retrieved 3 July 2016.

70. "Livestock Industry Opposed to Stricter Laws on Mad Cow Prevention". January 2003. Retrieved 3 July 2016.

71. Healthy People 2010 Home Page

72. "Preliminary FoodNet data on the incidence of infection with pathogens transmitted commonly through food—10 states, 2007". MMWR Morb. Mortal. Wkly. Rep. 57 (14): 366–70. April 2008. PMID 18401330.

73. "Codex Committee on Food Hygiene (CCFH)", European Commission, Retrieved April 7, 2015

CHAPTER 8

Impedance Microbiology

Chapter Contents

- **Introduction**
- **Principle of Operation**

Impedance microbiology is a rapid method that enables qualitative and quantitative tracing of microorganisms by measuring the change in the electrical conductivity. With direct impedance technology, the change in the conductivity of a liquid culture medium serves as a measuring parameter, whereas with indirect impediometry, the change in the electrical conductivity of a reaction solution, which occurs through the absorption of gases from the inoculated bacterial culture, is measured. Most investigations concerning the applicability of impediometry in food microbiology deal with the impedimetric detection or enumeration of Enterobacteriaceae, especially the detection of Salmonella.

INTRODUCTION

Impedance microbiology is a rapid microbiological technique used to measure the microbial concentration (mainly bacteria but also yeasts) of a sample by monitoring the electrical parameters of the growth medium. The ability of microbial metabolism to change the electrical conductivity of the growth medium was discovered by Stewart and further studied by other scientists such as Oker-Blom, Parson and Allison in the first half of 20th century. However, it was only in the late 1970s that, thanks to computer-controlled systems used to monitor impedance, the technique showed its full potential, as discussed in the works of Fistenberg-Eden & Eden, Ur & Brown and Cady.

PRINCIPLE OF OPERATION

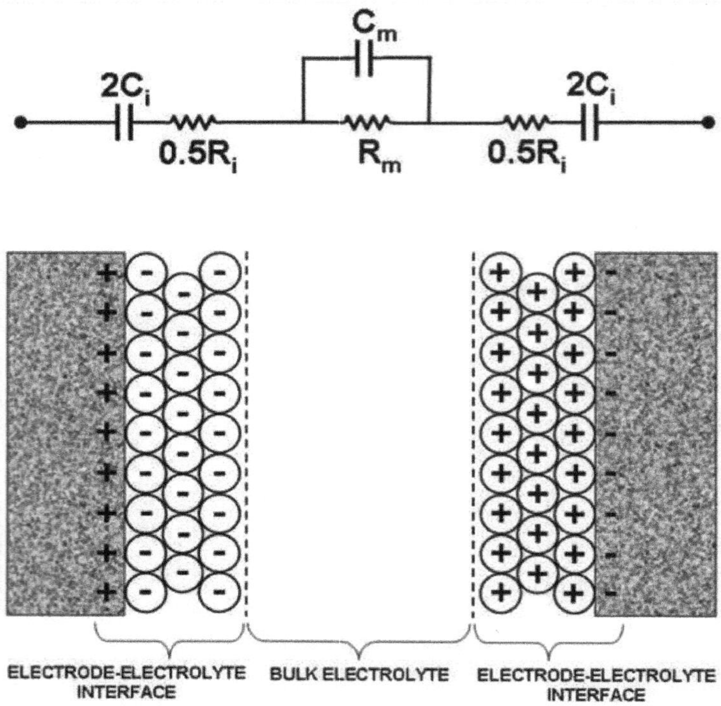

Equivalent electrical circuit to model a couple of electrodes in direct contact with a liquid medium

When a pair of electrodes are immersed in the growth medium, the system composed of electrodes and electrolyte can be modeled with the electrical circuit of Fig. 1, where R_m and C_m are the resistance and capacitance of the bulk medium, while R_i and C_i are the resistance and capacitance of the electrode-electrolyte interface. However, when frequency of the sinusoidal test signal applied to the electrodes is relatively low (lower than 1 MHz) the bulk capacitance C_m can be neglected and the system can be modeled with a simpler circuit consisting only of a resistance R_s and a capacitance C_s in series. The resistance R_s accounts for the electrical conductivity of the bulk medium while the capacitance C_s is due to the capacitive double-layer at the electrode-electrolyte interface. During the growth phase, bacterial metabolism transforms uncharged or weakly charged compounds of the bulk medium in highly charged compounds that change the electrical properties of the medium. This results in a decrease of resistance R_s and an increase of capacitance C_s.

Impedance Microbiology technique works this way:

- The sample with the initial unknown bacterial concentration (C_0) is placed at a temperature favoring bacterial growth (in the range 37 to 42 °C if mesophilic microbial population is the target) and the electrical parameters R_s and C_s are measured at regular time intervals of few minutes by means of a couple of electrodes in direct contact with the sample.
- Until the bacterial concentration is lower than a critical threshold C_{TH} the electrical parameters R_s and C_s remain essentially constant (at their baseline values). C_{TH} depends on various parameters such as electrode geometry, bacterial strain, chemical composition of the growth medium etc., but it is always in the range 10^6 to 10^7 cfu/ml.
- When the bacterial concentration increases over C_{TH}, the electrical parameters deviate from their baseline values (generally in the case of bacteria there is a decrease of R_s and an increase of C_s, the opposite happens in the case of yeasts).
- The time needed for the electrical parameters R_s and C_s to deviate from their baseline value is referred as Detect Time (DT) and is the parameter used to estimate the initial unknown bacterial concentration C_0.

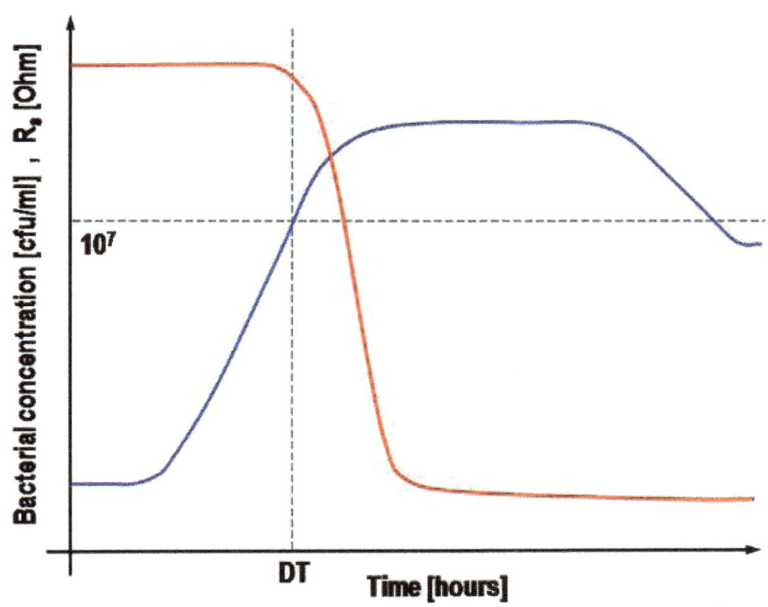

R_s curve and bacterial concentration curve as function of time

In Fig. 2 a typical curve for R_s as well as the corresponding bacterial concentration are plotted vs. time. Fig. 3 shows typical R_s curves vs time for samples characterized by different bacterial concentration. Since DT is the time needed for the bacterial concentration to grow from the initial value C_0 to C_{TH}, highly contaminated samples are characterized by lower values of DT than samples with low bacterial concentration. Given C_1, C_2 and C_3 the bacterial concentration of three samples with $C_1 > C_2 > C_3$, it is $DT_1 < DT_2 < DT_3$. Data from literature show how DT is a linear function of the logarithm of C_0:

$$DT = A \cdot \log_{10}(C_0) + B$$

where the parameters A and B are dependent on the particular type of samples under test, the bacterial strains, the type of enriching medium used and so on. These parameters can be calculated by calibrating the system using a set of samples whose bacterial concentration is known and calculating the linear regression line that will be used to estimate the bacterial concentration from the measured DT.

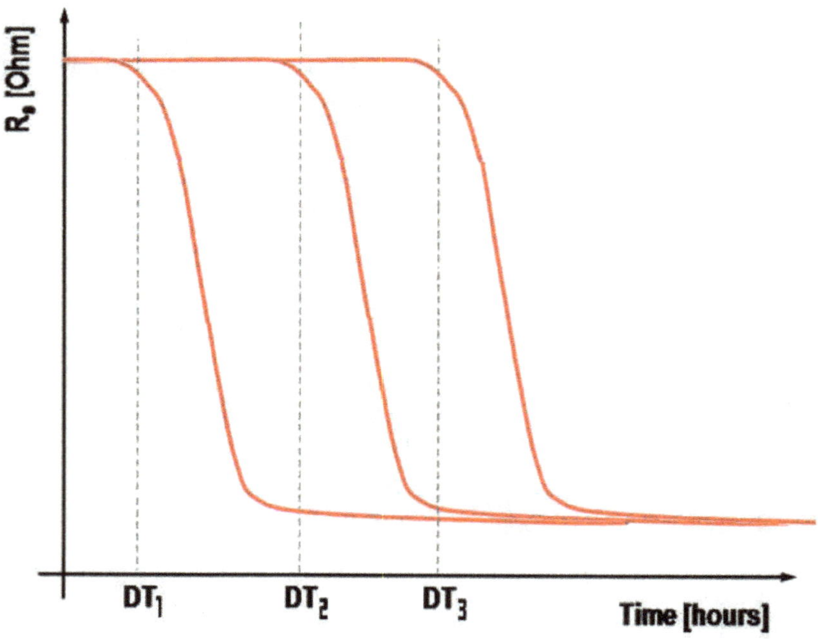

R_s curves for samples featuring different bacterial concentration as function of time

Impedance microbiology has different advantages on the standard Plate Count technique to measure bacterial concentration:

- It is characterized by faster response time. In the case of mesophilic bacteria, the response time range from 2 – 3 hours for highly contaminated samples (10^5 - 10^6 cfu/ml) to over 10 hours for samples with very low bacterial concentration (less than 10 cfu/ml). As a comparison, for the same bacterial strains the Plate Count technique is characterized by response times from 48 to 72 hours.
- Impedance microbiology is a method that can be easily automated, i.e. implemented as part of an industrial machine or realized as an embedded portable sensor, while Plate Count is a manual method that needs to be carried out in a laboratory by long trained personnel.

Instrumentation

Over the past decades different instruments (either laboratory built or commercially available) to measure bacterial concentration using impedance microbiology have been built. One of the best selling and well accepted instruments in the industry is the Bactometer by Biomerieux. The original instrument of 1984 features a multi-incubator system capable of monitoring up to 512 samples simultaneously with the ability to set 8 different incubation temperatures. Other instruments with performance comparable to the Bactometer are Malthus by Malthus Instruments Ltd (Bury, UK), RABIT by Don Whitley Scientific (Shipley, UK) and Bac Trac by Sy-Lab (Purkensdorf, Austria). A portable embedded system for microbial concentration measurement in liquid and semi-liquid media using impedance microbiology has been recently proposed. The system is composed of a thermoregulated incubation chamber where the sample under test is stored and a controller for thermoregulation and impedance measurements.

Applications

Impedance microbiology has been extensively used in the past decades to measure the concentration of bacteria and yeasts in different type of samples, mainly for quality assurance in the food industry. Some applications are, the determination of the shelf life of pasteurized milk and the measure of total bacterial concentration in raw-milk, frozen vegetables, grain products, meat products and beer. The technique has been also used in environmental monitoring to detect the coliform concentration in water samples, in the pharmaceutical industry to test the efficiency of novel antibacterial agents and the testing of final products.

REFERENCES

1. Stewart, G.N. (1899). "The changes produced by the growth of bacteria in the molecular concentration and electrical conductivity of culture media". Journal of Experimental Medicine. 4: 235–243. doi:10.1084/jem.4.2.235.
2. Oker-Blom, M (1912). "Die elektrische Leitfahigkeit im dienste der Bakteriologie". Zentralbl Bakteriol. 65: 382-289.
3. Parsons, L.B.; Sturges, W.S. (1926). "The possibility of the conductivity method as applied to studies of bacterial metabolism". Journal of Bacteriology. 11: 177–188.
4. Allison, J.B.; Anderson, J.A.; Cole, W.H. (1938). "The method of electrical conductivity in studies of bacterial metabolism". Journal of Bacteriology. 36: 571–586.
5. Fistenberg-Eden, R.; Eden, G. (1984). Impedance Microbiology. New York: John Wiley.
6. Ur, A.; Brown, D.F.J. (1975). Monitoring of bacterial activity by impedance measurements. New York: Chapter 5 in "New approaches to the identification

of microorganisms", edited by C. Heden & T. Illeni, John Wiley & Sons. pp. 63–71.

7. Cady, P. (1978). Progress in impedance measurements in microbiology. Springfield: Chapter 14 in "Mechanizing microbiology" edited by Anthony N. Sharpe & David S. Clark, Charles C. Thomas Publisher. pp. 199–239.
8. Grossi, M.; Lanzoni, M.; Pompei, A.; Lazzarini, R.; Matteuzzi, D.; Riccò, B. (June 2008). "Detection of microbial concentration in ice-cream using the impedance technique". Biosensors and Bioelectronics. 23 (11): 1616–1623. doi:10.1016/j.bios.2008.01.032.
9. Felice, C.J.; Valentinuzzi, M.E.; Vercellone, M.I.; Madrid, R.E. (1992). "Impedance bacteriometry: medium and interface contributions during bacterial growth". IEEE Transaction on Biomedical Engineering. 39 (12): 1310–1313. doi:10.1109/10.184708.
10. Grossi, M.; Pompei, A.; Lanzoni, M.; Lazzarini, R.; Matteuzzi, D.; Riccò, B. (2009). "Total bacterial count in soft-frozen dairy products by impedance biosensor system". IEEE Sensors Journal. 9 (10): 1270–1276. doi:10.1109/JSEN.2009.2029816.
11. Silverman, M.P.; Munoz, E.F. (1979). "Automated electrical impedance technique for rapid enumeration of fecal coliforms in effluents from sewage treatment plants". Applied and Environmental Microbiology. 37 (3): 521–526.
12. Priego, R.; Medina, L.M.; Jordano, R. (2011). "Bactometer system versus traditional methods for monitoring bacteria populations in salchichón during its ripening process". Journal of Food Protection. 74 (1): 145–148. doi:10.4315/0362-028X.JFP-10-244.
13. Jawad, G.M.; Marrow, T.; Odumeru, J.A. (1998). "Assessment of impedance microbiological method for the detection of Escherichia Coli in foods". Journal of Rapid Methods & Automation in Microbiology. 6 (4): 297–305. doi:10.1111/j.1745-4581.1998.tb00210.x.
14. "RABIT instrument".
15. "Bac Trac instrument".
16. Grossi, M.; Lanzoni, M.; Pompei, A.; Lazzarini, R.; Matteuzzi, D.; Riccò, B. (2010). "An embedded portable biosensor system for bacterial concentration detection". Biosensors & Bioelectronics. 26: 983–990. doi:10.1016/j.bios.2010.08.039.
17. Grossi, M.; Lazzarini, R.; Lanzoni, M.; Pompei, A.; Matteuzzi, D.; Riccò, B. (2013). "A portable sensor with disposable electrodes for water bacterial quality assessment". IEEE Sensors Journal. 13 (5): 1775–1781. doi:10.1109/JSEN.2013.2243142.
18. Bishop, J.R.; White, C.H.; Fistenberg-Eden, R. (1984). "Rapid impedimetric method for determining the potential shelf-life of pasteurized whole milk". Journal of Food Protection. 47 (6): 471–475.
19. Grossi, M.; Lanzoni, M.; Pompei, A.; Lazzarini, R.; Matteuzzi, D.; Riccò, B.

(2011). "A portable biosensor system for bacterial concentration measurements in cow's raw milk". 4th IEEE International Workshop on Advances in Sensors and Interfaces: 132–136. doi:10.1109/IWASI.2011.6004703.

20. Gnan, S.; Luedecke, L.O. (1982). "Impedance measurements in raw milk as an alternative to the standard plate count". Journal of Food Protection. 45 (1): 4–7.
21. Hardy, D.; Kraeger, S.J.; Dufour, S.W.; Cady, P. (1977). "Rapid detection of microbial contamination in frozen vegetables by automated impedance measurements". Applied and Environmental Microbiology. 34 (1): 14–17.
22. Sorrels, K.M. (1981). "Rapid detection of bacterial content in cereal grain products by automated impedance measurements". Journal of Food Protection. 44: 832.
23. Fistenberg-Eden, R. (1983). "Rapid estimation of the number of microorganisms in raw meat by impedance measurement". Food Technology. 37: 64–70.
24. Pompei, A.; Grossi, M.; Lanzoni, M.; Perretti, G.; Lazzarini, R.; Riccò, B.; Matteuzzi, D. "Feasibility of lactobacilli concentration detection in beer by automated impedance technique". MBAA Technical Quarterly. 49 (1): 11–18. doi:10.1094/TQ-49-1-0315-01.
25. Evans, H.A.V. (1982). "A note on two uses for impedimetry in brewing microbiology". Journal of Applied Bacteriology. 53: 423–426. doi:10.1111/j.1365-2672.1982.tb01291.x.
26. Colquhoun, K.O.; Timms, S.; Fricker, C.R. (1995). "Detection of Escherichia Coli in potable water using direct impedance technology". Journal of Applied Microbiology. 79 (6): 635–639. doi:10.1111/j.1365-2672.1995.tb00948.x.
27. Strauss, W.M.; Malaney, G.W.; Tanner, R.D. (1984). "The impedance method for monitoring total coliforms in wastewaters". Folia Microbiologica. 29 (2): 162–169. doi:10.1007/bf02872933.
28. Gould, I.M.; Jason, A.C.; Milne, K. (1989). "Use of the Malthus growth analyzer to study the post-antibiotic effect of antibiotics". Journal of Antimicrobial Chemotherapy: 523–531. doi:10.1093/jac/24.4.523.

Index

A

adenosine triphosphate (ATP) 53
Altenuene (ALT) 208
Alternariol (AOH) 208
anthropogenic global warming potential (AGWP) 59
Antimicrobial preservatives 154
Archaeal Richmond Mine acidophilic nanoorganisms (ARMAN) 45
Archaeal Richmond Mine Acidophilic Nanoorganisms (ARMAN) 60

B

Bacterial food cultures 164, 165
Bacteriophages 34

C

carbon dioxide (CO2) 145
Center for Disease Control (CDC) 157
colony-forming units (CFU) 213

D

deoxynivalenol (DON) 209
Detect Time (DT) 225
diacetoxyscirpenol (DAS) 209

E

Endosymbiotic gene transfer (EGT) 79
enterohemorrhagic (EHEC) 205
enteropathogenic (EPEC) 205
Equivalent electrical 224
European Food and Feed Cultures Association (EFFCA) 167
European Food Safety Authority (EFSA) 167

F

Fermentation 2
first in first out method (FIFO) 153
Foodborne illness 204, 205, 221
Food preservation 137
Food sampling 3, 4

G

generally recognized by experts as safe (GRAS) 167

H

Hurdle technology 147

I

Impedance microbiology 223, 226, 227
Impedance Microbiology technique 225
International Dairy Federation (IDF) 167

L

lactic acid bacteria (LAB) 147
Lactic acid fermentation 153, 157, 158, 159, 161

Lactobacillus 40, 41, 118, 122, 123, 124, 125, 126
Leukoencephalomalacia (LEM) 208
Limit of Reporting (LOR) 209

M

Microbial food cultures 163, 164, 167

O

Ochratoxin A (OTA) 209

P

polymerase chain reaction (PCR) 45
Polymerase Chain Reaction (PCR) 5
Poly-γ-glutamic acid (γ-PGA) 3
Pulsed electric field (PEF) 145

Q

qualified presumption of safety (QPS) 167

R

Radicinin (RAD) 208
ribosomal RNA (rRNA) 45

S

Salmonella typhimurium 40
serial endosymbiotic theory (SET) 78
Several microbially 2
Sexual organisms 33
Sodium hydroxide 141

T

Tenuazonic acid (TeA) 208

W

World Health Organization (WHO) 138